The First Half Second

The First Half Second

The Microgenesis and Temporal Dynamics of Unconscious and Conscious Visual Processes

edited by Haluk Öğmen and Bruno G. Breitmeyer

The MIT Press
Cambridge, Massachusetts
London, England

MIT Press books may be purchased at special quantity discounts for business or sales promotional use. For information, please email special_sales@mitpress.mit.edu or write to Special Sales Department, The MIT Press, 55 Hayward Street, Cambridge, MA 02142.

This book was set in Times by SNP Best-set Typesetter Ltd., Hong Kong.
Printed and bound in the United States of America.

Library of Congress Cataloging-in-Publication Data

The first half second: the microgenesis and temporal dynamics of unconscious and conscious visual processes / Haluk Öğmen and Bruno G. Breitmeyer, editors.
    p. cm.
  Includes bibliographical references and index.
  ISBN 0-262-05114-1 (alk. paper)—ISBN 0-262-65107-6 (pbk. : alk. paper)
    1. Visual perception. 2. Consciousness. 3. Neuropsychology. I. Öğmen, Haluk. II. Breitmeyer, Bruno G.
QP481.F57 2006
152.14–dc22

                                                                    2005047868

10 9 8 7 6 5 4 3 2 1

Contents

Preface

The most readily apparent and intriguing aspect of normal human vision is that it is accompanied by a rich phenomenology. Less apparent but also puzzling is that a considerable level of behaviorally relevant information processing occurs at unconscious levels not accessible to phenomenological report. The 1990s, the "Decade of the Brain," witnessed major advances in the study of visual cognition and consciousness. An impressive array of techniques—neurophysiological, neuroanatomical, neuropsychological, electrophysiological, psychophysical, computational, and brain imaging—were developed to specifically address these areas. As a result, major strides in the study of visual cognition and consciousness as well as attention were achieved. However, most of these advances—with the exception of Libet's (2004) groundbreaking work and work on how temporal synchronization of 40-Hz or gamma-range neural activity might relate to consciousness (Crick & Koch, 1990; Llinás & Pare, 1996; Singer, 1994)—have dealt with the steady-state properties of visual processing. The common theme has been to identify types, levels, or sites of neural activity that correlate with conscious and unconscious aspects of visual processing (e.g., Crick & Koch, 1995; Sheinberg & Logothetis, 1997). To complement this approach, it would be highly desirable to bring together the current state-of-the-art in research probing the *dynamic* aspects of conscious and unconscious visual processing and to chart promising directions for future research in this area. To achieve this goal, we organized a workshop entitled "The First Half Second: The Microgenesis and Temporal Dynamics of Unconscious and Conscious Visual Processes," which was held in Houston, Texas, November 1–3, 2003. This book is the outcome of the presentations and the discussions that took place at that workshop. We expect this book to appeal to a broad audience from graduate students to advanced researchers with expertise in cognitive psychology, neuropsychology, neuroscience, neuroengineering, computational intelligence, and philosophy of the mind.

Acknowledgments

The workshop leading to this book was supported by grant R13 MH068548 from the National Institutes of Health. We would like to thank Dr. Dennis Glanzman from the National Institute of Mental Health for his advice and assistance throughout this project. We would like to thank several University of Houston components for supporting the workshop: The Office of Vice President for Research, Colleges of Engineering, Liberal Arts and Social Sciences, Natural Sciences and Mathematics, Center for Neuro-Engineering and Cognitive Science, and Texas Learning and Computation Center and the Departments of Electrical & Computer Engineering and Psychology. We would like to thank Barbara Murphy and Kate Blakinger from MIT Press for their help and support in putting this book together. Emre Çilingiroğlu helped us in all aspects of editing and formatting the manuscript. Finally, special thanks go to the anonymous reviewers for their timely and insightful reviews and feedback.

The First Half Second

1 Introduction

1.1 Microgenesis and Temporal Dynamics of Conscious and Unconscious Processing

The objective of this book is to probe in detail the dynamic aspects of conscious and unconscious visual processing. This involves looking at the time course of visual processes from the moment a stimulus is presented until it registers in a behavioral response or in consciousness a few hundred milliseconds later. Following Werner's (1940) terminology, we use the term *microgenesis* to describe the development of visual processes from their beginnings immediately after the presentation of the stimulus to their state at the time at which they lead to conscious registration and/or behavioral responses (see chapter 2 for an in-depth discussion of the term).

The title of the book was chosen for several reasons.

1. Humans are mobile visual explorers, and because we frequently shift our gaze when we inspect the world of objects and events, vision is, by definition, a highly dynamic process. Given the usual two to four fixations per second, behaviorally relevant as well as phenomenally rich representations must be modified or newly constructed by the visual system in a period of time lasting from about 250 to 500 ms. Thus, even the manifest steady-state properties of visual experience during a fixation period rely on highly dynamic underlying neural processes that must be updated several times per second.

2. Recent evidence has accumulated from the study of neurologically impaired as well as normal subjects showing that separate visual pathways support conscious perception and unconsciously controlled behaviors and emotional responses (de Gelder et al., 2001a; Milner & Goodale, 1995; Weiskrantz, 1997). The dynamic, temporal properties of these different pathways have not yet been explored extensively. Such exploration may prove useful in differentiating these pathway activities.

3. A number of sophisticated techniques have been developed separately by psychophysicists, electrophysiologists, neuroscientists, engineers, and computer

scientists to investigate the dynamic, time-dependent behavior of individual neurons or networks of neurons. However, a clear interdisciplinary dialogue has not been attempted nor has such an interdisciplinary approach been formulated.

The objective of the book is to provide a venue for laying out the most important conceptual, methodological, and empirical issues and problems that have to be addressed when investigating, in an interdisciplinary manner, the temporal dynamics of activity in the visual system related to unconscious and conscious cognitive processes.

It is widely accepted that attention and consciousness are intimately related (Posner, 1994). Recently published work focused on the temporal aspects of attentional control (Shapiro, 2001) without however relating them to conscious and unconscious processes, while other recent work highlighted the differences between conscious and unconscious visual processes (Metzinger, 2000; de Gelder et al., 2001a) without looking at the temporal dynamics or how they relate to attention. This book is combining the topics of attention and of conscious and unconscious processes in visual cognition within the context of its temporal dynamics.

The investigation of the temporal dynamics can shed significant light on various processes in vision. For example, the recordings of cortical visual evoked potentials (CVEPs) demonstrate that different aspects of attentional and other task-relevant processing correlate with different epochs and waveforms of the CVEPs (e.g., Vogel et al., 1998). Later components are usually taken to correspond to higher level processes than are earlier components. The related work of neuroscientists has detailed the functional and structural properties of these early and late cortical levels (Desimone & Ungerleider, 1989; Zeki, 1993). These approaches, when combined with psychophysical work that carefully determines the temporal sequence and dynamics of visual processing, promise to uncover the levels and types of cortical activity involved in unconscious and conscious visual processes (Breitmeyer & Öğmen, 2000).

Determining these stages or levels of visual processing and their timing is also useful for biomedical engineering in developing improved or new methods for recording and analyzing brain activity, such as the electroencephalogram (EEG), the magnetoencephalogram, functional magnetic resonance imaging (fMRI) and others. Such improvements would have important implications for diagnosis and treatment. For example, since deficits in the temporal processing are characteristic of a number of special populations such as schizophrenics (Green et al., 1999) and neurological patients, the study of the temporal dynamics of unconscious and conscious processing can shed light on the abnormalities in visual processing associated with these various diagnostic categories.

We believe that the recent research emphasis on the dynamics of information processing in neurophysiology and psychophysics provides the necessary framework to achieve the synthesis required to lay the foundations of the aforementioned goals. We hope that the book will stimulate a more inclusive approach to the study of visual information processing that integrates known steady-state properties of vision in a meaningful way with its dynamic aspects. Such an approach will provide useful information to the fields of visual neuroscience, cognitive psychology, neuropsychology, and neuroengineering and help chart new integrative and interactive directions in brain research that focus on the flux of information processing characterizing ongoing, real-time visual behavior.

1.2   Organization of the Book

The book consists of six parts that follow the topical organization of the workshop.

Part I. Conceptual issues in studying conscious and unconscious visual processes. This part provides a general foundation for the book by focusing on conceptual, methodological, and historical issues. It contains two chapters, the first one emphasizing microgenetic aspects and the second one emphasizing conscious versus unconscious aspects of visual processing. The first chapter gives a historical introduction to the science of perceptual microgenesis with an in-depth discussion of different types of perceptual microgenesis, namely, representational and phenomenal. It outlines pertinent experimental approaches and phenomena, which appear in subsequent chapters of the book. This chapter also introduces a neurophysiological architecture that the author uses to explain several aspects of perceptual microgenesis. A notable aspect of this architecture is the role played by subcortical nonspecific pathways in modulating real-time processes that take place in cortical modules.

The second chapter provides a review that probes the neural correlates of conscious (NCC) and the neural correlates of unconscious (NCU) vision. The chapter introduces conceptual issues, from the definition of consciousness to how it relates to neural structures and processes. During the last decade, consciousness became a scientific question of interest to researchers in a variety of disciplines, and a multitude of studies, from neurophysiological to behavioral, have been conducted to search for its underpinnings in brain structures and processes. The chapter provides an integrative review of these findings, culminating in several proposals for NCC and NCU. To provide the necessary framework for the theme of the book, a section is devoted to the temporal properties of conscious and unconscious vision with a discussion of several experimental techniques that are used in the subsequent chapters of the book.

Part II. Neurophysiological correlates of dynamic processing in vision.   The second part consists of three chapters. From the *neuroanatomical* point of view, the first chapter discusses distinctions between dorsal and ventral neural streams, the second chapter focuses on visual areas in the ventral stream, and the third chapter focuses on inferotemporal (IT) cortex, considered to be the "endpoint" of the ventral stream.

From the *functional* point of view, the first chapter analyzes the distinctions between perception and action systems associated with the ventral and dorsal systems, respectively. The second chapter considers the distinctions between edge detection and scene segmentation. The third chapter analyzes conscious versus unconscious perception.

Following the theme of the book, all chapters highlight the aforementioned functional distinctions along the time dimension. The first chapter proposes that the action system (dorsal stream) works in *real time* and lacks memory. Memory, on the other hand, is considered essential for the computations carried out in the perception system (ventral stream). It uses the priming technique to test this prediction. The second chapter reviews "classical" and "surround" receptive field organization of neural connectivity and argues the need for recurrent processing, in particular, for scene segmentation. One of the supporting arguments is based on the timing properties of horizontal versus cortico–cortico (interareal) connections. This proposal is tested by use of EEG and fMRI experiments in humans. The third chapter uses the technique of backward masking by pattern to investigate the timing of information in the IT cortex and to relate the temporal dynamics of neuronal firing to conscious versus unconscious perception. The results indicate that a backward pattern mask shortens the duration of neuronal firing, thereby reducing the amount of information available in the spike trains. On the basis of signal timing, the chapter argues that top-down feedback processing is not likely to be a prerequisite for conscious perception. The chapter also argues against stimulus-dependent synchrony as a correlate for conscious perception. Instead, it is suggested that neural activities need to exceed a threshold level for conscious registration of stimuli.

Part III. Visual masking and the dynamics of vision.   Visual masking is the reduction in the visibility of one stimulus, called the *target*, due to the presence of another stimulus, called the *mask*. Visual masking has been used extensively to probe *static* and *dynamic* properties of vision, typically by use of long- and short-duration stimuli, respectively. A survey of papers published in a representative set of psychological journals during a 15-year time period showed that 11% of articles used masking as a methodological tool (Bachmann, 1994). Typically, a mask is introduced to "curtail," "interrupt," or "terminate" the processing of other stimuli. Mask stimuli are also used to prevent conscious registration of stimuli, thereby allowing a systematic study of conscious versus unconscious processing. The interpretation of the data obtained from these studies depends on our understanding of the visual masking phenomenon itself. Visual masking has been studied as a topic in itself (e.g., 3 percent of the articles in the aforementioned survey by Bachmann, 1994, studied masking as the scientific topic), and a broad taxonomy of masking emerged (reviewed by Bachmann, 1994; Breitmeyer, 1984). Visual masking has also been extensively studied at the mechanistic level with a long tradition of computational modeling (e.g., Landahl, 1967; Weisstein, 1968; Bridgeman, 1971; Anbar & Anbar, 1982; Öğmen, 1993; Francis, 1997; Di Lollo et al., 2000).

The chapters in this part address three questions: What are the mechanisms of visual masking? What can visual masking tell us about the operation of the normal brain? What can visual masking tell us about the operation of the abnormal brain? The first chapter addresses *how* masking operates. Several computational models are analyzed, and a common mechanism, namely, mask blocking, is identified as a common characteristic shared by several models. The chapter presents data that test a prediction of models using a mask blocking mechanism. The following two chapters address *why* masking occurs, *how* it operates, and *what* it can tell us about the dynamics of visual information processing in normal observers. In the second chapter, masking is embedded into a general reentrant (recurrent, feedback) processing theory of visual processing, and a unified view of visual masking, object substitution, and response priming is presented and related to reentrant information processing principles. The third chapter argues that delays and positive feedback loops in recurrent neural architectures can lead to unstable behavior (which may not be apparent in time-limited simulation of models). It presents a dual-channel model—the retinocortical dynamics (RECOD) model—where masking is an emergent property. The chapter presents a unified view of dissociation phenomena in masking and relates these phenomena to the dynamics of perceptual epochs in visual processing. The last chapter in the section uses the masking paradigm to probe the dynamics of visual processing in the abnormal brain (schizophrenia). It provides a review of backward masking deficits in schizophrenia and presents recent findings using electrophysiological and imaging studies that supplement previous neuropsychological approaches. The studies are guided by and related to the theoretical approaches presented in the previous chapters.

Part IV. Temporal aspects of attention. Attentional mechanisms play an important role both in the selective deployment of processing resources during the first half second of visual processing and in the consolidation of stimulus representations in consciousness and memory. This part of the book focuses on the dynamics of attentional mechanisms from electrophysiological, behavioral, and modeling perspectives. The first chapter starts with a tutorial on electrophysiological techniques, in particular event-related potentials (ERPs), used to determine temporal characteristics of attention-related processes during the first half second following stimulus presentation. A wide range of experimental findings are reviewed, culminating in a mapping of various attentional processes on the temporal dimension. The second chapter uses the rapid serial visual presentation (RSVP), where brief images are presented in rapid succession in order to probe dynamical aspects of task-related processes. When two target items are inserted in an RSVP stream, the performance for the second target item is hampered if it follows the first target item by about 500 ms, a phenomenon known as *attentional blink* (AB; Raymond et al., 1992). The chapter uses the AB paradigm to investigate the dynamics of attentional processes within the context of a two-stage competition model. The model consists of a stage of detection and identification followed by a stage of short-term memory consolidation. The third chapter in this section uses the EEG technique, in particular the lateralized readiness potential (LRP) and the N2pc components of ERPs, to probe how masked stimuli can affect attention and response tendencies. The LRP is used as a neural marker for *response selection*. The N2pc component, on the other hand, is used to track the deployment of attentional processes for *stimulus selection*. The chapter also discusses a clinical application of the ERP findings, namely, pathological hemineglect.

Part V. Temporal characteristics of feature and object perception. The visual system is organized in anatomically identifiable areas that contain neurons tuned to different stimulus features such as color, orientation, and motion. This part of the book focuses on the timing and the dynamics of processes whereby various features of the stimuli are detected and "bound together" to form higher level object representations. The first chapter discusses processing asynchronies for different stimulus features as revealed by perceptual mismatches that occur for rapidly changing stimulus features. It focuses on two visual illusions, the flash-lag phenomenon and the color-motion asynchrony, and provides a unified explanation and a qualitative model based on task-dependent differential latencies in neural processing. The next chapter addresses the question of how features are bound together to form objects and how objects are segregated from the background by using feature-inheritance and shine-through effects in masking. *Feature inheritance* refers to the perception of features of a masked target as part of the mask stimulus. *Shine through* is a complementary perceptual state where the target stimulus is visible as a superimposed object on the mask stimulus. The chapter analyzes how the spatial configuration of the mask stimulus can affect feature inheritance and shine through, and it relates the findings to the dynamics of feature binding and figure–ground segregation. The chapter also provides an application of these effects to the study of neural processing deficits in schizophrenia. The final chapter in this part presents a model using a theoretical framework wherein the dynamics of perceptual processing are construed as a process of real-time hypothesis testing, in particular following a Bayesian-like formalism. The model is applied to feature-inheritance and shine-through effects, and a unified view including backward masking and temporal integration is offered.

Part VI. The dynamic relation of unconscious and conscious processes in vision. The chapters in the previous parts provide a rich empirical and theoretical foundation for a distinction between conscious and unconscious processes. The last part of the book revisits many of the themes—such as masking and priming—introduced and discussed in the previous sections and elaborates further on the dynamics of conscious and unconscious processes. The first chapter studies the effects of masked primes on stimulus-dependent motor responses using the eye-movement system. It addresses the questions of how the effects of a masked prime unfold in time and which processes they modulate. By analyzing the effects of masked primes on saccade latencies and trajectories, the authors present an extended version of their accumulator model. They also provide a neurophysiological mapping for real-time effects of masked primes on decision making, response preparation, and motor execution. The second chapter uses masked primes to investigate differences between conscious and unconscious processing of form and surface attributes of objects. It draws distinctions between stimulus- and percept-dependent levels and activities and shows how the effect of masked primes can change depending on the level at which they operate. The chapter reviews the distributed architecture of the visual system and adds another dimension to this architecture, namely, a hierarchy of unconscious and conscious information-processing stages within functional units of the architecture. The last chapter builds upon many of the themes presented in the previous chapter and reviews additional findings from patients with neuropsychological deficits as well as from experiments using the transcranial magnetic stimulation (TMS) technique on normal observers. TMS and masking are complementary techniques that can be used to suppress conscious registration of stimuli. While masking operates through visual signals delivered by the afferent pathways, TMS operates by magnetic fields delivered directly to the cortex via the scalp. A synthesis is offered according to which unconscious vision is fast, is direct, and is bottom-up while conscious vision is slower, is indirect, and includes top-down feedback processing.

Overall, the reader will find common as well as contrasting views in different chapters of the book. In the Epilogue chapter, we will revisit these themes to discuss promising areas for future research. Terms are defined in the glossary at the end of the book.

I CONCEPTUAL ISSUES IN STUDYING CONSCIOUS AND UNCONSCIOUS VISUAL PROCESSES

2 Microgenesis of Perception: Conceptual, Psychophysical, and Neurobiological Aspects

Talis Bachmann

2.1 Introduction

. . . Here are some of his prices:

Ear chawed off $ 15

Leg or arm broke   19

Shot in leg   25

Stab   25

Doing the big job   100 and up

Sometimes, to keep his hand in, Eastman personally carried out a commission.

Even from this excerpt of Jorge Luis Borges's *A Universal History of Infamy* (1979, p. 55), it is clear that humans have always had a strong urge to systematize things, keep them in order and typologized. If this urge applies even to infamous undertakings, then, in the somewhat more noble field of scientific research, it has to be irresistible. And indeed it is, as evidenced by innumerous attempts including those of Linnaeus, Darwin, Mendeleyev, and the unravellers of the genomes. Researchers of visual microgenesis are no different . . .

In what follows I will provide a brief conceptual introduction to the science of perceptual microgenesis, list the most pertinent experimental approaches, and outline some basic regularities of microgenesis found in perception and attention research. Finally, I will suggest a metatheoretical synthesis allowing integration of the different approaches and phenomena established within the microgenetic, perceptual-information-processing research. I will supplement the activity of the mechanisms of microgenesis, which is usually described exclusively from within the domain of sensoria-specific cortical levels of representation, with the contribution of the so-called nonspecific thalamic modulation systems, considered to be necessary for conscious perceptual experience (Magoun, 1958; Bachmann, 1984, 1994; Crick, 1984; Bogen, 1995; Llinás, 2001; Rees et al., 2001; Schiff & Purpura, 2002; Crick & Koch, 2003).

If we take the contribution of the "contentless" thalamic modulation systems for conscious vision that are well-known in neurobiology and adopt it for the purposes of research of explicit perception in psychophysics, then a need emerges for a new psychological concept. It should stand for the information-processing operation that is dedicated for transforming the implicit representational activities into the explicit, consciously experienced format. My term of choice for representing this function used to be *perceptual retouch* (Bachmann, 1984) but eventually developed into *pertention* (Bachmann, 1999). I will deal with pertention in the last part of this chapter.

2.2   Conceptual and Foundational Aspects of Microgenesis

The simple fact that all behavioral and mental responses to pertinent stimulation emerge only after a "silent" delay, termed *latency*, has long been recognized—it was known to such authorities as von Helmholtz, Donders, Wundt, Cattell, and many others. It took some time to realize that mental responses that occur after the latent time interval do not appear in their final, fully formed character as sudden "anti-catastrophes" with infinitesimally small times of formation. Instead, mental responses themselves are subject to development that is characterized by definite successive stages (Lange, 1892a, 1892b, 1892c, 1892d; Sander, 1962; Werner, 1940, 1956; Undeutsch, 1942; Flavell & Draguns, 1957; Hanlon, 1991). Thus there are at least two aspects to the psychological latencies—(1) the time it takes for any specified psychological state or reaction to become first detectable or registered and (2) the time it takes for a psychological state or representation to develop from its initial manifestation up to the full-blown stabilized state that no longer develops further (and may decay or be replaced by another psychological entity). The mental microdevelopmental processes that are characterized by the second variety of latency were termed *microgenesis* by Heinz Werner (1956). Although there are neuropsychological (Brown, 1977, 1988), developmental (Wapner & Kaplan, 1983), and psychodynamic (Kragh & Smith, 1970) approaches to microgenesis, our present concern will be perceptual microgenesis in its psychophysical, computational, and neurobiological aspects.

In a less theory-laden sense, *microgenesis can be defined as a short-term formation of a psychological process*. It can be a percept, provided a respective object or event that ultimately becomes represented in its entirety in a subject's mind is sampled by his or her senses; it can be an emotional response to a visual stimulus; it can be formation of an action targeted at some object. Here, we must distinguish between two interpretations of perceptual formation as microgenesis. First, there is *representational microgenesis* (RMG) that stands for formation of an active mental representation of an object, scene, or event which is the object matter (OM) of cognition. This formation is based on specialized neurobiological processes and constitutes the succession of the necessary stages in mental activity that will guarantee that the information about a particular OM becomes a psychological reality that allows a person implicitly or explicitly to understand the properties and the meanings of the OM, to respond to or act upon it, and to store this information in memory (to use it in responses, actions, and thoughts in future). We can deal with the notion of RMG irrespective of its relation to whether what is (actually becoming) represented is reflected in consciousness or not. There is plenty of documented evidence for us to be convinced that quite specific information about physical properties, meanings, emotiogenic qualities, numerical characteristics, and action-guiding alternatives is processed, represented, and stored by the brain preconsciously (Dixon, 1981; Marcel, 1983; de Gelder et al., 2001a; Dehaene & Naccache, 2001; Naccache & Dehaene, 2001; Jaśkowski et al., 2002; Moutoussis & Zeki, 2002; VanRullen & Koch, 2003c; Kinoshita & Lupker, 2003). A gross technical analogue for RMG would be the photographic process where a negative image of a scene stands for OM and the physical–chemical processes taking part within the emulsion layer of the photographic paper after it has been stimulated by the light pattern from the negative image stand for RMG.

The second interpretation of perceptual formation relates to *phenomenal microgenesis* (PMG). This concept refers to the unfolding or formation of an active mental representation of OM in the directly experienced, phenomenally explicit format (Bachmann, 2000). PMG necessarily requires RMG as its prerequisite, but not vice versa. A gross technical analogue for PMG would be the photographical process where the photochemically structured information from the negative image within the emulsion layer of the photographic paper becomes developed into the pattern of reflectance gradients on the surface of the paper after it has been immersed into the developer liquid. While in photography the directly observable picture development usually takes dozens of seconds, in mental (perceptual) microgenesis the process unfolds within the first half second, that is, it lasts about 0.1–0.3 s (Breitmeyer, 1984; Bachmann, 2000). That is why it is very difficult to obtain authentic phenomenal descriptions of PMG. Many of the facts and the phenomenology of PMG are yet to be discovered and/or agreed upon.

The transfer rules or transformation rules between RMG and PMG are far from clear. Basically, PMG helps to explicate RMG contents for consciousness. But are the preconscious contents within the evolving RMG transformed into explicit format quantally as distinct successive stages that replace each other, or is this transform a continuous change between the developing states of the original "primordial" representation? Is the process of PMG serial (complete one stage, terminate it, and then go to the next) or accumulative, where the continuously updated gist about OM is gradually complemented by the additional experienced information? What are the mandatory and optional steps in the transition between RMG and PMG? Does the phenomenal status of representational contents play any further necessary role for RMG, or is phenomenality just an epiphenomenal property of RMG, and so forth? On the other hand, there are serious methodological difficulties and pitfalls for PMG to be studied, as discussed in the respective research on consciousness (Revonsuo & Kamppinen, 1994; Metzinger, 1995; Bachmann, 2000; Churchland, 2002; Erdelyi, 2004). The first and foremost is the difficulty in crossing the explanatory gap between the subjective phenomenal realm and the third-person domain of objective responses and descriptions that are inevitable if we want to speak about the science of microgenesis. Thus, it is safer and easier to deal with RMG, with experimental evidence based on psychophysical procedures that require objective responses. On the other hand, it is more intriguing and philosophically fundamental to understand the transfer rules between RMG and PMG. In one way or another, we cannot avoid collegial postulates and assumptions about certain minimum levels of intersubjective veridicality of the reports that subjects produce in psychophysical experiments.

It seems that it is easier to find cases where unfolding of PMG can be directly observed from the first-person perspective and "online" if instead of invariant perceptual objects perceptual events are considered. Such cases include binocular rivalry, the flash-lag effect, and the line-motion illusion (e.g., Hikosaka et al., 1993; Wilson et al., 2001; Bachmann et al., 2003). The irony is that in the extremely rapid process of PMG within a fraction of a second and with static, spatially invariant or overlapping objects or scenes, the representational content of the percept at the later stages of its development tends to replace or substitute for the representational content proper to the perceptual act at the earlier stages (Bachmann & Allik, 1976; Michaels & Turvey, 1979; DiLollo et al., 2000; Schlag & Schlag-Rey, 2002). Elsewhere, I have called this *autoclitic masking* (Bachmann, 1987), a problem still without any good solution.

To take apart the actual, however largely hidden process of microgenesis, several methods for probing the microgenetic stages or "freezing" microgenesis at one or another stage of its perceptual development have been used. One can list at least the following experimental strategies and paradigms:

1. Backward masking and metacontrast with the idea to interfere with target microgenesis at different time epochs after target presentation (e.g., Werner, 1935; Breitmeyer, 1984; Bachmann, 1994; Wilenius-Emet et al., 2004; Herzog, this volume; Öğmen & Breitmeyer, this volume; Francis & Cho, this volume; Wynn & Green, this volume). This can be done by systematically changing the stimulus onset asynchrony (SOA) between target and mask onsets.

2. Presentation of hierarchical images (e.g., Navon, 1977; Stoffer, 1993) or hybrid images (e.g., Schyns & Oliva, 1994, 1999; Hughes et al., 1996) with the idea to check out the relative time course of microgenesis of coarse (or global) levels of image description and detailed (or local) levels of description. This can be done by measuring and comparing reaction times to fine-scale/local and coarse-scale/global characteristics of stimulus images or by determining which aspects of the compound image determine identification at short and long exposures or, alternatively, in the conditions of orthogonally varied coarse versus fine and preceding versus succeeding pairings of the stimulation subsets.

3. Perceptual priming of the succeeding stimulus by the preceding, often masked, stimulus (e.g., Calis et al., 1984; Leeuwenberg et al., 1985; Bachmann, 1989; Sanocki, 1993; Hoeger, 1997; Morris et al., 1998; Naccache et al., 2002; Wong & Root, 2003; Scharlau & Neumann, 2003; Vorberg et al., 2003; Scharlau, 2004; Breitmeyer and Öğmen, this volume). This paradigm allows to see what types and aspects of the preceding stimulation pertaining to incomplete MG can facilitate and what types and aspects impair perception of the succeeding stimulation.

4. Presentation of target stimuli within the rapid serial visual presentation (RSVP) streams in order to disclose interaction of feature processing, token processing, individuated object processing, and attentional and short-term memory processes involved in detecting single or multiple targets (e.g., Lawrence, 1971; Potter, 1975; Potter, this volume; Reeves & Sperling, 1986; Broadbent & Broadbent, 1987; Raymond et al., 1992; Chun & Potter, 1995; Seiffert & Di Lollo, 1997; Visser et al., 1999).

5. Spatiotemporal analysis of the components and intracranial distribution of the foci of event-related potential (ERP), magnetoencephalogram (MEG), or functional magnetic resonance imaging responses that are selectively associated with processing one or another type of information inherent in stimulation (e.g., Tong et al., 2000; Sagiv & Bentin, 2001; Liu et al., 2002; Johnson & Olshausen, 2003; Di Russo et al., 2003; Ruz et al., 2003; Proverbio et al., 2004). The idea is to describe the time course of cognitive processes and relate it to specific brain systems.

6. Registration of single-cell activities in response to features, objects, or events with the idea of tracking the time course of respective representational processes at the neuronal level (e.g., Zipser et al., 1996; Lamme & Spekreijse, 1998; Lee et al., 2002; Kreiman et al., 2002; Supèr et al., 2003; Gail et al., 2004).

7. Intervention into brain processes at different sites and different time epochs after visual stimulation onset by administering transcranial magnetic stimulation in order to probe the succession and the mechanisms of the microgenetic stages (e.g., Amassian et al., 1989; Kamitani & Shimojo, 1999; Pascual-Leone & Walsh, 2001; Kammer et al., 2003; Ro et al., 2003; Overgaard et al., 2004).

The most typical support for RMG has been found in the time course functions of perceptual recognition with increasing SOA in backward masking, in the latency operating characteristics (i.e., increase in the precision of perceptual reports with increase in reaction time), and in the temporal dynamics of the successive ERP or MEG components that are known to be related to different information-processing functions within the brain.

In a more theory-laden conceptualization, microgenesis can be interpreted as dynamic perceptual unfolding and differentiation in which the "germ" of the final experience is already embodied in the early stages of its development; later stages do not replace the earlier ones but are founded on them, carrying on their basic contents by refining and supplementing them (Rosenthal, 2004; Bachmann, 2000). Here, microgenesis as a descriptive concept has changed into microgenesis as an explanatory concept (Froehlich, 1984). The key developmental regularities in microgenetic processes are as follows:

1. From less differentiated to more differentiated content.

2. From dynamic and unstable content to stabilized content.

3. From eidotropic to ontotropic qualities ("from appearance to essence").

4. Instead of the stimulus-driven format, microgenesis essentially is an exploratory, search activity striving for the organismic–environmental, adaptively expedient interpretation of stimulation.

Similarly, Crick and Koch (2003) suggested that consciousness functions to provide the best current interpretation of the stimuli. Environmental conditions are not just the "stimulus" but also the constraints within which an organism has to carry out its exploratory and adaptive activity. To accomplish this, the visual system has to rely on a set of different types of specialized and hierarchically organized neurons: (1) the drivers located mostly in the back of the cortex that signal the presence of specific features of stimulation and thus carry the basic content of stimulation; (2) the modulators located in the front of the cortex and in the subcortical structures that increase or decrease the activity of drivers according to situational or contextual pertinence and importance; (3) enabling neurons that function to provide necessary background activity for explicit representation (consciousness) to be possible at all; and (4) penumbra that themselves do not participate directly in the encoding, enabling, or modulating functions but that are necessary as a support and maintenance system. To understand the neurobiological meaning of microgenesis, we have to understand the computational functions and processing algorithms of the basic types of neurons in dealing with sensory data. In the last part of this article I will discuss this problem in a bit more detail.

When addressing the topic of microgenesis, we inevitably try to answer several basic questions that prevail in perception research in general, however concentrating on the time-course aspect. From the microgenetic point of view, we want to know (1) how features are integrated into objects in real time or, alternatively, how the perceptual system extracts and differentiates among the features involved initially in a holistic, undifferentiated entity; (2) how the gist of a scene (or proto-object or token of a thing) develops into its detailed and differentiated representation (or how the object token is individuated); (3) whether RMG is a process where activity is successively transferred between different modular systems that are *located in different brain areas* or this is a change in the *modus of activity* within the *same* neurobiological representational units; (4) how attention influences RMG and PMG and what happens to perceptual microgenesis of one object if attention is engaged with processing of another object; (5) whether it is sufficient to use exclusively feed-forward models of microgenesis to adequately mimic its neurobiological implementation or reentrant activity is inevitably necessary (or whether the solution of this dilemma depends on the task a subject has to solve); (6) what the differences are between the data contents and control functions of RMG and PMG; (7) whether each separate object requires an RMG of its own or there are interactive microgenetic processes that are interchangeable between the different OMs (e.g., microgenesis starting for one object's data but continuing on the data provided by another object, avoiding the redundant steps already executed); (8) how action microgenesis and perceptual microgenesis interact; (9) to what extent, if any, event microgenesis, object microgenesis, and scene microgenesis are carried out by the same processes and based on the same mechanisms, and if there are respective different microgenetic subtypes, how they interact; and (10) what the most adequate algorithms and computational models are for describing microgenetic processes as they unfold within the real neuronal networks in the brain.

Before we are able to provide a satisfactory answer to these more or less fundamental questions, we need to know about more simple properties and characteristics of microgenesis. Pertinent experimental research has already offered some knowledge.

2.3 Psychophysical Regularities of Visual Microgenesis

In what follows, a selection of research results will be discussed, with general implications for the microgenetic domain explicitly stated.

2.3.1 Successive form Recognition (Mutual Masking)

Two successive and spatially overlapping targets (small geometric forms T1 and T2) are presented for 10 ms each and with varying SOAs; both targets have to be recognized. Typical experimental results are depicted in figure 2.1 (adapted from Bachmann & Allik, 1976). With very short SOAs, forms blend into one noisy entity

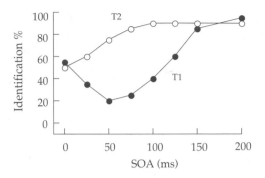

Figure 2.1
Correct perceptual identification of successive target stimuli (T1 and T2) as a function of stimulus onset asynchrony (SOA). With the shortest SOA, targets blend into a composite perceptual object and discrimination is impaired (about 50% correct). With intermediate SOAs, T2 dominates and T1 is rarely perceived. From 150 ms onward both targets are successively identified. (Adapted from Bachmann & Allik, 1976)

and both of them cannot be perfectly identified. With intermediate SOAs around 40–80 ms, perceptibility of T1 drops essentially to the chance level of recognition while T2 becomes almost perfectly perceived. When the SOA reaches about 150 ms, T1 becomes also perfectly recognizable and both targets are clearly and successively perceived. In a follow-up study (one of the experiments in Bachmann, 1994) a task was changed so as to obtain more data about PMG in addition to RMG. Subjects had to manipulate SOA (without knowing the actual value of it) so as to obtain finally a visual experience corresponding to the subjective criterion set for each particular block of trials. T1 had higher intensity than T2 ($200 \, cd/m^2$ vs. $100 \, cd/m^2$). When subjects had to find an SOA that would result in the blending of T1 and T2, to a maximum extent, the actual SOA distribution between subjects centered around 32 ms. When the criterion was to find a condition that would lead to maximum absence of a distinct *visual sensory* (i.e., direct visibility related) quality for T1, combined with distinct visibility of T2, then the distribution of SOA adjustments centered around 67 ms. If the task was to find the SOA that would satisfy the criterion of seeing contrasted T1, however without sufficient time to read out the full alphabetic content of the trigram T1, then the adjusted SOAs grouped around 170 ms. The threshold of full release from visual *and* cognitive masking was set to 244 ms on the average.

We can conclude that (1) in microgenesis, subsequent input tends to prevail over the preceding input; (2) it takes about 150 ms for the stabilized, finalized visual-microgenetic process to complete (given few object alternatives and an absence of extra noise besides targets) and about 240 ms for visual and conceptual microgenesis; (3) with very short time intervals, very brief stimulus objects (e.g., 10 ms each) become perceptually integrated into one blended object (features of two objects bound into one object); (4) separate perceptual object formation takes about 100 ms or more; (5) higher level cognitive contents of an object may require more time to reach end stages of PMG compared to strictly sensory-objective microgenesis. It is important to note that even though the contrast and intensity of T1 considerably exceed those of T2, at intermediate SOAs T2 nevertheless dominates and T1 is deprived of the efficient PMG (Bachmann, 1994). It is important to mention that for T1, the recognition function (masking function) resembles the J-shaped or U-shaped functions that are typical for metacontrast (Werner, 1935; Breitmeyer, 1984): T2 acts as a mask for T1.

Even more important is to acknowledge the importance of attention in modulating the effects of mutual masking. When subjects were asked to report whether a stimulus that was predesignated as target for that particular trial was presented, the U-shaped function for T1 disappeared and T1 and T2 were perceived with virtually the same efficiency (Bachmann & Allik, 1976). Thus, perceptual microgenesis can be modulated by the attentional processes (see also Ramachandran & Cobb, 1995).

If T1 consists of a single letter and T2 is a pair of mutually identical letters (but different from T1), then the result of mutual masking depends on the relative spatial position of the letters, but only if the SOA is short or intermediate (Bachmann et al., 2005a). With shorter time intervals a pair of T2 letters masks the T1 letter more strongly if T1 is flanked by T2 tokens as in a typical crowding display and similarly to metacontrast masking, compared to the conditions where T1 itself is one of the flanking stimulus letters. With a long SOA of 100 ms, there is no difference in the masking level between the flanking and flanked conditions for T1, although masking is still very strong at about 30% correct identification. Thus, with longer SOAs object competition, instead of sensory characteristics of the stimulus objects, is what matters (figure 2.2).

Taken together, the results from mutual masking experiments suggest that in the microgenesis of successive sensory input pertaining to localized perceptual objects first there is spatiotemporal integration (where intensity relationships and camouflage capacity strongly contribute to the probability of correct perception and where intrachannel inhibition occurs—cf. also Öğmen & Breitmeyer, this volume; Francis & Cho, this volume), followed by visual object formation (allowing some form of interchannel inhibition or object substitution if the objects compete), which in turn gives way to attentional focusing (allowing switching from the first object to the second object, provided there has been enough time to form separate successive objects). In the absence of attentional focus, object substitution can take place, only whereby the second replaces the first in consciousness (see also Enns et al., this volume).

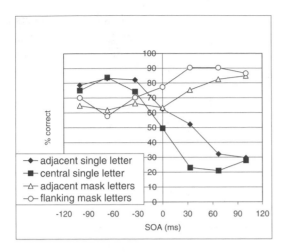

Figure 2.2
Correct perceptual identification of successive targets (single letter and a pair of identical letters) as a function of stimulus onset asynchrony (SOA) and spatial arrangement of the stimuli. Positive values of SOA refer to the conditions where the single-letter target is presented before the double-letter target. With shorter SOAs up to 60 ms, when a single-letter target is backward masked by bilaterally flanking two letters of the double-letter target, masking is stronger than masking when the single-letter target itself is a flanking stimulus. However at an SOA of 100 ms, where strong backward masking continues spatial arrangement does not matter anymore. (Adapted from Bachmann et al., 2005a)

2.3.2   Masking by Spatially Quantized Images

What are the relative roles of features, configurations of feature tokens, and spatial frequencies in microgenesis? We carried out face-identification experiments where images of faces (targets) were masked by spatially quantized masks that were derived from (1) same faces as targets, (2) different faces than targets, and (3) Gaussian random noise with the spectra similar to typical faces (Bachmann et al., 2004a, 2005b). In forward masking, provided that spatial quantization was coarse, the strongest impairment of target perception was obtained with the noise mask; however, both quantized different face mask and quantized same face mask allowed relatively high-level and equally efficient target identification. We conclude that at the early stages of RMG the visual system builds up a kind of proto-object representation where detailed characteristics of identity are not represented as yet; however, a coarse configuration that can be shared between the different specimens of the same general visual category of objects (e.g., faces) sets the foundation of object microgenesis. With fine-scale quantization, same-face masks produced virtually no masking (naturally, because T1–T2 integration just emphasizes target identity) and noise masks produced intermediate-level masking (about 65% correct), while the different-face masks caused strong masking (about 40% correct). Object feature configuration seems to be the decisive characteristic at the early stages of microgenesis, leaving local features and generalized spatial-frequency content with secondary roles. This conclusion rests on the following arguments. First, forward masking (compared to backward masking) is known to have its effect at the early contrast- or luminance-integrative stages of stimulus processing (Turvey, 1973; Breitmeyer, 1984; Bachmann, 1994). Second, the spatial-frequency contents of noise masks and face masks preset at the same quantization level are equal; local features are "dissolved" within the squares of quantized image, however image configurations differ. Third, with more and more fine-scale quantization different-face masks produce increasingly stronger masking while fine-scale quantization of noise masks does not increase masking.

In backward masking with the same types of quantized masks we found equally strong masking (about 25% correct) at short SOAs with different-face and noise masks and weak masking (about 70% correct) with same-face masks. With the largest SOAs around 100 ms, strong backward masking by a different-face mask was sustained, but masking by a noise mask became weaker (about 45% correct). (See figure 2.3.) Because spatial-frequency contents of the different types of quantized masks were equal, but configural properties vis-à-vis target faces were different, we conclude that backward masking at longer SOAs cannot be explained exclusively by spatial-frequency masking (Rogowitz, 1983) or transient-on-sustained, interchannel inhibition (see also Öğmen & Breitmeyer, this

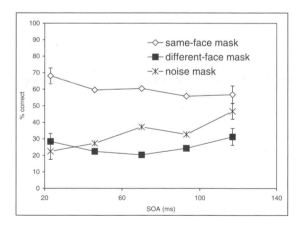

Figure 2.3
Correct perceptual identification of stimulus faces backward masked by three types of spatially quantized ("blocked") masks as a function of stimulus onset asynchrony (SOA). With shortest SOAs, different-face mask and noise mask produce equally strong masking; however, with longer SOAs above 60 ms different-face mask exerts a significantly stronger masking effect than noise mask, which acts at a level close to the effect of same-face mask. (Adapted from Bachmann et al., 2005b)

volume). The contribution of configurational and attentional processes should be acknowledged.

Generally stated, the results of these studies suggest that (1) if the first appearing structured stimulus is coarsely similar to S2, it can serve as an input for the proto-object stage of interactive RMG where S1 and S2 can be regarded as aspects of the same microgenetic event and S2 processing essentially begins on the basis of pre-processed S1 data (S1 allows "surrogate microgenesis" to begin for S2); (2) later stages of microgenesis are governed by meaningfulness and attention-capturing capacity of the formed/forming perceptual objects; and (3) with more advanced stages of microgenesis the local features are replaced by integrated configural objects (scenes?) as the primary OM of microgenesis and microgenetic competition.

2.3.3 Proactive Facilitation Between Successive Forms

In this paradigm, two successive spatially overlapping or closely adjacent visual forms (S1 and S2) are presented. The delay with which S2 becomes visible is measured by temporal order judgment (TOJ) or other methods and compared to the delay in the control condition where S2 is presented at the target location alone or preceded by some different stimulus than S1. It appears both that S2 subjective contrast is increased (Bachmann, 1988) and its perceptual latency is decreased (Bachmann, 1989; Aschersleben & Bachmann, submitted; Scharlau & Neumann, 2003; Vorberg et al., 2003; Scharlau, 2004) if a prime (S1) precedes S2. Importantly, the proactive facilitation effect occurs even though S1 is backward masked to invisibility. Whether the above-described economy in time of microgenesis is a consequence of the process of facilitation (increase in the gain of neural responses) that originates from a nonspecific source of facilitatory modulation (e.g., pertentional retouch from the thalamus) or a result of time saving due to "surrogate" preliminary steps of microgenetic percept development within the specific systems (e.g., exclusively within the domain of driver neurons) remains an unsolved problem.

It also appears that a higher contrast stimulus among the rapidly alternating stimuli tends to be evaluated as the later occurring one despite its actual order relative to the other stimulus (Bachmann et al., 2004b). At the present stage of our knowledge, it is difficult to say whether the illusory effects of stimulus order are truly visual effects (e.g., microgenesis of S2 completed before the microgenesis of S1) or whether they originate from purely nonsensory decision-making stages as response biases.

In conclusion, (1) a spatially overlapping or nearby stimulus can speed up and increase the resultant saliency of RMG and PMG for the succeeding stimulus; (2) facilitative effects of the preceding stimulation originate also from the primes that remain preconscious; (3) masked primes can influence motoric responses to later stimuli even if masked to invisibility; (4) in the PMG of brief visual events the higher contrast stimuli tend to be evaluated as the later occurring ones; (5) in the finalized microgenesis of extremely rapid visual events consisting of successive exposures, veridical temporal order of stimulation may be transformed.

2.3.1 Perception of Targets Presented Within RSVP Streams of Invariant Items

In ecologically valid sensory environments we rarely meet blank backgrounds with one or two brief stimuli presented against them. To bring microgenetic research a bit closer to more ecovalid circumstances, it is important to present experimental stimuli within streams of sensory input items. The research based on RSVP techniques somewhat fulfills this purpose (Potter, 1975, this volume; Reeves & Sperling, 1986; Raymond et al., 1992). However, in RSVP streams all successive stimulus items typically represent mutually different objects (e.g., different letters). This creates a situation that tends to lean toward the other extreme: We rarely meet ecovalid environments where within a second a dozen or more spatially overlapping, however mutually different objects are presented. There are almost no studies with "proto-streams," that is, with streamed input that consists of samples of the same stimulus object in continuous succession.

It appears that target objects (e.g., the letter *Z*) within streams of unchanging items (e.g., the letter *I*) tend to be perceived before the replicas of the same targets that are simultaneously presented out of stream, in isolation (Bachmann & Põder, 2001; Bachmann et al., 2003). The perceptual speeding up of microgenesis of the samples of in-stream stimulation accumulates and sampling obtains its maximum perceptual speed within the first 150 ms from the stream onset (the temporal advantage of the in-stream target perception over the isolated target perception amounts to 60–80 ms). In-stream temporal facilitation somewhat subsides at the subsequent epochs but persists with the value of about 30 ms up to and over the stream epochs that are characteristic for the attentional blink (see Potter, this volume) and for repetition blindness (figure 2.4). The time values and the essence of the in-stream facilitation effect permit us to consider this effect as a variety of the well-known flash-lag effect (FLE; see Nijhawan, 1994; Krekelberg & Lappe, 2001; Eagleman, 2001; Whitney, 2002). In both cases the isolated presentation of the target is juxtaposed experimentally with the continuously changing stimulus (a moving object that changes its spatial position or an object that continuously changes its color or spatial frequency). In both cases, also, perception of the "flashed" (i.e., isolated, out-stream) object lags behind perception of the object that is undergoing continuous change or is presented within the continuously presented stream of sensory input.

We can conclude that (1) microgenesis of in-stream objects is facilitated, (2) the most conspicuous temporal facilitation takes place between 100 and 150 ms after stream onset, (3) in-stream facilitation is sustained at the epochs of stream presentation that are typically associated with attentional blink (200–400 ms), and (4)

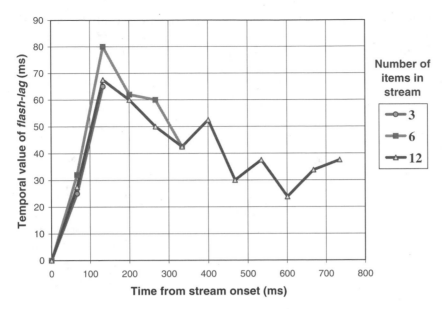

Figure 2.4
Temporal value of the flash lag for the targets presented out of the stream of invariant, spatially unchanging stream items with regard to the targets presented within the stream. Flash-lag is shown as a function of time from stream onset. Relative in-stream facilitation is maximized within 150 ms of stream onset and decreases thereafter; however, it is sustained at least for almost 1 s. (Adapted from Bachmann & Oja, 2003)

temporal values of in-stream microgenetic acceleration are compatible in static and dynamic displays of streamed input. Our recent observations have shown that beta-frequency (20-Hz) presentation of the stream items is no less favorable for in-stream facilitation compared to a higher gamma-frequency rate (e.g., 60 Hz) of presentation.

2.3.5 General Conclusions

It is realistic to assume that in microgenesis a representation is "computed" at the proto-object stage that will be used for further updating and individuation at later stages (cf. "tokens" and "types"; Kanwisher, 1987). Updating of the evolving microgenetic object is faster than creating a new representation for the newly appearing object ab ovo. Proto-objects at the early stages of microgenesis are sufficient in order to provide the "gist" of stimulation for the higher cognitive levels before the full-blown PMG has been completed. In microgenesis, gist precedes the detailed and individuated perceptual object (Bachmann, 2000; Crick & Koch, 2003; Edelman & Tononi, 2000; Rensink, 2000; Hochstein & Ahissar, 2002; Lamme, 2003). Both specific data-processing operations by drivers and nonspecific processes of facilitative modulation are involved in predetermining the dynamics of RMG and PMG.

2.4 Hypothetical Neurobiological Mechanisms Subserving Microgenesis

As is always the case in developing areas, in microgenetic research there are more unanswered questions than firmly established regularities and principles. Is the succession of microgenetic stages based on successive transfer of the processing focus between separately located cortical modules, or is it primarily a change in state and activity patterning over the global distributed network of active neurons? Is feedforward activity upstream from lower to higher levels sufficient for PMG, and thus the later reentrant processes (if ever needed at all) are just the useful, but not necessary supplement to the feedforward processes? Or, alternatively, maybe reentrant activity from higher order nodes is absolutely necessary for PMG to become completed? Do nonspecific thalamic and reticular systems that are often considered to be just an enabling factor for PMG play a causally necessary role in microgenesis proper? How might binding mechanisms in the brain (e.g., feature binding; cf. works of Treisman (1988), Singer (1994), Engel et al. (1992), and others) and the processes of RMG and PMG be related? Is microgenesis essentially a time-consuming binding process?

Despite the many unanswered questions, combined neuroscientific and psychophysical research from the last half century makes it possible to describe a general neural architecture that allows for implementation of basic principles of visual data processing (both implicit and explicit) and to suggest an interdisciplinary metatheory. Hence, psychophysical microgenetic phenomena are explained on the basis of the activities of this architecture. I will rely primarily on the accounts of conscious visual processing suggested by Crick and Koch (2003), Lamme (2003), and Bachmann (1994, 1999).

The generalized neural processing architecture is shown in figure 2.5. When an organism is actively searching his or her environment, reacting to the impinging stimulation, and building up or reactivating the informational model of the surroundings and the situation (its representation), the following subtasks of information processing have to be carried out:

1. *Sensing*, where specialized modular systems in the back of the cortex (e.g., V1, V2, V3, V4, MT, and inferotemporal and temporal cortices) including selectively tuned driver neurons (having small receptive fields) become activated so as to extract and encode specific features inherent in the actual sensory input. This system provides the elementary featural contents, the "what it is" type of information of what will be perceived—location, color, brightness, size, edges, orientation, spatial

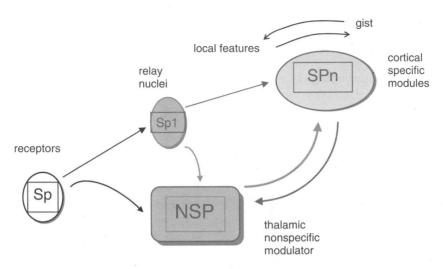

Figure 2.5
Generalized neurobiological architecture of visual information processing combining the contributions of specific sensory systems (SP; including driver neurons) and nonspecific thalamic modulation systems (NSP). The specific processing stream begins from receptors, passes via relay nuclei to the cortex at the sites where local features are encoded, and sends information further to the higher cortical levels representing the gist of the stimulation. The nodes at the gist-related levels send reentrant signals back to the features level. SP provides the contents of explicit perception, but its necessary activity is insufficient for conscious perception. For the SP contents to become upgraded to conscious status, facilitatory modulation from the thalamic NSP system is needed, the process termed *pertention*. (Adapted from Bachmann, 1994, 1999)

frequency, motion—and also some integrated (complex and hypercomplex) characteristics combined on the basis of simple features—visual forms and patterns. This system receives input from receptors, conveys the signals via the relay nuclei (e.g., lateral geniculate) up to the back of cortex, and activates the drivers that are selectively tuned to their particular features. Two main cortical streams, ventral and dorsal, originate from this feedforward flow (see also Goodale et al., this volume). The contact with the designated drivers can be effected very quickly—for instance, within 10–40 ms (Rolls & Tovée, 1994; Lamme, 2003; Bachmann, 1994). The activity of this specific system (SP) is necessary for providing the elementary constituents of the contents of perceptual images, however insufficient for the explicit status ("conscious quality") to be acquired for this data. Sensing means finding a code for the feature type of computation implemented mainly by the activity of drivers and their penumbra.

2. *Perceiving*, where feature-level drivers send their signals upstream to the advanced temporal, parietal, and prefrontal modules of SP, specifying the gist of the sensory content (e.g., an image of a scene or object). Higher level nodes become

activated. Generalized visual categories, proto-object level of input specification, and meaning of the stimulation are specified (suggested and "hypothesized"?). However, the initial stages of this process are characterized by ambiguity, instability, and lack of invariant integration. Computational pluralism, with less probable interim outcomes of computation still being uninhibited and available for further operations at par with the most probable computational variants, characterizes this state. It takes about 50–100 ms to fulfill neural computations up to this stage. The following stage in perceiving requires that reentrant (backpropagating, reverse-hierarchical) signals from the generalized, gist-related nodes arrive back to the early levels in the back of the cortex, providing necessary modulations that help to disambiguate and individuate the perceived objects and scenes. This is done, therefore, by integrating the gist representation (proto-object representation) related activity in the more advanced cortical sites with the activity in the back of the cortex that stands for the local detailed features. The eidotropic and ontotropic functions of RMG are thus satisfied jointly. Top-down signals from the front of the cortex to the back of the cortex act as modulators of the early activity that help to shape the structuring of the neuronal pool that stands for the invariant, active, detailed representation of the actual input. This process takes about 100–150 ms at least, which is definitely longer than the time it takes to carry out the initial feedforward contact with drivers at the beginning of sensing. For Victor Lamme, Shaul Hochstein, Francis Crick, and Christof Koch the reentrant modulation within SP (i.e., within the cortical tissue) seems to be sufficient for PMG of stimulation. For me (and probably for Gerald Edelman, Giulio Tononi, Joseph Bogen, and Rodolfo Llinás), top-down modulation from the front of cortex is necessary but insufficient for explicit representation to be created. The activity within SP should be synchronized with or at least modulated by the subcortical activity from the nonspecific thalamic nuclei (the NSP), such as intralaminar nuclei, *nucleus reticularis thalami*, and pulvinar, and possibly brainstem reticular activating afferents. Perceiving means integration of multifeatured data carried by a multitude of drivers under the supervision of the category-specific nodes higher up in the hierarchy and possibly by the coordinated bottom-up and top-down activity involving reentrant signaling.

3. *Attending*, where a subset of designated drivers, specified according to receptive field location, sensory features, conceptual categories, or other preselected characteristics, becomes singled out and selectively facilitated (or filtered out from among the inhibited competitors) under the control of higher level nodes in parietal and/or frontal parts of the cortex. *Attending* means selecting a domain or place and concentrating processing resources on the selected representations. Modulators fulfill the control functions. It has been quite convincingly argued that attention cannot be equated with consciousness (Baars, 1997; Naccache et al., 2002; Crick & Koch, 2003; Lamme, 2003; Kentridge et al., 2004). First, maximum concentration of

undistracted attending does not guarantee awareness of information that is in the focus of attention. Second, selective attention also improves processing of preconscious and subconscious information. Third, attention can select between different objects or stimuli that are already consciously perceived. Fourth, neurobiological structures that control attention are different from neurobiological structures that are necessary for phenomenal consciousness, although there is a notable overlap, of course (cf. works of Scheibel (1981), Posner (1994), LaBerge (1995)). Attention is selective activity and presetting priorities irrespective of whether the *result* of this activity also implies clear and enhanced conscious apprehension. Yet most of what is unattended remains out of explicit perception. It takes from 100 up to 400 ms in most cases to preset and effect attentional focusing.

4. *Generating conscious status* for perceptual processed data, where (a) enabling neurons in the ascending reticular activating system and nonspecific thalamus set the activity of cortical neurons at the level that is necessary for alertness, and (b) modulating neurons in the thalamus (and possibly in the front of the cortex) modulate the activity of drivers so that preconscious sensory and perceptual information encoded and represented by these drivers becomes explicitly experienced (conscious). As mentioned above, I had earlier used the concept of perceptual retouch for this purpose (Bachmann, 1984, 1994), but more recently I have suggested a special term for the psychophysiological process that has the function of transforming preconscious perceptual (representational) information into an explicitly sensed/perceived form (Bachmann 1999): *pertention*. This neologism was created by combining *perception* and *attention*; however, in terms of meaning it serves the same function as *perceptual retouch*. It is my firm belief that a lot of controversies and disagreements in neuroscience and psychology originate from the absence of a special concept for the operation of transforming preconscious into conscious information. Using terms such as *attention* and *perception* instead just creates a lot of confusion—not least because perception can be preconscious and attention does not guarantee consciousness for the objects in attended locations. While attention is typically under the subject's direct control, pertention is always a spontaneous operation. Although pertention serves an important function to feed working memory with explicated perceptual information, it is a different concept from working memory because pertentional functions and working memory functions can be dissociated (e.g., Yi et al., 2004).

The basic neural mechanism that works as the basis of pertention involves efferent fibers from subcortical thalamic (featurally nonspecific!) neurons that project onto apical dendrites of cortical driver neurons, respective synapses, and local circuitry that carries out the functions of increase in the gain of driver responses and coincidence detection (and thus synchronization) between the activity of driver neurons in SP and modulating neurons in NSP. (Whereas Crick & Koch, 2003, interpret cortical frontal neurons as the main mechanism of [top-down] modulation and render to intralaminar and other thalamic neurons the role of the enabling factor, I believe that NSP-thalamus sends its modulating efferent impulses upstream to the cortical drivers and thus fulfills the function of pertention (see Bachmann, 1994, 1999, for the arguments in favor of NSP as the modulator that is necessary for perceptual consciousness). Importantly, it is known that signals within SP that travel from receptors to cortical drivers and signify the presence of specific features (the stimulation content) are insufficient for the conscious awareness of this content. Modulation from NSP-thalamus is a necessary addition in order for the SP contents to become explicitly perceived. Moreover, afferent arrival of signals that carry specific content is much faster (cortical latencies are about 20–50 ms) than the thalamic nonspecific modulation that is evoked by actual stimulation via collaterals that bypass classical sensory relays. The latter process takes about 80–200 ms to be shipped to cortical levels where the content-specific drivers reside. Also, receptive fields of the NSP modulator neurons are much larger than receptive fields of the drivers in SP. Among other things, nonspecific efferents from the thalamus branch widely in cortical areas containing SP neurons.

The standard local effect of the afferents from NSP-thalamus is to quantally increase the excitatory postsynaptic potentials (EPSPs) of the driver neurons. This leads to (1) an increase in the cumulative and/or epoch frequency of firing of the driver neurons that carry the specific contents of stimulation (and, consequently, increase in the signal-to-noise ratio of respective information and higher probability of inclusion in the widespread global active assemblies), (2) a decrease in the latency with which a driver begins to discharge, and (3) an increase in the flow of synaptic mediator substances associated with activation and alertness. The more global effect, based on local presynaptic gain effects and coincidence detection, involves (re)setting the global coherence of activity in the neurons that represent the currently most important input. This process is under the NSP control that is capable of synchronizing the activity of mutually distant pools of neurons (Edelman & Tononi, 2000; Llinás, 2001; Ward, 2003). PMG can be conceptualized as resetting coherence (adjusting the relative phase of the oscillatory envelope of the firing activity) in a selected subset of SP drivers subjected to NSP modulation.

Now, what about microgenesis in the light of this architecture, provided we use psychophysical stimulation described in the second part of this chapter? Let me explain the typical effects and phenomena on the basis of the workings of the SP + NSP architecture.

1. *Mutual masking.* The dominance of T2 over T1 at intermediate SOAs is explained as a result of association of the delayed (slow) NSP modulation that was

evoked by T1 with the arrival of the maximized, initial activity from T2 at the respective cortical drivers. As a result, the gain and spiking frequency for the carriers of T2 information exceed respective values of the carriers of T1 information and pertention is more salient for T2, which becomes the prime matter of attention. The fact that even a more intense T1 can be effectively masked by a weaker T2 owes to the importance of the NSP process that was evoked by T1 in explicating T2. This is an example of interactive microgenesis where a preceding object processing participates in the succeeding object processing and can be considered as a surrogate initial microgenetic operation for the latter.

2. *Metacontrast.* The explanation is the same, but simply because NSP neurons have larger receptive fields than SP drivers, the spatially adjacent preceding stimulus can cause NSP modulation that spatially covers also receptive fields of drivers that stand for sensory input originating from the neighboring *specific* receptive field. Two different specific receptive fields reside within a common overlapping *nonspecific* receptive field. The known neurobiology of sensory SP and NSP systems allows this conceptualization to be realistic (Brooks & Jung, 1973; Gusel'nikov, 1976).

3. *Substitution masking.* The otherwise inefficient ("weak") masks that cannot have a masking effect on targets when attention is prefocused on target location nevertheless produce severe masking if distractors are presented together with the target. Distractors disperse attentional resources, and masking gets stronger (Di Lollo et al., 2000; Enns et al., this volume). If we assume that NSP resources (mediator substances, number of parallel channels available) are sensitive to the number of objects displayed, it is natural to assume that it would take longer for pertention to highlight SP input from the target locus when distractors are displayed. Consequently, pertention becomes effective only later when most of what is there to be transformed into explicit format is SP information that pertains to the mask. Moreover, if the substitution-masking theory of DiLollo and Enns necessarily assumes reentrant processing for explaining substitution of S1 by S2, the NSP modulation account can explain the dominance of S2 over S1 simply in feedforward terms (for another feedforward account of substitution, see, e.g., Neill, Hutchison, & Graves, 2002).

4. *Proactive facilitation of S2 by the preceding S1.* The same general logic also applies here. Without S1, the information in SP for S2 has to persist long before the slow-latency pertentional activity from NSP arrives at the critical drivers in SP. Respective drivers that stand for S2 begin spiking late. On the other hand, if S1 has already set the NSP modulation in motion, S2-specific signals become upgraded by presynaptic NSP impulses earlier and visual latency for S2 decreases. Nothing changes in principle if S1 itself remains preconscious. Alternatively, the RMG for S1 within SP can be considered as a surrogate RMG for S2, and as soon as S2-

specific signals arrive, some preprocessing has become redundant and S2 microgenesis catches up halfway, thus reaching an explicit and stabilized state faster than it would have done without the S1.

5. *In-stream facilitation in RSVP and FLE.* Again, at the onset of the stream, it takes some time until NSP modulation becomes optimized, and sampling of information from the first items in the stream for PMG is slow. With ever more advanced epochs of stream (up to about 100–200 ms postonset), the NSP modulation has been better and better prepared and the SP information about the items in the stream becomes explicated by pertention faster than the items that appear as the first ones in the stream or that are presented in isolation ("flashed").

6. *Attentional blink.* When pertentional activity becomes associated with setting or holding T1-related information in working memory (e.g., 200–300 ms after T1 onset), which requires extra afference from NSP, there will be insufficient pertentional resources left for T2 to be upgraded enough to capture attention. This means that working memory uses not only attentional resources but also pertentional resources.

7. *Line-motion effect.* Visible expansion along the length of a line that is presented as S2, with expansion starting from the locus of a preceding S1 presented at one end of the S2, could well exemplify the visible spatiotemporal gradient of pertention as it unfolds online with NSP modulation. The data about S2 that were encoded preconsciously by drivers become continuously upgraded to explicit format by spatially spreading presynaptic activation. It was first instigated at the receptive field centered on S1 but gradually spreads to more advanced locations specified by the SP content of S2.

Why do we need an extra mechanism, the NSP, in order to process visual information for explicit perception? Why can functions of consciousness not be fulfilled exclusively or primarily by the SP subsystems of perceptual processing? Should not it be more parsimonious that just SP systems would suffice? It seems to me that there are several adaptively useful properties in the pertentional system. The existence of a special, dedicated mechanism for consciousness (i.e., for explicating implicit perception) is justified by the following:

1. In the course of RMG, the representational state supported by the active driver neurons is initially noisy, ambigous, and nonstabilized. A subject should not *see* this as far as we stick to the conceptualization of consciousness as the best current interpretation of the environmental stimulation. (Cf. also the saccadic suppression effect that guarantees that a smear of image resulting from eye movements will not be explicitly perceived.) Only when the disambiguated and stabilized RMG representations have emerged does PMG become effective. If the consciousness property of

perception were to accompany all SP processes (and were interim computations included), noisy and unexplicable states would be experienced. We have not evolved to see noise.

2. In order to carry out SP computations regarding features and objects quickly and with minimum occurrence of errors, it would be desirable to avoid burdening the system of specific data processing with an additional task—for instance, the task of generating consciousness. For this purpose, a special (however "nonspecific" in terms of computing the contents) process termed *pertention* is used.

3. Consciousness property per se as a characteristic of mental information-processing systems has to be unspecific, invariant to specific contents, if it is expected to keep the function of providing subjective unity and consistency to conscious cognition from the first-person perspective. The neurobiological means that bring together a variety of qualitatively different sensory contents as the experiences of the same person have to be themselves general and lacking any sensory specificity. This may be understood via a comparison: A mirror that is expected to reflect equally well everything patterned and qualia laden and do this independently from how this patterning and quality communicating is instantiated should itself carry no patterning. For this, a special, general-purpose system of pertention is needed.

4. It is parsimoneous to carry out some processing without concomitant consciousness being associated with that which is processed. Some tasks are better left as preconscious activities. The SP system should and can do this, being specific to informational contents. But this also means that there should be some additional mode of activity reserved for processing up to the consciously explicated level.

5. If Richard Gregory (1998) is correct in suggesting that one of the prime functions of consciousness is to define the present moment (as different from past and future), then almost by definition there should be some process specialized for consciousness. This is because computation of the sensory-perceptual content of the stimulation within SP is heavily dependent on information stored in memory, the effects of dispositional, need-related factors included. As taken exclusively from within SP processing, it may happen that the sense of past, present, and future appear as hopelessly confused. However, for the pertentional process that has a privileged position to associate the highest explicit saliency of the processed perceptual information with what is actually there, stimulating the receptors is just a suitable means of flagging the present. Adaptively sensible reacting very much depends on distinguishing between past information and present information. Remember the difficulties Luria's patient S. encountered when his imagination, remembering, and perception were compatible in terms of sensory salience (Luria, 1969). (In the cases of illusory presence, as in night dreams, pertention may work only to upgrade the memory-based sensory contents.)

To end the introductory story of microgenesis, let us think about an imaginary famous hero named Westman. He, similarly to the infamous Eastman who appeared at the outset of this article, feels an irresistible urge to set the system and carefully preplan things. However, *his* job is related to microgenetic research. What would he list as the proper jobs to do? I think one central job would be to understand how RMG and PMG interact and what the best experiments are to use for this purpose. Another important job would be to make clear what the relative roles of feedforward and reentrant processes are within the processing architecture that is used to describe the time course of perceptual microgenesis. Further, he would try to understand what constitutes the proto-object level of microgenesis, where in the brain the structures responsible for proto-object representation reside. Are proto-objects and finalized (detailed, individuated) objects encoded in different brain locations or, alternatively, in the same locations, however at different time epochs featuring different types of activity (i.e., structural code vs. processing-mode code)? And how do within-level microgenesis (e.g., from coarse-scale object to fine-scale object representation) and between-levels microgenesis (e.g., from features to objects to concepts and back again) interrelate? But what is the big job? I hope my highly esteemed colleagues in the following chapters help approach the answer to this question.

Acknowledgments

The preparation of this article was partly supported by Estonian Science Foundation Grant 4967.

3 Neural Correlates and Levels of Conscious and Unconscious Vision

Bruno G. Breitmeyer and Petra Stoerig

3.1 Introduction

The last 15 to 20 years have increasingly revealed the material beauties and workings of the brain and have also spawned a resurgent interest in the study of its fellow traveler, veiled in the complex and intricate pattern of its electrochemical events. On the right side of the body–mind concept, somewhere between the subjectively obvious and the objectively mysterious, consciousness has become a prized quarry pursued by a motley party of cognitive scientists including among others physicists, chemists, engineers, computer scientists, neurobiologists, psychologists, and philosophers. Our survey deals mainly with topics relevant to the latter four categories of researchers, for whom the neural correlates (or causes) of consciousness (NCCs) currently present an especially important field of inquiry (e.g., Baars, 1988; Block, 1996; Crick & Koch, 2003; Dehaene & Naccache, 2001; Dennett, 1991; Edelman, 2003; Metzinger, 2002). Moreover, we limit ourselves to the most extensively studied system, the visual system, hoping that the organizational principles governing conscious registration there may also apply in other sensory or cognitive systems. A key operative assumption adopted by most neuroscientists studying the NCCs in vision is that consciously represented neural activity (the visual "homunculus") is in some identifiable way distinct from other simultaneously ongoing activities that are not represented in this form (the visual "zombie"). In animals possessing a central nervous system (CNS), neural activity is assumed to be a prerequisite of conscious experience, although in humans, as well as in the most extensively studied other mammals, the vast majority of neural processing appears not to be consciously represented.

Several important, interrelated issues arise when searching for the NCCs in vision (and in any other sensory or cognitive modality). As noted by Stoerig (2002), consciousness can be regarded both as a global state of an organism and as a trait of particular cognitive contents such as a perception, memory, thought, desire, or intention. A second, more problematic issue is how to conceive of, and specify, the locus and the functional architecture of the NCCs (Frith et al., 1999). For instance, if all losses of consciousness resulted from a corresponding necessary loss of, or damage to, the same minimal set of structures in the CNS, one could take that set to comprise the hypothetical NCCs. In this case the site and architecture of the NCCs would be highly specifiable, even if we still must search for the neurons or neuronal activity patterns that mediate the experience of sensations. Alternatively, if consciousness is an emergent, holistic property of overall brain activity (Sperry, 1969, 1970), any such specification is problematic. A third issue of interest is to what extent trait consciousness is unified or diverse and separable into several types. Phenomenal and access consciousness are examples of such types, with the first referring to the "feely" aspect of conscious experience such as color, warmth, and softness, and the second to the operations we can perform consciously on the basis of the phenomenal representations, such as recalling the smell of a rose, counting the number of red patches in an array, or reporting the result of such a process (Block, 1995, 1996; Nelkin, 1996). Moreover, the multitudes of different qualia—in vision alone, color, motion, depth, brightness—may have specific neural networks or modules (Zeki, 1997, 1998; Zeki & Bartels, 1999). A fourth issue is that the term *NCC* can be used in different ways. With regard to vision, the NCCs, when defined broadly enough, can be found along the entire retino-geniculate-cortical tract and, for instance, could even include retinal receptor activity correlated with the perception of color. Despite this, very few would seriously argue that consciously represented neural processes reside at the level of the retina, lateral geniculate nucleus, or other subcortical retinorecipient nuclei; even the role of the primary visual cortex is discussed controversially (Crick & Koch, 1995; Pollen, 1999). If processing at higher cortical levels is required, this activity, with or without its being broadcast via these higher cortical levels' reentrant backprojections to lower cortical visual areas (Edelman, 1987; Edelman & Tononi, 2000; Hochstein & Ahissar, 2002; Pascual-Leone & Walsh, 2001; Stoerig & Brandt, 1993; Zeki, 1993), would form an essential set of the NCCs. Since conscious representations depend on the organism's being in a conscious state, this set must additionally rely for its upkeep on modulatory activity from subcortical, sensorily nonspecific areas of the brain (Bachmann, this volume; Bogen, 1995, 1997; Hobson & Steriade, 1986; Moruzzi & Magoun, 1949; Stoerig, 2002). As a fifth issue, if vision proceeds from early, precortical and unconscious stages to later cortical and conscious stages of processing, the information being processed must pass from an unconscious to a conscious representation. We know neither when nor where this occurs (Libet, 1993, 2004). To become behaviorally relevant, however, information need *not* achieve the status of a conscious representation. Ample evidence from studies of neurologically impaired patients (Milner & Goodale, 1995; Stoerig, 1996; Stoerig & Cowey, 1997; Weiskrantz, 1997), as well as healthy subjects (see Breitmeyer & Öğmen, this volume; Goodale et al., this volume; Schwarzbach & Vorberg, this volume), indicates that a significant amount of sophisticated and behaviorally relevant visual information can be processed, without being consciously perceived, by what Koch and Crick (2001a) recently called the *visual zombie*. Elucidating the differences between conscious and unconscious vision may not only help us identify the differences in structures, timing, network properties, cell types, and neurotransmitters involved in the processing of conscious vision but may also go some way in explaining what conscious representations are good for.

3.2 Consciousness as State and Trait

Neuroscientific study of consciousness is not a novel discipline, although its various recent expressions have found new fertile ground in a number of allied disciplines, among them philosophy (Block, 1995, 1996; Dennett, 1991), paleoanthropology (Mithen, 1996), religious studies (D'Aquili & Newberg, 1999), and the arts (Solso, 2003; Zeki, 1999). Each of these fields may have its own more or less clear notion of consciousness or simply takes the existence of consciousness, however defined, as an obvious datum. The problem for especially the scientific, empirically based study of consciousness is that an inherently subjective and private experience, not empirically observable by or directly accessible to the (similarly private) experiences of other individuals, constitutes its starting point. Although each one of us clearly knows what it is like to be conscious, none of us, including neuroscientists, have a very clear definition of what constitutes consciousness. Despite dismissive assertions by some neuroscientists to the contrary (Crick, 1994), the definition and the existence of consciousness remains a durable problem for science as well as philosophy. Arriving at clear and empirically accessible and acceptable definitions of consciousness, a task in which philosophy can be most helpful, thus provides important starting points for its scientific study.

Although there is as yet no generally accepted definition of consciousness, the distinction between consciousness as a state and as a trait, as previously noted, provides a useful starting point. Searle (1992) proposes that consciousness be defined as that which you lose while in a coma or during general anesthesia and what you gain upon recovery from either. This definition takes consciousness to be a *state* of an organism. Healthy individuals undergo state changes diurnally through the sleep–waking cycle. When awake, what they are conscious of depends much more on external stimulation than when asleep because sleep inhibits the central processing of sensory information. Accordingly, levels of activation that change endogenously during sleep and waking life are more subject to exogenous events during waking. For instance, in the intermediate range of activation, a person may be fully alert during midmorning after a light breakfast and coffee, somewhat drowsy during midafternoon after a generous two-cocktail luncheon, and briefly overaroused after narrowly escaping a fender bender during rush hour. While these biological state changes involve the ascending reticular activating system, the pontine nuclei, the locus coeruleus, the raphe, the dorsal tegmental nuclei, and the thalamus and its reciprocal connections with the cortex (Bogen, 1995, 1997; Hobson, 1989; Hobson & Steriade, 1986; Moruzzi & Magoun, 1949; Steriade, 2000; Steriade & McCarley, 1990), pathology- and anesthesia-induced state changes are not easily attributed to particular neural networks. The pharmaceutical agents used to induce general anesthesia are chemically very different, suggesting that the conscious state may be affected by quite different neurochemical processes; and comatose states, and, in their wake, vegetative states are caused by drastic toxic, traumatic, degenerative, metabolic, vascular, and anoxic conditions. Despite the consequent variation in brain lesions as assessed by postmortem pathology (Plum & Posner, 1982) or brain imaging in vivo, a strong preponderance of bilateral damage to the thalamus has recently been reported while cortical damage appeared less severe (Jennett, 2002). As some converging evidence on commonly used clinical anesthetics also implicates regionally enhanced deactivation of the thalamus (Alkire et al., 2000), it is presently the favorite core structure for modulating the conscious state. Its dense connections with brainstem, hypothalamus, and cortex may explain dysfunctions of consciousness even in cases in which it is not primarily affected.

The state of consciousness is characterized by a lack of specificity, since an organism is conscious regardless of the specific contents of its consciousness. For this reason, Searle (2000) regards consciousness as a *state* as having priority over its contents. Consciousness as state provides the preexisting field in which various transient perturbations express themselves as the contents in the flow of conscious experience. In contrast to this approach, consciousness can be regarded primarily as a *trait* of specific sensory, cognitive, emotive, or volitional representations that we experience as perception, thought, desire, or intention. From this perspective, conscious contents have priority over conscious state (Dennett, 1991), with each fleeting, richly endowed macrostate of consciousness derived from the transient compositions of separable, content-specific, and continually modifiable modular consciousnesses (Dennett, 1991; Zeki, 1997, 1998; Zeki & Bartels, 1999). Since one or more of those may be lost due to circumscribed brain lesions (Meadows, 1974; Zeki, 1993; Gelb & Goldstein, 1922; Zihl et al., 1983), we have good evidence that the physiological underpinnings of the phenomenal modules are modular too.

We assume that there are important interdependencies between the contents and the state of consciousness. For instance, sensory deprivation (of representational contents) and the anesthetic ketamine not only affect conscious experience by yielding progressively more and stronger hallucinations but also induce altered states of consciousness. Specific contents such as the perception of events associated with a potential or actual threat to the well-being of an organism raise the general level of alertness. Neurophysiological evidence points to such interaction as, for example, between the nonspecific intralaminar thalamic nuclei and the reticular formation, on the one hand, and specific thalamic and cortical responses, on the other (Jasper, 1949; Munk et al., 1995). Moreover, recent work (Jones, 1998) has shown that nonspecific and specific neurons are quite intermingled, indicating that interactions between specific and nonspecific systems are more common than previously suspected. Defined as either a state of an organism or a trait of a mental representation, consciousness readily yields to further, empirically rich investigations. Since most of current research in visual cognition and neuroscience focuses on visual contents, we now take consciousness as a state to be a necessary given and, for the remainder of the chapter, proceed to focus on the contents of visual consciousness.

3.3   Criterion Content, Linking Hypotheses, NCCs, and Neural Correlates of Unconscious Processing

If one defines perception as the phenomenal registration of sensory input, one can, as mentioned above, find neural correlates of visual perception almost anywhere along the visual tract. For example, for years the functional properties of antagonistically organized receptive fields found in the retina or lateral geniculate nucleus have been correlated with the perceptual awareness of simultaneous brightness contrast, illusory Mach bands, and illusory Hermann grid patterns (Jung, 1973; Rossi & Paradiso, 1999; Spillmann, 1971) and thus would qualify as NCCs, although we know that conscious representations cannot reside at these early levels.

However, even at higher cortical levels, NCCs must, from a third-person perspective, relate to some observable indicator response. Here, consideration of the distinct types of visual information providing the contents of consciousness is of prime importance. For example, color and motion information may be processed by neural activities in different cortical pathways (Livingstone & Hubel, 1988; De Yoe & Van Essen, 1988). Besides specifying such informational criterion contents (Breitmeyer, 1984; Bridgeman et al., 1979; Kahneman, 1968), one must carefully state the hypotheses that link a psychophysical measure of visual performance to the underlying neural responses (Teller, 1984). Similar distinctions can be made with regard to the unconscious visual control of behavior (Goodale & Milner, 1995; Ro et al., 2004; Stoerig, 1996; Weiskrantz, 1997). Here one can speak of neural correlates of unconscious processing (NCUs) as the necessary neural activity that forms the immediate substrate of, and thus has direct influence on, visually guided behavior. These NCUs are the putative basis for the unconscious visuomotor abilities attributed to the visual zombie (Crick & Koch, 2003).

To tell NCCs and NCUs apart, two major approaches have been used. The first is the neuropsychological studies of patients or animals with circumscribed brain lesions that have revealed the modular architecture of conscious vision. The second uses healthy subjects whose visual functions are challenged by experimental manipulations that make it difficult to detect some aspect of a target either by psychophysical procedures or by the application of transcranial magnetic stimulation (TMS) or electrical stimulation of the brain. These approaches are complementary: Neuropsychology has the advantage of studying subjects who have permanently lost a particular aspect of visual function; inducing "experimental blindness" of some type in normal subjects, in contrast, either is very transient, lasting at most a few seconds, as in metacontrast masking or the attentional blink (AB; Francis & Cho, this volume; Ogmen & Breitmeyer, this volume; Potter, this volume) or can be corrected by instruction, as in change blindness (Rensink et al., 1997). Moreover, subjects often report sensing or detecting something even if they cannot see the target or change, which makes it difficult to get at the basis of conscious vision as such rather than at specific criterion contents involved in target or change perception. On the other hand, brain lesions affect not only the neurons directly destroyed but also neurons that projected onto them or received their output, as well as fibers of passage, making it difficult to localize function solely on the basis of lesion effects. Tools ranging from functional neuroimaging to single-cell physiology are used with both approaches to link psychophysics and behavior to brain processes.

3.4   Functional Architecture (Levels and Loci) of Unconscious and Conscious Vision

3.4.1   Varieties of Conscious Vision

A leading question in neurophilosophy is whether consciousness is unitary or manifold, and correspondingly a leading question in visual neuroscience is whether there is a single cortical locus for conscious representation or many such sites and levels of processing (Block, 1996; Dennett, 1991; Rosenthal, 2002; Stoerig, 1997, 2002; Stoerig & Brandt, 1993; Zeki, 1997, 1998; Zeki & Bartels, 1999). For instance, on the basis of—among other phenomena—a reported case of "reverse Anton's syndrome" (Hartmann et al., 1991), Block (1996) distinguishes between phenomenal awareness as subjective experience, on the one hand, and access consciousness as a kind of control of cognitive behavior (e.g., reasoning, recognition, identification, verbal reporting, motor response), on the other. Moreover, Block (1996) maintains that access consciousness, at least in limited form, is independent of phenomenal consciousness or may simply include it as one of its particular forms. In contrast, Rosenthal (2002) argues against separate consciousnesses and thus for a single unitary type of consciousness.

In a related vein, Dennett (1991) argues against a cortical "Cartesian theater" where everything in consciousness converges and rather refers to highly fluid and evanescent "multiple drafts" associated with spatiotemporally dynamic and distributed cortical processes. Somewhat compatible with this view is that of Zeki (1997, 1998) and Zeki and Bartels (1999), who downgrade the significance and role of central, hierarchical "executives" where "things come together" in consciousness and emphasize instead the importance of multiple parallel and independent "microconsciousness nodes." While Cartesian dualism and the attendant notion of a homunculus viewing the action in a Cartesian theater are outdated (Ryle, 1949), some neuroscientists (e.g., Craik et al., 1999; Pribram, 1999; Vogeley et al., 1999) nonetheless posit the existence and functional role of a central "convergence zone." In particular, the dorsolateral prefrontal cortex has access to a wide range of inputs and control over a wide range of outputs. Posner (1994) notes that, as part of the anterior attention system, the dorsolateral prefrontal cortex appears to be involved in activities that collectively might be termed "executive function" and that one function of such an "executive" is to be informed about the processes occurring within the cortical organization. To discharge this function, the prefrontal cortex provides a site for rich convergence of multisensory inputs (Pandya & Barnes, 1987). Regarding vision, Rao et al. (1997) and Young (1992) have shown that, among other areas in the prefrontal cortex, area 46 is one convergence zone of activities from the ventral "what" and dorsal "where" streams (Van Essen et al., 1992) of cortical visual processing.

The second executive function of the prefrontal cortex is to exercise some control over the rest of the cortical system (MacDonald et al., 2000). In relation to vision, such control may be provided through reentrant pathways (Edelman, 1987; Edelman & Tononi, 2000) whereby activity at a higher level of neural processing, via feedback, modulates activity at a lower level. Attention may be one such control mechanism. Indeed, Posner (1994) notes that attention under executive control can amplify activity within a particular cortical area not only by amplifying its initial afferent feedforward activity but also by subsequently reentering that area. If the dorsolateral prefrontal cortex—specifically area 46—provides such reentrant modulation to lower visual areas, it may qualify as a site for "executive oversight and control." Such access to sensory information by prefrontal executive functions is a key feature of the account of visual consciousness advocated by Crick and Koch (1998). Although executively controlled, access to and outflow of information, as every real-life executive who knows how to delegate responsibility will attest, may be indirect as well as direct. Such indirection leaves a lot of leeway for distributed multiple-drafts activity (Dennett, 1991) or activity at multiple microconsciousness nodes in lower levels of cortical information processing (Zeki, 1997, 1998; Zeki & Bartels, 1999).

Another cortical visual convergence zone identified by Young (1992) is the superior temporal polysensory area, which receives input from the posterior parietal cortex (Baizer et al., 1991). This region and the dorsolateral prefrontal area 46 may, respectively, be part of the posterior and anterior attention systems (Posner & Petersen, 1990) and allow for conscious report of such contents. It may be more than coincidence that several recent studies using functional magnetic resonance imaging and event-related potentials have shown that content- and category-specific cortical areas are activated by stimuli even when they are rendered invisible by binocular rivalry suppression or visual masking, whereas dorsal prefrontal and parietal areas are activated significantly only when the stimulus is accessible to report (Beck et al., 2001; Dehaene et al., 2001; Lumer et al., 1998). However, dorsolateral prefrontal activation is also found when subjects assertively report a stimulus that was not presented (Pessoa & Ungerleider, 2004), indicating that the executive may be misled and that in addition to imaging studies studies of single neurons and their networks are required (Thompson & Schall, 2000).

However, even if cortical convergence zones and their executive functions play a major role in visual consciousness, neuropsychological evidence shows that although frontal lesions impair the use of consciously represented information, it is only destruction of the primary retino-geniculo-striate cortical system that produces total, and of predominantly extrastriate cortical areas that produces visual feature-specific, blindness (e.g., Wilbrand & Saenger, 1900). Regarding content, there thus is no single correlate or locus of consciousness (Stoerig, 1996; Zeki, 1997, 1998; Zeki & Bartels, 1999). Selective lesions in higher areas of the cortical visual system affect correspondingly selective aspects of visual perception such as color (Meadows, 1974), motion (Zeki, 1991), or object recognition (Benson & Greenberg, 1969; Grüsser & Landis, 1991). Nonetheless, the lower areas, V1/V2, play a pivotal role in conscious vision, since their destruction leads to near total blindness even though the higher visual centers are intact. Whether this is due to their providing necessary inputs to the higher centers, to their receiving reentrant signals from them, or to their establishing or recruiting reverberating intra- and interareal network activities is still not known.

On the basis of studies of neurological patients, one can distinguish several levels of conscious vision. Here we identify at least three (Stoerig, 1996): (1) phenomenal vision yielding a qualia-endowed image; (2) segmenting of foreground and background, and binding of image components into distinct visual objects or aspects of visual scenes; and (3) the categorical recognition and identification of an object or scene and its meanings in relation to one's history, experience, intentions, and knowledge (recognition memory). The phenomenal level is lacking in patients with destruction of the geniculostriate pathway. Very likely it is a prerequisite of object vision and recognition (Stoerig, 1996) and may provide what Gestalt psychologists (Koffka, 1935) referred to as a *primitive unit formation* based on first-order luminance, wavelength, or motion differences in the optic array. While some grouping of these distinct areas may rely on low-level sensory qualia of color, brightness, and motion, it is known that much of the second, object-level vision relies also on second-order groupings based on texture, motion, and disparity differences (Braddick, 1993; Julesz, 1972; Nothdurft, 1992). Object vision is lacking or defective in patients with apperceptive agnosias, resulting from extrastriate cortical damage, which commonly affects the various object-specific areas such as the lateral occipital complex, the fusiform face area, and the parahippocampal place area. While these patients are aware of qualia, they are unable to segment the primitive unity into foreground and background or to fuse its spatially distributed elements into coherent shapes and objects. Conversely, patients who lack certain sensory qualia such as color nevertheless may exhibit form and object vision, although they obviously cannot group elements on the basis of color. The third level of conscious vision allows one to associate the object or scene with cognitive categories and to recognize its meaning based on one's unique prior experience and history. Cortical damage to visual memory-related structures in the temporal cortex and the limbic system or their afferents (Albert et al., 1979) may result in loss of the ability to classify an object (Lissauer, 1890; Farah, 1990) or additionally in the loss of the object's individuality and meaning (Teuber, 1968; Damasio et al., 1982).

3.4.2   Varieties of Unconscious Vision

Although consciousness has acquired pride of place in current cognitive science, much of visual processing that has survival value or is behaviorally relevant proceeds unconsciously (Goodale et al., this volume; Milner & Goodale, 1995; Stoerig, 1996). Moreover, given the numerous selective lesion–induced forms of blindness in neurological patients and the experimentally induced phenomena of inattentional blindness (Mack & Rock, 1998), change blindness (Rensink et al., 1997), the AB (Potter, this volume), and masked priming (Breitmeyer & Öğmen, this volume; Dehaene et al., 2001; Schwarzbach & Vorberg, this volume), and TMS in normal subjects, the search for not only NCCs but also NCUs in vision is of clinical and theoretical interest. Based on findings from studies of neurological patients as well as normal observers, several types and levels of unconscious visual responding can be discerned.

   If we consider first the data based on studies of pathological cases, absolute or total blindness occurs with certain congenital conditions as, for example, in the very rare cases of a baby born prematurely without eyes. Short of that, there are four levels of blind visual responding: neuroendocrine responses, reflexes, effects of unconscious visual processes, and "informed" guesses regarding the presence or attributes of stimuli that are not consciously seen (Stoerig, 1996). The closest to nearly total blindness is what is observed in patients with destruction of the retinofugal projections except for the pathway to the hypothalamus. Although the pupillary reflex and any vestige of even crudest light perception are lacking, these patients may still suppress the secretion of melatonin when exposed to bright light (Czeisler et al., 1995). Hence, the very rudimentary endocrine functions regulated by diurnal and seasonal changes of ambient illumination may still be (partially) intact. The next level of unconscious vision is reflexive and includes the pupillary light reflex, the photic blink reflex, and optokinetic nystagmus. Somewhat compromised, these reflexes can be elicited in comatose patients lacking any perception of light (Keane, 1979) and in patients with destruction of retinal input to the geniculostriate projections but with spared retinofugal pathways to the extrageniculate nuclei known to mediate the visual reflexes (Barbur, 1995). A third, still more inclusive, level of unconscious vision occurs in patients with destruction or denervation of part or all of the primary visual cortex. Besides maintaining (compromised) reflex functions, such blindsight patients, despite absence of conscious perception in the blind area of the visual field, exhibit two methodologically distinct types of visual function. In the first type, a visual stimulus presented in the blind area affects the response to a second stimulus presented in the sighted area of the visual field (Cowey et al., 2003; Marzi et al., 1986; Poeppel, 1986; Richards, 1973). In the second type, significantly better-than-chance performance is obtained when stimuli are presented within the visual field defect and the patients are "forced" to guess whether a stimulus was presented, where a stimulus was presented, or which stimulus was presented. Among the indices of preserved visual functions are (1) discriminating the presence of a briefly flashed stimulus from its absence (Stoerig et al., 1985), (2) localizing a stimulus presented at variable locations in the blind area of the visual field via saccades or hand pointing (Poeppel et al., 1973; Weiskrantz et al., 1974), (3) discriminating among speeds and directions of moving stimuli (Perenin, 1978; Azzopardi et al., 1998), (4) rudimentary wavelength discrimination (Cowey & Stoerig, 2001; Stoerig & Cowey, 1989, 1992), (5) temporal and spatial attentional cuing (Cowey & Stoerig, 2004; Kentridge & Heywood, 2001), (6) coarse orientation and low-spatial-frequency pattern discrimination (Weiskrantz et al., 1974; Trevethan & Sahraie, 2003), and (7) responses to facial emotional expressions (de Gelder et al., 2001b). Exactly where and how in the visual system these residual abilities are expressed is not certain, although it appears that subcortical pathways including the superior colliculus and pulvinar are involved.

In healthy observers, a stimulus can be rendered invisible via a number of experimental techniques. One of the most potent techniques relies on the use of binocular-rivalry suppression (Blake, 1998; Blake & Logothetis, 2002), whereby the stimulus presented to one eye is perceptually suppressed by an incompatible, rivalrous stimulus presented to the other eye. There is debate about how and where in the brain binocular rivalry occurs and how it interacts with global pattern rivalry (Blake & Logothetis, 2002; Lee & Blake, 2004; Kovács et al., 1996; Tong, 2001; Tong & Engel, 2001). However, while global pattern rivalry may involve high-level cognitive processes that govern the perception of coherent patterns (Kovác et al., 1996), the local areas within the pattern remain subject to low-level interocular rivalry (Lee & Blake, 2004), which single-cell physiology has shown to be resolved in superior temporal sulcus and inferotemporal cortex (Sheinberg & Logothetis, 1997). Under conditions of binocular rivalry, observers report no phenomenal awareness of the stimulus presented to the suppressed eye. Despite this, evidence points to unconscious processing of stimulus attributes processed at early levels in the cortical or subcortical visual system. These attributes include orientation (Blake & Fox, 1974), apparent motion (Wiesenfelder & Blake, 1991), and emotional facial expressions (Pasley et al., 2004; Williams et al., 2004), the last of which may be accessed through subcortical pathways, via the pulvinar (Jones & Burton, 1976), accessing the amygdala. In contrast, higher level processes such as semantic and picture priming do not survive binocular rivalry suppression (Cave et al., 1998; Zimba & Blake, 1983), nor, as preliminary results from one of our labs indicate, does metacontrast masking when the eye stimulated by the mask is suppressed (Breitmeyer, Öğmen, & Koç, unpublished observations).

Visual masking (Breitmeyer, 1984) and generalized flash suppression (Breitmeyer & Rudd, 1981; Wilke et al., 2003) also can be used to render a stimulus phenomenally invisible. Nevertheless, a host of past and recent studies have shown that several lower level properties of a stimulus, including its presence/location, its chromatic features, and its form features, although unavailable for phenomenal report, are accessible to unconscious visual information processing (see Breitmeyer & Öğmen, this volume). Even high-level aspects such as the form and meaning of a masked word appear to be accessible to unconscious visual processing (Dehaene et al., 2001) as are the emotional expressions of masked faces and the emotional valence of masked stimuli (Dimberg et al., 2000; Morris, Öhman, & Dolan, 1998; Whalen et al., 1998; Wong & Root, 2003). While TMS-induced suppression of visual stimuli can be readily obtained (Corthout et al., 1999a, 1999b; Ro, this volume), it is not clear what sorts of unconscious visual information processing are spared. Recall, however, that during binocular rivalry suppressed motion and emotional facial expressions appear to be accessible, and that this has also been shown for patients with fields of cortical blindness (de Gelder et al., 2001b). Since TMS pulses applied to the occipital pole can suppress vision in circumscribed regions of the visual field and hence in retinotopically organized V1 and V2, it seems reasonable that, here, motion and emotional facial expressions should also be accessible via alternative projections involving the amygdala and possibly somatosensory cortex (Anders et al., 2004).

3.5 Temporal Properties of Unconscious and Conscious Vision

In his extensive studies of the temporal dynamics of conscious perception and voli-tion, Libet (1985) has devised a mixture of an "external" (stimulus-driven) and an "internal" (endogenously generated) psychophysics of consciousness. While this attempt has faced major criticism on conceptual and methodological grounds (Breitmeyer, 2002; Churchland, 1981; Dennett & Kinsbourne, 1992; Pockett, 2002; see also commentaries on Libet's, 1985, article), it has paved the way for the current approaches. By focusing on the dynamics of neural networks and consciously or unconsciously represented information flow in the visual system, one can experi-mentally tag temporal properties and stages of processing that map onto functional levels in a reliable and interpretable manner (e.g., Breitmeyer & Öğmen, this volume; Luck, this volume; Ro, this volume; Verleger & Jáskowski, this volume). At the neural level, temporal properties, in terms of both response latency (Maunsell, 1987; Nowak et al., 1985) and response synchronization (Engel et al., 1992; Singer, 1994), can provide important information about intra- and interareal cortical inter-actions governing the speed and spatiotemporal coherence or grouping of visual information processing. In contrast, although binocular rivalry is a dynamic state (Blake, 1998; O'Shea & Crassini, 1984), the dominance-suppression switches tend to be too irregular to yield precise estimates of the temporal locus of conscious pro-cessing. Leopold and Logothetis (1999) used the stochastic switches between per-cepts to argue that behavior-related frontal areas challenge the visual processing areas to provide a consistent interpretation in cases of ambiguous input. Whenever this is impossible because the system is faced with rivalrous input, perceptual switches occur whose timing resembles that of a variety of exploratory behaviors. A route to including this paradigm into the ones that can yield information about time to consciousness is opened by flash suppression. Here a monocular stimulus is rendered temporarily invisible by the sudden onset of an incompatible stimulus in the other eye, giving the experimenter control over the perceptual state of the subject (Wilke et al., 2003). Other paradigms especially amenable for the study of temporal properties of unconscious and conscious processing include TMS masking, visual masking, attentional cuing, and the AB. Of these, TMS and visual masking share several properties but also differ in others (Breitmeyer et al., 2004b). With TMS stimulation applied to the occipital pole over a range of stimulus onset asynchronies (SOAs) relative to the visual target stimulus, Corthout et al. (1999a, 1999b) have identified at least two epochs of target suppression, the earlier one corresponding to the initial feedforward sweep of cortical activity and the later one to activity depending on reentrant feedback (Lamme et al., 2000). In a comparison of visual and TMS masking, Breitmeyer et al. (2004b) argue that these early and late epochs of TMS masking correspond to the optimal SOA intervals obtained in paracontrast and metacontrast masking, respectively. Moreover, Breitmeyer et al. (2004a; see also Breitmeyer & Öğmen, this volume) have shown that unconscious stimulus processing may occur not only at very early but also at later stages of cortical processing. These findings are confirmed by the work of Dehaene et al. (2001) with regard to the processing of word form and meaning and by demonstrations of implicit processes at all stages of processing in neuropsychological patients suffering from blindsight to higher levels of cerebral color blindness and prosopagnosia. Since the psychophysical techniques described above also yield distinctive types of suppression (e.g., visual masking and binocular rivalry) that might reveal correspondingly distinctive levels of processing, experimental regimens that combine two or more of the psychophysical techniques described above can provide useful ways of establishing functional hierarchies of unconscious as well as conscious processing. Although the combination of psychophysical paradigms with evoked potentials in humans (Niedeggen et al., 2001; Pins & ffytche, 2003; Wilenius-Emet et al., 2004) and physiological recordings from awake behaving monkeys (Super et al., 2001) promises to advance our understanding of the temporal dynamics of brain processes mediating visual awareness, as yet we do not know when exactly a visual stimulus is first seen.

3.6   A Complex Problem

A wealth of hypotheses and data reported to support them have been put forward to attribute conscious vision to particular brain structures. The main contenders are the visual cortices by themselves (Zeki, 1997) or in combinations that include V1/V2 and allow concerted activity, whether by means of reentrant signals (Cowey & Stoerig, 1991; Lamme et al., 2000; Super et al., 2001) and/or temporal synchronization (Singer, 1994). Alternatively, primarily dorsal frontoparietal regions (Beck et al., 2001; Lumer et al., 1998; Pins & ffytche, 2003) or nonspecific thalamic nuclei (Bachmann, this volume) are assumed to be necessarily activated in addition to visual cortex. We think identifying the contributions that these structures make to conscious vision will require more precise differentiations among varieties of conscious vision. At present, we have good reasons to think that different visual cortical regions are involved in rendering different visual qualia, based on evidence from lesion studies and studies of single-cell physiology, functional neuroimaging, and TMS. We also have good reasons to think that nonvisual brain structures influence the activity of visual cortical neurons. This is true for changes in the structures mediating the level of arousal (Munk et al., 1996), sleep (Yamada et al., 1988; Czisch et al., 2002), and the conscious state (Martin et al.; Laureys et al., 2002), but also the networks mediating attention. Attentional effects are seen on the single-cell level (Moran & Desimone, 1985), in regional activation changes detected in functional neuroimaging even in the absence of stimuli (Kastner et al., 1999), and on the perceptual level where attention may alter appearance (Carrasco et al., 2004) as well as prevent detection when overtaxed as in the AB. A further factor not sufficiently parceled out concerns the subjectivity of experience: In order to know whether a subject has consciously seen something, we need some kind of report, whether verbal or nonverbal. When a report is requested in experiments designed to discern conscious and unconscious vision, this implies a possible confounding of neural activations related to phenomenal vision and those related to report, the latter of which involve not only the motor system including its frontal planning areas but also working memory–related structures. Only recently have some studies systematically begun to use stimulus- and response-contingent analysis to define activations related to correct and false responses and to distinguish them from stimulus-driven activation (Pessoa & Ungerleider, 2004; Thompson & Schall, 2000). Unraveling the above-noted complexities will require further studies differentiating percept- from response-contingent activations as well as differentiating attentional processes from, and relating them to, the NCC and the NCU.

II NEUROPHYSIOLOGICAL CORRELATES OF DYNAMIC PROCESSING IN VISION

4 Grasping the Past and Present: When Does Visuomotor Priming Occur?

Melvyn A. Goodale, Jonathan S. Cant, and Grzegorz Króliczak

4.1 Introduction

Humans are able to use vision to generate and control an impressive array of skilled actions. Much of this control presumably depends on processing within the intricate network of visual areas (more than 30) that have been charted in the cerebral cortex (for recent reviews, see Kaas, 2000; Grill-Spector & Malach, 2004; see also Felleman & Van Essen, 1991). Despite the bewildering complexity of the interconnections between these cortical visual areas, two broad "streams" of anatomically distinct visual projections have been identified in the macaque monkey brain: a ventral stream, projecting from area V1 to the inferotemporal cortex, and a dorsal stream, projecting from area V1 to the posterior parietal cortex (Ungerleider & Mishkin, 1982). These regions also receive inputs from a number of other subcortical visual structures, particularly the superior colliculus, which sends prominent projections to the dorsal stream (via the thalamus). Although some caution must be exercised in generalizing from monkey to human, recent neuroimaging evidence suggests that the visual projections from primary visual cortex to the temporal and parietal lobes in the human brain involve a separation into ventral and dorsal streams similar to that seen in the monkey (for review, see Culham & Kanwisher, 2001; Tootell et al., 2003; Van Essen et al., 2001).

Although the anatomical distinction between the ventral and dorsal streams of visual processing has been recognized for some time, the different functions of the two streams have undergone various interpretations. In their seminal paper, Ungerleider and Mishkin (1982) argued that the ventral stream plays a critical role in the identification and recognition of objects, while the dorsal stream mediates the localization of those same objects. Some have referred to this distinction in visual processing as one between "what" versus "where." Although the evidence for this distinction initially seemed quite compelling, recent findings from a broad range of studies in both humans and monkeys has forced a reinterpretation of the division of labor between the two streams.

According to Goodale and Milner's (1992) reinterpretation of the functions of
the two streams, the ventral stream plays the major role in constructing the perceptual representation of the visual world and the objects within it, while the dorsal
stream mediates the visual control of actions directed at those objects (figure 4.1).
In contrast to the "what versus where" model put forward by Ungerleider and
Mishkin (1982), Goodale and Milner argued that the structural and spatial attributes of an object are being processed by both streams, but for different purposes.
In the case of the ventral stream, information about a broad range of object parameters is transformed for perceptual purposes; in the case of the dorsal stream, some
of these same object parameters are transformed for the control of actions. This is
not to say that the distribution of visual inputs does not differ between the two
streams, but rather that the main difference lies in the nature of the transformations
that each stream performs on those two sets of inputs.

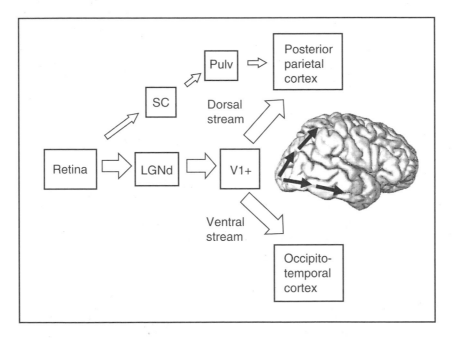

Figure 4.1
Schematic representation of the two streams of visual processing in human cerebral cortex. The retina
sends projections to the lateral geniculate nucleus, pars dorsalis (LGNd), in the thalamus, which projects
in turn to primary visual cortex (V1). Within the cerebral cortex, the ventral stream arises from early
visual areas (V1+) and projects to regions in the occipitotemporal cortex. The dorsal stream also arises
from early visual areas but projects instead to the posterior parietal cortex. The posterior parietal cortex
also receives visual input from the superior colliculus (SC) via the pulvinar (Pulv). The approximate locations of the pathways are shown on the left side of the three-dimensional reconstruction of the pial
surface of the brain made from an anatomical magnetic resonance image. The routes indicated by the
arrows involve a series of complex interconnections.

4.2 Frames of Reference for Perception and Action

According to Goodale and Milner (1992), the two separate streams of visual processing evolved because of the different transformations required for vision for perception and vision for action. For one to be able to grasp an object successfully, for example, it is essential that the brain compute the actual size of the object—and its real distance and position with respect to the observer. In addition, these computations will take into account only the dimension of the goal object that is relevant for action, such as its width, for example, while ignoring other dimensions, such as its length, that may not be immediately useful in performing the task at hand (e.g., Ganel & Goodale, 2003). Moreover, the information about the orientation and position of the object must be computed in frames of reference that take into account the orientation and position of the object with respect to the effector that is to be used to perform the action (i.c., in *egocentric frames of reference*). In addition, because observers and goal objects often do not stay in a static relationship with one another, the required coordinates for action are most effectively computed immediately before the movements are initiated, that is, in *real time*. A corollary of real-time visuomotor transformation is that neither the coordinates for a particular action nor the resulting motor program need to be stored in memory. Indeed, such storage could create interference between competing action plans for multiple objects in the visual array, or between action plans to the same object following a change in the spatial relationship between target and actor. In fact, there is a good deal of evidence that object-directed actions, such as grasping, that are initiated *after* the goal object has been removed from view are qualitatively different from the actions that are programmed while the object is visible (for a review, see Goodale et al., 2003). As we shall see, these findings suggest that the control of actions to remembered objects may depend heavily on earlier perceptual processing—processing that does not typically intrude on the control of visually guided actions operating in real time.

In contrast to the vision-for-action system, the vision-for-perception system computes the size, location, shape, and orientation of an object primarily in relation to other objects and surfaces in the scene. In other words, the metrics of perception are inherently relative and the frames of reference are largely scene-based, which explains why we are so sensitive to size-contrast illusions and other visual illusions that depend on comparisons between different objects in the visual array (for reviews, see Goodale & Haffenden, 1998; Goodale & Milner, 2004; Goodale et al., 2003). Encoding an object in a scene-based frame of reference (sometimes called an *allocentric frame of reference*) permits a representation of the object that preserves the relations between the object parts and its surroundings without requiring precise information about the absolute size of the object or its exact position with respect to the observer. Because of this reliance on allocentric computations, individual features of objects cannot be perceived in isolation. For example, explicit judgments of the width of an object cannot help but be affected by the length of that object (Ganel & Goodale, 2003) or by the apparent width of other objects in the scene (Hu & Goodale, 2000).

Vision for perception also operates over a much longer time scale than that used by vision for action. We can recognize objects we have seen minutes, hours, days— or even years—before. In fact, object recognition would not be possible unless perceptual information about previously encountered objects were stored in memory—and an allocentric representation system is ideal for storing this information. As we indicated earlier, there is evidence that the vision-for-perception system is recruited when a goal object is no longer visible at the moment an action is initiated. In other words, the programming and control of memory-driven actions make use of information that was processed and encoded earlier by vision for perception. As a consequence, memory-guided actions tend to be based on the relative rather than the absolute metrics of the target object. Indeed, there is evidence that grasping movements that are programmed and initiated after a goal object has been removed from view are qualitatively different from the actions programmed while the target remains visible (Goodale et al., 1994; Hu & Goodale, 2000; Milner et al., 1999; Milner & Goodale, 1995; Westwood & Goodale, 2003). This reliance on allocentric scene-based representations for guiding memory-driven or "offline" actions is presumably much more efficient than the use of a stored egocentric encoding of the target (or a stored motor program) that would have to be continuously updated as the observer's position with respect to the target changed during the delay.

To reiterate: Vision for action and vision for perception require fundamentally different frames of reference and temporal scales—which helps to explain why two separate visual pathways have evolved in the primate cerebral cortex. Visually guided actions, it appears, depend on pathways that engage relatively encapsulated visuomotor mechanisms in the dorsal stream. These dedicated visuomotor mechanisms, together with related networks in the premotor cortex and brainstem, compute the absolute metrics of the target object and its position in the egocentric coordinates of the effector used to perform the action. Such real-time programming is essential for the production of accurate and efficient movements in a world where the location and disposition of a goal object with respect to the observer can change quickly and often unpredictably. In contrast, the perceptual mechanisms in the ventral stream (and associated cognitive structures) use relative metrics and scene-based or allocentric coding. Such computations make it possible not only to recognize objects but to plan and execute actions upon objects long after they have vanished from view.

4.3 Neurological Studies of Timing in Perception and Action

Studies with neurological patients have demonstrated clear temporal limits on the ability of the isolated dorsal system to guide manual prehension. Consider, for example, the case of D.F., a young woman who suffered damage to her ventral-stream pathway as a result of anoxia from carbon monoxide poisoning (Milner et al., 1991). Even though D.F. is unable to indicate the size, shape, and orientation of an object, either verbally or manually, she shows normal preshaping and rotation of her hand when reaching out to grasp it (Goodale et al., 1991). For example, even though D.F. was unable to report the width of objects that varied in their dimensions from trial to trial, she showed excellent size scaling of her grasp in flight as she reached out to pick up each object. On the basis of this dissociation between perceptual report and the visual control of action, Goodale and Milner (1992) argued that D.F.'s dorsal stream was still functioning relatively normally despite the apparent damage to her ventral stream, a conclusion that was recently confirmed in a neuroimaging study of D.F. (James et al., 2003). It appears that her ventral stream can no longer process form information for perception but her dorsal stream remains sensitive to form information about objects that are the targets of visually guided grasping movements. However, despite the fact that D.F. can pick up objects accurately in real time, she demonstrates extremely poor size scaling of her grip when she attempts to pick up objects that are no longer visible (Goodale et al., 1994).

Thus, when a delay of only 2 s was introduced between D.F.'s viewing a goal object and the instruction to initiate her grasping movement, the aperture of her grasp in flight showed no correlation at all with the size of the object. D.F.'s deficit contrasts sharply with the performance of normal participants in the same task, who showed only subtle differences in their visually guided and delayed grasping movements. The dissociation between D.F.'s ability to perform real-time actions and her inability to perform memory-driven actions suggests that D.F., unlike normal subjects, cannot use her memory of the goal object to program her delayed grasping movements. Since visual memory for object features depends on the perceptual mechanisms that reside in the ventral stream, which we now know is damaged in D.F. (James et al., 2003), she was precluded from setting up such memories. In other words, she had no memory of the object's dimensions because she failed to perceive those dimensions in the first place. Her damaged ventral stream meant that she did not form a percept of the object's form when she was exposed to it initially. In the same experiment, however, D.F. was able to pantomime grasping movements to familiar objects such as a pea or a tennis ball, on verbal instruction, presumably because the size information in this case could be retrieved from her long-term memory of these objects. Taken together, these results suggest that (1) the dorsal system normally operates in real time, accessing transient visual signals about the target object at the time of movement programming, and (2) the ventral stream is required for creating the object representations that are maintained in memory for the control of later actions. These conclusions are supported by evidence from other neurological patients who have damage to the dorsal rather than the ventral stream. These patients show the opposite pattern of deficits and spared visual abilities from those seen in D.F. (a double dissociation). The optic ataxia patient A.T., for example, is quite unable to scale her grasp when reaching to unfamiliar objects—even though the objects remain visible both before and during the action. Presumably, this deficit arises because such actions are normally generated exclusively on the basis of online visual processing of the objects' features—processing that is thought to take place in the dorsal stream, which is damaged in this patient. A.T. shows much better scaling of her grasp when she reaches to familiar objects, however, where the appropriate actions can be programmed on the basis of stored semantic information about the object that is derived from long-term memory (Jeannerod et al., 1994). The memory is presumably triggered by her visual recognition of the familiar object using the intact perceptual mechanisms in her ventral stream—which she can then use to shape her grasp. But what about actions directed to unfamiliar objects that are no longer visible, objects whose features cannot be accessed from long-term memory but must instead be stored in short-term memory? If, as suggested earlier, the control of such memory-driven movements depends not on the visuomotor mechanisms of the dorsal pathway but rather on the perceptual mechanisms of the ventral pathway, then one might expect a patient with optic ataxia to show a paradoxical improvement in performance if the grasping movement is delayed until the goal object has been removed from view. In this situation the patient would be forced to rely on a stored representation of the target object, laid down moments earlier by the perceptual mechanisms of the ventral stream, rather than an online computation of the object's features, which would normally engage the visuomotor mechanisms in the (damaged) dorsal stream.

This is exactly what happened in a recent experiment with the optic ataxia patient I.G. (Milner et al., 2001). Like other patients with optic ataxia, I.G. is quite unable to open her hand and fingers appropriately when reaching out to pick up objects of different sizes. Yet despite this deficit in real-time grasping, I.G. showed good grip scaling when "pantomiming" a grasp for an object that she had seen earlier but that was no longer present. In fact, after some practice, I.G. was able to scale her grip when grasping a real target object that she had previewed 5 s earlier—even though the object was visible during the movement. In other words, despite the presence of real-time vision, her performance improved by virtue of the preview. By interposing catch trials in which a different object was covertly substituted for the original object during the delay between the preview and the grasp, the experimenters were able to show that I.G. was using memorized visual information to calibrate her grasping movements. In other words, on these catch trials, her grip scaling reflected the size of the object she had previewed earlier rather than the size of the object that was now in front of her, in contrast to what happened with normal participants. These findings again provide compelling support for the idea that the control of grasping movements made after a delay depends on information derived from earlier perceptual processing of the object by mechanisms in the ventral stream. As will become evident in the next section, this ventral-stream perceptual processing plays a significant role in the apparent priming of some kinds of visuomotor responses by earlier exposure to the target stimulus.

4.4 Can the Visuomotor System be Primed?

The more recently we have seen an object, the easier it is to recognize when it is presented again, even when we cannot recall having seen the object earlier. The improvement in recognition from earlier presentation of the target stimulus, which is often called *priming*, has been the subject of extensive behavioral research over the last 2 decades. Although it is clear that the perceptual processing of a visual stimulus and/or access to various semantic associations, such as its name, show evidence of priming (e.g., Thompson-Schill & Gabrieli, 1999), it is not clear that this would be the case for visuomotor processing for actions directed at that same object. Indeed, the perception–action dissociation put forward by Goodale and Milner (1992) would suggest that such priming should not occur. As was discussed earlier, according to their account, the dorsal "action" system works in real time and does not make use of memory for the computations that are carried out in programming an object-directed action. Memory-guided actions, it seems, are mediated instead by the ventral "perception" mechanisms and thus make use of visual information that is quite distinct from that used to control real-time actions.

Despite these arguments, one recent study claims that visuomotor priming can and does occur. Craighero et al. (1996) demonstrated that the time to initiate a grasping response was reduced when participants viewed a priming stimulus (presented 100ms earlier) that was congruent in orientation with the target object (as compared to their response on trials in which an incongruent or neutral priming stimulus was presented). They interpreted this improvement in reaction time as evidence for a visuomotor priming effect, suggesting that earlier exposure to the congruent prime reduced the amount of processing required to program the goal-directed action. On the face of it, this idea is completely inconsistent with Goodale and Milner's view that visuomotor computations are made immediately before the movement is made, with no computations being stored in memory that can be used to execute subsequent goal-directed movements. How, then, can the results of Craighero et al. be explained in light of this real-time view of visuomotor transformation?

A critical aspect of the Craighero et al. (1996) study was that the target object was *never visible* to the participants. Participants were told by verbal instruction at the beginning of the trial what the orientation of the target object would be—and this instruction was always correct. Only later was the visual "prime" presented (just before the grasping movement was initiated). This meant, of course, that participants would have had to plan their action from memory rather than from direct visual input. As discussed earlier, memory-guided actions appear to engage quite different visuomotor mechanisms from those used by visually guided actions (and are, in fact, quite different from our everyday interactions with objects—in that we usually see the object that we wish to pick up). Thus, the fact that Craighero et al. used a memory-driven grasping movement—a movement that presumably is programmed using information derived from the perceptual processing in the ventral stream—might explain why they found evidence of priming in their task. However, what is needed to test this directly is a direct comparison of priming in memory-driven and visually driven grasping.

4.4.1 Visuomotor Priming with Novel Objects

Cant et al. (2005) recently conducted a series of experiments to address this issue. In their first experiment, they compared priming of memory-guided and visually guided grasping using a paradigm similar to that of Craighero et al. (1996). The prime and target objects were presented on a turntable (figure 4.2), which could be rapidly rotated after participants had viewed the prime, and viewing time was controlled by LCD goggles that could quickly be made transparent or opaque. In both the memory-guided and the visually guided tasks, participants were instructed to grasp the target object (a long, rectangular block) as quickly as possible upon hearing an auditory cue. Each trial began with an auditory verbal cue that indicated the orientation of the target object (i.e., the word *left* when the far end of the block was oriented 45° leftward from the participant's midline, or *right* when it was oriented 45° rightward). After a 1,500-ms interval, the goggles became transparent and revealed the prime object for a duration of 500 ms. The goggles then were occluded for a randomly varied interstimulus interval (ISI) of 1,250, 1,500, or 1,750 ms. During the ISI, the turntable was rotated in order to position the target object in the work space. After the ISI, an auditory signal cued participants to respond. In the visually guided task, the goggles were made transparent coincidentally with the auditory cue and then vision was occluded either when the response was initiated or after 500 ms, whichever came first. Thus, participants received direct visual information about the target object during the movement-programming phase but not during

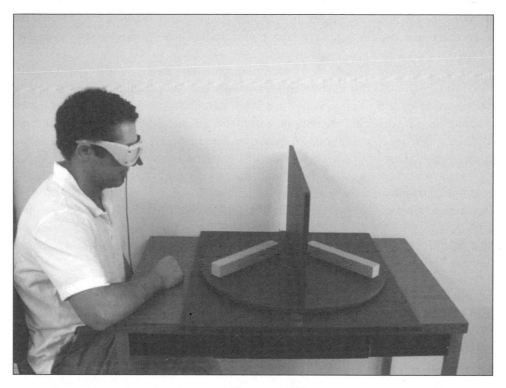

Figure 4.2
Turntable apparatus used to present the prime and target objects to the participants. (Reproduced with permission from Cant et al., 2005)

the online control phase. In the memory-guided task, the goggles remained occluded after the auditory cue, so participants received no direct vision of the target object at any time.

In both tasks, grasping movements were made under four different priming conditions (congruent, incongruent, no-prime, and neutral), which were randomly interleaved. In the congruent and incongruent conditions, a rectangular prime object, identical in shape to the target, was presented in either the same or different orientation with respect to the target object. In the no-prime condition, no object was presented during the prime-viewing period; this condition was included to determine a baseline reaction time for visually guided and memory-guided grasping. In the neutral condition, a circular disk was presented during the prime-viewing period; this condition was included to determine whether or not viewing any object at all—even one that bears no visual similarity to the upcoming target object—could influence the speed with which a grasping movement is initiated. A similar condition was also used by Craighero et al. (1996).

As figure 4.3 indicates, the results from this first experiment were clear: Memory-guided, but not visually guided, grasping movements were primed. In the memory-guided grasping task, participants initiated their grasp to the target significantly faster after viewing a congruent prime than after an incongruent prime. The fact that visually guided grasping movements were completely unaffected by the earlier presentation of the priming condition is consistent with the idea that dedicated visuomotor networks that mediate object-directed movements operate in real time, and the necessary computations are based on information derived directly from the retina rather than from memory of earlier presentations. When the object is not visible, however, the grasping movement has to be based on stored information—and this is presumably the reason that presenting congruent or incongruent stimuli just before the memory-driven movement was initiated had an effect on response latency. This latter finding, of course, replicates the Craighero et al. (1996) study—and indicates that "visuomotor" priming may in fact be limited to memory-guided actions.

Even so, it has to be acknowledged that the paradigm that Cant et al. (2005) adapted from Craighero et al. (1996) is somewhat unconventional. In most perceptual priming studies, no advance information is given about the features of the upcoming target stimulus. Yet in the Craighero et al. experiment (and in Cant et al.'s replication), participants were given accurate verbal information about the

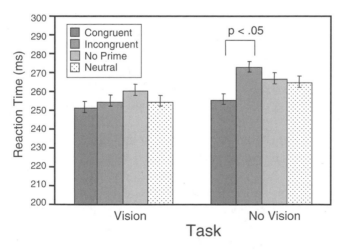

Figure 4.3
Reaction times for each experimental condition in the visually guided and memory-guided tasks used in the first experiment by Cant et al. (2005). Reaction times for visually guided grasping were not significantly different for the four conditions. For memory-guided grasping, however, reaction times for the congruent prime–target trials were significantly faster than those for the incongruent trials. In all cases, Bonferroni pairwise comparisons were used. (Reproduced with permission from Cant et al., 2005)

target's orientation well before the so-called priming stimulus was presented. Under these conditions, Cant et al. found no evidence for visuomotor priming (for visible targets). It is possible, however, that a priming paradigm of the sort known to produce robust priming in a naming task with visible objects (e.g., Wiggs & Martin, 1998) might result in visuomotor priming—even in a visually guided grasping task. Cant et al. explored this possibility in an additional experiment that made use of a more conventional priming paradigm.

In this experiment, each trial consisted of a prime stimulus followed a short time later by the target object, and the effects of presenting the prime were explored in both a visually guided grasping task and a naming task. As figure 4.4 illustrates, four novel objects that varied in shape were used; each object afforded the same whole hand grasp in which the thumb opposed the finger pads of three or four of the remaining digits. Participants were first taught to associate a name with each of the four shapes (*kiff*, *fid*, *tam*, and *sup*). Following this training period, the participants were tested in both the naming and the grasping tasks. In each task, the prime stimulus was presented for 500 ms and then the target was presented following a variable ISI (1,250, 1,500, or 1,750 ms). On some trials, the prime and the target were identical in shape and orientation. On others, they had the same shape but different orientations, or vice versa. On still other trials, they differed in both orientation

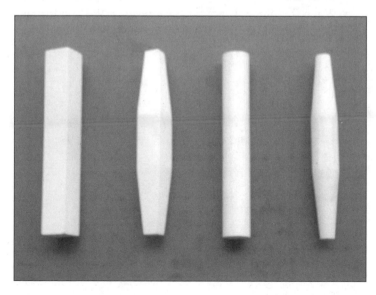

Figure 4.4
Stimuli used in the second experiment by Cant et al. (2005). Each object was given a nonsense name (i.e., *kiff*, *fid*, *tam*, and *sup*). The shape of the blocks varied on two dimensions: cross-section (circle vs. square) and tapering (tapered vs. nontapered). (Reproduced with permission from Cant et al., 2005)

and shape. Finally, there were "baseline" trials in which no priming stimulus was presented at all. All these different trials were randomly interleaved.

In the naming task, participants were faster to name the target when its shape was the same as the prime—but there was no effect of orientation (figure 4.5). This demonstrated that the paradigm could reproduce the standard priming effects on naming that have been reported many times in the literature. However, despite the robust effect on naming, the reaction time for grasping was completely unaffected by the orientation or the shape of the prime (see figure 4.5). This clear difference between naming and grasping confirmed that the null effect of priming on visually guided grasping in the first experiment was not due to the peculiarities of that particular paradigm.

It could be argued, however, that priming was not found in the grasping tasks because the visuomotor circuitry underlying visually guided grasping was not sufficiently engaged during the priming phase (whereas some sort of covert naming could have occurred). Thus, in a final experiment, Cant et al. (2005) required participants to grasp the prime before grasping the target object. Again, reaction time remained unaffected by the prime stimulus. This inherent lack of priming (for all visually guided grasping tasks across all three experiments) is entirely consistent with the real-time view of visuomotor control. To reiterate, the initial programming of visually guided grasping appears to be determined more by what is on the retina than by what is in memory. When the object is not visible, however, the "real-time" dorsal visuomotor circuitry is circumvented and the initiation of the subsequently

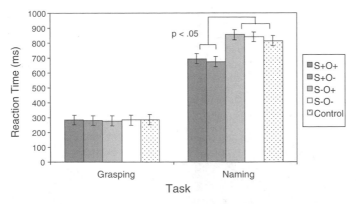

Figure 4.5
Reaction times for each experimental condition in the grasping and naming tasks used in the second experiment by Cant et al. (2005). Reaction times for grasping were not different for the five experimental conditions. For naming, reaction times were reduced for conditions in which prime and target objects were the same shape. S+, same shape; S−, different shape; O+, same orientation; O−, different orientation. (Reproduced with permission from Cant et al., 2005)

"blind" grasping movement is executed by the perceptual circuitry in the ventral stream.

4.4.2 Visuomotor Priming with Familiar Objects

But can priming ever affect the visuomotor system? Behavioral studies supporting the idea of the online nature of visuomotor control (including the experiments by Cant et al., 2005) have used simple wooden blocks and/or nonsense objects. Such objects have no particular function—and thus there is no stored representation of function that could be "primed" and later used by the vision-for-action system. Perhaps the situation would be very different for familiar objects, such as tools, that invoke functional hand postures in anticipation of their use.

There is certainly evidence that functional objects engage the visuomotor system in a rather different way than meaningless objects do. In a series of elegant experiments, for example, Creem and Proffitt (2001) showed that the processing of functional components of the grasp operates independent of the more metrical aspects of grasp scaling. In their studies, participants were presented with a series of tools and implements, such as a hammer, a toothbrush, and a screwdriver, with the handle turned away from them. When the participants reached out to pick up these objects, they grabbed the handle even though this meant adopting an uncomfortable posture. If, however, they were required to carry out a paired-associate memory task at the same time, the participants picked up the object as if blind to its function. Nonetheless, although they grasped the objects inappropriately, they still picked them up deftly, showing well-calibrated grasp postures. In other words, vision-for-action circuits in the dorsal stream were still doing their job as well as ever. Only the functional elements of the grasp were missing. They were missing presumably because the paired-associate task was placing heavy demands on the high-level cognitive processes needed to retrieve the functional information about the object and thus the appropriate grasp to use. Indeed, Creem and Proffitt showed in another experiment that tasks that did not have a large semantic component but that were nevertheless attentionally demanding did not interfere with the functional aspects of their grasps.

All of this suggests that it might be possible to prime the grasping of functional objects. Garofeanu et al. (2004) carried out a series of studies designed to investigate just this possibility. The motivation was twofold. First and foremost, the studies were designed to test whether or not priming of grasping would occur when familiar objects are used as goal objects. (Rare studies that have investigated facilitation of visuomotor responses with such objects—e.g., Tucker & Ellis, 1998; see also Tucker & Ellis, 2004—have used mainly depicted objects as stimuli and/or a button-press response as a measure of reaction time, a response that may depend more on initial ventral rather than dorsal-stream processing.) Second, the Garofeanu et al.

studies explored whether or not grasping and naming of familiar objects would be differentially affected by the nature of the priming event. (Behavioral studies of visual priming with familiar objects have concentrated almost entirely on recognition tests limited to line drawings or photographs, e.g., Williams & Tarr, 1999; Liu & Cooper, 2001; see also Biederman & Gerhardstein, 1993, and/or the stimuli often consisted of verbal [semantic] material, e.g., Thompson-Schill & Gabrieli, 1999; for a review, see Schacter & Buckner, 1998.)

Garofeanu et al. (2004) measured reaction time when participants grasped and/or named objects in a repetition-priming paradigm. In such a paradigm, an object is first presented during a study phase and then presented again during a test phase, along with other objects that were not presented before (see Schacter, 1987; Tulving & Schacter, 1990; Toth, 2000). The effects of earlier exposure on later performance— for example, decreased latency and/or better object identification for old as compared to new objects—are measured. If any effects are found, they are assumed to depend on implicit memory of that previous encounter. It is thought that implicit memory must be involved because the experimenter never makes any reference to the prior occurrence of the stimulus, and participants are never explicitly required to remember the studied objects for later recall or recognition tests.

In their first experiment, Garofeanu et al. (2004) looked at the effects of prior grasping on later grasping or naming of the same objects and at the effects of prior naming on later naming or grasping. In other words, there were two within-task conditions in which priming could occur (grasping–grasping and naming–naming) and two cross-task conditions (naming–grasping and grasping–naming). Forty common objects (from several superordinate categories, such as household objects, personal care objects, and tools) were presented. All the objects had a prominent axis of elongation and required a specific hand posture during grasping. These objects were presented one at a time at a distance of 60 cm in front of the participant, 20 of them at an orientation of 0°, where the handle pointed away from the participant, and the other 20 at an orientation of 135°, where the handle pointed to the right and toward the participant (for examples, see figure 4.6). In the study phase, participants were shown only 20 of the objects (half at an orientation of 0° and the other half at an orientation of 135°) and were asked either to grasp or to name them. In the later test phase, the same 20 objects were presented randomly interleaved with the 20 new objects—and again the participants were asked to either grasp or name all the objects. The orientation of the old objects did not change from study to test. In a second experiment, Garofeanu et al. manipulated the orientation of the object; on some blocks of test trials the orientation of the old objects was changed from study to test, and on others the orientation remained the same. In this second experiment, the two orientations were mirror symmetrical (135° vs. 225°) and demanded quite different hand postures. From the point of the view of the participants in both these

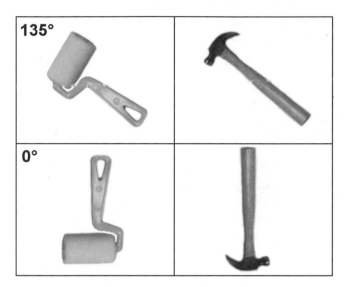

Figure 4.6
Examples of the objects used in the first experiment by Garofeanu et al. (2004). The objects were presented in one of two different orientations during the study and test phase of the experiment. (Reproduced with permission from Garofeanu et al., 2004)

experiments, however, there was no real difference between the study phase and the test phase, except that the latter lasted longer.

No priming of grasping was found in either experiment. In other words, the latency to grasp studied objects did not differ from the latency to grasp new objects (figures 4.7 and 4.8). Of course, in those cases in which the orientation of the object changed from study to test, it was perhaps not surprising that there was no reduction in latency, since the required hand movement would be quite different and an earlier encounter with the object would not be that helpful. However, even when the orientation of the object was maintained from study to test, there was no latency advantage for the studied over the new objects.

The complete absence of priming in this study is surprising given that the objects to be grasped were tools and implements—objects that are associated with particular functions and thus particular hand postures. Even though one might not expect the metrical aspects of the grasping movement to be subject to priming, one might still think it possible that the generation of function-appropriate hand postures might be subject to priming (by virtue of the fact that the identification of the object—and thus its function—was almost certainly primed). The absence of priming suggests that the visuomotor system has quick and automatic access to functional components of the grasp well before the programming of the reach-to-grasp

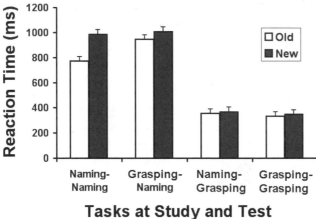

Figure 4.7
Reaction times in the object-naming and object-grasping tests in the first experiment by Garofeanu et al. (2004). There were four conditions: naming–naming, grasping–naming, naming–grasping, and grasping–grasping (at study and test, respectively) under which the old (studied) objects were encountered. The new (nonstudied) objects were named or grasped only in the test phase. Participants showed significantly faster naming of the objects they had named and grasped earlier. Participants did not grasp the studied objects any faster than they did the new objects, irrespective of whether the old objects had been named or grasped earlier. (Reproduced with permission from Garofeanu et al., 2004)

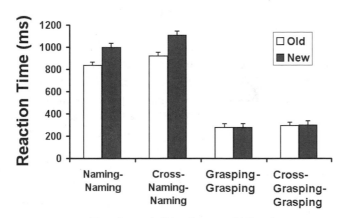

Figure 4.8
Reaction times in the object-naming and object-grasping tasks, with and without the change in object orientation. Irrespective of whether the orientation was maintained or changed (crossed) from study to test, the objects previously named were named significantly faster than new objects. The objects previously grasped were not grasped faster. (Reproduced with permission from Garofeanu et al., 2004)

kinematics is completed or even initiated. It could be the case, for example, that the specification of the metrical components of grasping—movement amplitude and grip scaling, for instance—is more computationally demanding than selection of the particular functional hand posture to be used. To put it another way, if the kinematics of a reach-to-grasp movement are specified de novo on every occasion an action is generated, but the functional components of the grasp can be accessed efficiently, and perhaps in parallel, then no priming of grasping might be evident.

In contrast to what they observed with grasping, Garofeanu et al. (2004) found that naming an object showed evidence of robust priming (see figures 4.7 and 4.8). In other words, objects that had been named during the study phase were named significantly faster than new objects. This was true irrespective of whether the orientation of the object was maintained or changed from study to test. The fact that priming of naming did not differ as a function of object orientation converges with the results of many studies that have found viewpoint independence in object identification and discrimination, particularly with mirror symmetrical presentations (e.g., Biederman & Gerhardstein, 1993; Cant et al., 2005; James et al., 2002). However, naming was also primed by previous grasping of the same objects. That is, even if the object was only grasped at study, its naming was then significantly faster at test. (As was already discussed, the opposite was not true: Grasping was not faster when preceded by naming.) Further tests also showed that naming was faster regardless of the method of examination used in the study phase. It did not really matter whether, during study, participants named the object, grasped the object, matched the orientation of their arm to the object, or simply observed the object; subsequent naming of these objects at test was always faster as compared to the naming of objects that had not been seen before (although explicit naming during the study phase did produce the best priming).

Even though Garofeanu et al. (2004) found no evidence for visuomotor priming, they did find some improvement of performance over the course of the experiment. Participants were faster at initiating their grasping movements to the target objects during the test phase than during the study phase—independent of whether or not the objects were old or new. In other words, participants got better as they became more experienced with the task. Practice helps with visuomotor performance, as anyone who has learned to ride a bicycle can attest to. Nevertheless, there is little evidence that the storage of specific visual information has much of a role to play in the programming of movements directed at visible targets. In contrast, visual memory appears to play a much bigger role in perceptual processes, such as object recognition and identification.

4.5   The Role of Visual Memory in the Control of Action

The results of Cant et al. (2005) and Garofeanu et al. (2004) demonstrate that prior perceptual/semantic processing of objects (including their orientation) does not prime later grasping of those objects. Even when a "transfer-appropriate" paradigm is used, in which the objects are grasped during both the study phase and the test phase, there is no indication of priming. Yet, at the same time, any kind of prior interaction with the objects, cognitive or visuomotor, appears to prime later naming of those objects. These findings converge nicely with a broad range of findings in both neurological patients and normal observers discussed earlier showing that the dedicated visuomotor mechanisms in the dorsal stream do not make use of visual information that is presented *prior* to the programming of a target-directed action. Indeed, recent work by Westwood and Goodale (2003) has shown that for information about target size, for example, to be reflected in the scaling of a grip aperture during a grasping movement, that information must be present on the retina during the programming of the grasp.

Nevertheless, in setting out this real-time account of how visuomotor processing occurs, we do not mean to imply that visual memory does not have a role to play in some aspects of visuomotor control. Visual memory contributes quite directly to certain aspects of motor programming, notably those that depend on information that cannot be derived directly from the retina. One example is the calibration of the initial grip and lift forces that are applied to an object when it is picked up. When people pick up familiar objects, the force they apply to the object is scaled appropriately for the object's weight (and other characteristics) from the moment their hand makes contact, well before any somatosensory feedback is available (Gordon et al., 1993). This means that they must have retrieved the information about the object from memory, information that could be activated only when they recognized the object. Such recognition is presumably mediated by visual mechanisms in the ventral, not the dorsal, stream. At present it is not clear how this information is communicated to the motor system, although a number of plausible accounts have been put forward (for a discussion of this issue, see Goodale & Haffenden, 2003).

When people reach out and pick up objects they have not encountered before, they have to make an estimate of the object's weight—an estimate that is presumably based on previous experience with similar objects. Thus, when people reach out to pick up objects that "look" heavy, such as objects that appear to be made of stone or metal, they apply more force than they do to objects that look as though they are made of lighter materials, such as polystyrene. Moreover, when participants are presented with objects of different sizes that are made of the same material, they typically apply more force to the larger object than they do to the smaller objects— even when the objects are actually the same weight (Gordon et al., 1991). When participants heft such objects, they typically experience what has been called the "size–weight illusion" and conclude that the smaller object is heavier than the larger one. Even though it has been often assumed that the size–weight illusion is a consequence of the mismatch between applied force and the actual weight of the object, it turns out that this is not the case (Flanagan & Beltzner, 2000). When participants make repeated lifts of a set of objects that have the same weight but different sizes, they eventually apply the same initial lift force to all the objects. Nevertheless, the size–weight illusion is not at all diminished by this recalibration of lift force. In other words, participants continue to believe that the smaller object is heavier than the larger one even though they apply to same initial lift force to both.

Despite this apparent dissociation, there are good reasons to believe that both the calibration of the lift forces and the maintenance of the size–weight illusion depend on object recognition systems in the ventral stream that activate specific memories and/or related information about those particular objects. First of all, if the objects to which the observers have recalibrated their lift forces are replaced with new objects (with different surface features), which like the original objects have different sizes but the same weight, the observers now revert to applying less force to the smaller object in the new set (J. R. Flanagan, personal communication). Second, the patient D.F., who has visual form agnosia from ventral-stream lesions, does not show any evidence of a size–weight illusion when she picks up cylindrical objects of different sizes (but the same weight) using a handle attached to the top of the cylinders. In other words, when the only information that D.F. has about the size of the object is derived from vision, she correctly reports that the cylinders are the same weight. Moreover, unlike normal participants, D.F.'s grip and lift forces on the initial trials are not correlated with the size of the cylinder; that is, she does not apply greater force to the larger object (McIntosh, 2000). In contrast, when she picks up the cylinders across their diameter with either her eyes open or her eyes closed, she does show the size–weight illusion. In other words, when she has kinesthetic information about the size of the cylinders, she incorrectly perceives the smaller cylinders as weighing more than the larger ones. A similar dissociation between visual and kinesthetic size–weight illusions has recently been observed in patient S.B., who also has ventral-stream lesions (Dijkerman et al., 2004). Taken together, these findings suggest that stored information about objects that is activated by ventral-stream mechanisms plays an essential role both in computing the required forces for a successful grasp and in generating and maintaining the size–weight illusion.

As we saw earlier, the perceived function of an object can also determine the nature of the hand posture that we select to use when picking it up. Thus, we pick up screwdrivers and hammers by the handle rather than the "business end"—often adopting an awkward posture to accomplish this. And as we also reviewed earlier, there is evidence that these functional components of grasping depend on high-level cognitive processing, which presumably makes use of object recognition circuitry in the ventral stream (Creem & Proffitt, 2001).

There are other aspects of our interactions with familiar objects in which visually driven memories can play an important role. For example, we typically pick up the same toothbrush and the same coffee cup every morning. As a consequence, non-metrical features of these objects, such as their color, can become associated with metrical properties such as their size and shape—and these reliable associations could then be used to program grip aperture. To put it another way, just as we apply the appropriate forces to pick up familiar objects, we can also use learned associations to scale our grasp to familiar objects. Using perceptual information to recover a motor routine could theoretically reduce the need for bottom-up computations of the metrics of the target object, thereby increasing the overall efficiency of the programming. That is, the incorporation of stored parameters such as grip aperture could reduce considerably the computational load on the visuomotor system. Thus, even though the grasp would have to be fine-tuned and adjusted to the particular situation, information retrieved from memory could provide the initial parameters for selecting the posture and scaling the grasp. In short, perceived object features such as color, which have no inherent link to the control of goal-directed actions, could through association provide a cue for the programming of such control. Nevertheless, experiments that have explored these learned associations have shown that the conditions under which such "shortcuts" are used are heavily constrained. For example, if the position of the familiar object is changed randomly from trial to trial, participants are less likely to make use of such learned motor routines (Haffenden & Goodale, 2002b). Moreover, the learned associations are more likely to be based on global cues derived from the entire surface of the object than on specific cues provided by isolated symbols or shapes on the object's surface (Haffenden & Goodale, 2000a, 2002a). Nevertheless, there is clearly a role for visual memory in some aspects of visuomotor programming and control—particularly with respect to those features of the goal object that remain relatively constant over time, such as size, shape, weight, compliance, and surface friction.

However, despite the fact that many aspects of our everyday actions can be influenced by prior experience, the evidence from the priming studies reviewed earlier suggests that many of the kinematic parameters of object-directed reaching and grasping movements are programmed in real time on the basis of current sensory information—with little influence from earlier encounters with the goal object. This reliance on bottom-up input rather than stored information makes good sense, particularly with respect to features such as the orientation and location of the goal object, since it is unlikely that the disposition of the object with respect to the observer would remain constant over time. But even apparently immutable features such as size or shape might not be expected to show evidence of priming either. After all, when the egocentric position of an object is changed, the affordance offered by that object can also change. In other words, the size of the grip and the configuration of the grasping fingers required to pick up an object are functions of the disposition of that object with respect to the hand. For this reason, then, prior information about the size or shape of a goal object in the real world should not be expected to affect the efficiency of movement programming—if that object is actually present and visible when the movement is programmed.

Although repetition priming has little effect on grasping, there is a long history of work showing that manipulation of attention to particular spatial locations can indeed reduce the response latency of orienting movements. In other words, precuing a particular location can speed up orienting responses to that location when the target is presented there. At present, it is not clear what the neural substrates are for this advantage, although there has been much speculation about what the circuitry might be (for a review, see Findlay & Gilchrist, 2003). The temporal parameters of this kind of spatial attention deployment are quite different from those involved in typical repetition-priming studies.

In summary, the visuomotor modules in the dorsal stream appear to work largely in real time—and earlier exposure to goal objects appears to have no apparent effect on the programming of the visually guided actions. The reliance of the dorsal stream on visible rather than stored information is clearly adaptive. In a world where the disposition and affordances of goal objects (with respect to the actor) can change from one moment to the next, it makes little sense to rely on visual memory. Only when vision of the goal object is not available at the time the movement is programmed does information from memory become useful. When this happens, offline information that was originally processed by the ventral stream is brought to bear on the programming of the memory-guided movement. In short, the two streams play complementary roles in the control of behavior.

5 The Cortical Processing Dynamics of Edge Detection and Scene Segmentation

H. Steven Scholte, Jacob Jolij, and Victor A. F. Lamme

5.1 Introduction

Visual perception can be subdivided in many different stages of processing. It is widely believed that edge detection and scene segmentation are among the earliest of these processes to occur in terms of both time (within the first 80–240 ms) and space (involving mainly early visual cortex). This chapter begins with an overview of research into edge detection and scene segmentation.

Together, edge detection and scene segmentation result in figure–ground segregation. In this chapter we will argue that activity related to edge detection is mainly a result of the anatomical wiring of horizontal connections relayed from lower tier to higher tier visual areas and that activity related to scene segmentation is a result of recurrent processing between the different visual areas. This latter process is particularly interesting because it appears to reflect part of the perceptual interpretation of a scene and appears to covary with visual awareness. We will end this chapter with an example of how we are currently studying these processes in human subjects.

5.2 Edge Detection and Scene Segmentation

Edge detection consists of detecting local discontinuities in the visual image on the basis of "primitive qualities" such as orientation, color, motion, or luminance. Scene segmentation consists of grouping parts of the visual scene that share these "primitive" qualities (Julesz, 1981; Treisman & Gelade, 1980; Nothdurft, 1985; Rock & Palmer, 1990; Caputo, 1998). Together these processes result in a surface representation of the visual image in which some surfaces of the visual scene are denoted as figure and other surfaces are denoted as ground (Koffka, 1935). This figure–ground relation has the following characteristics: (1) The figure appears to be located in front of the ground, (2) the local discontinuity between figure and ground is perceived as belonging to the figure (the figure has "border ownership"), and (3) the ground appears to continue behind the figure (Nakayama et al., 1989; Nakayama & Shimojo, 1992).

Theoretically, the processes of edge detection and scene segmentation may be related in two different ways. Edge detection could precede scene segmentation, or vice versa. For the stimuli displayed in figure 5.1A this would mean that first a boundary is formed on the basis of local orientation discontinuities; this is followed by "filling in" of the regions inside the boundaries. Alternatively, scene segmentation might precede edge detection when based on grouping, where boundaries are encoded implicitly at locations where different groups meet.

There are many studies on edge detection and scene segmentation at the psychological level (Nothdurft, 1985, 1991; Saarinen et al., 1997; Elder & Zucker, 1998), although the results appear to be inconsistent with each other. The first view is supported by experiments on, for example, brightness perception. The perception of brightness of a white patch, presented on a dark background, seems to evolve from the edge inward (Paradiso & Hahn, 1996; Rossi & Paradiso, 1996). A similar observation has been made for the process of texture segregation (Caputo, 1998). Moreover, it seems that local discontinuities, like those present in figure 5.1A, are more important in texture segregation than similarity of the features within the segregated surface (Nothdurft, 1985, 1992; Landy & Bergen, 1991). The view that scene segmentation precedes edge detection is supported by findings that global similarity influences the strength of local feature discontinuities in texture segregation

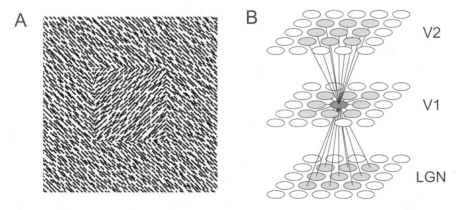

Figure 5.1
(*A*) Example of a texture-defined stimulus. It is possible to perceive a figure in this display because the line elements in the region in which a figure can be perceived have a different orientation than the line elements of the background. (*B*) A V1 neuron receives input via the lateral geniculate nucleus (LGN; feedforward), from lateral connections in the same cortical column (dark-gray disk), surrounding cortical columns (light-gray disk), and higher tier areas.

(Enns & Rensink, 1990) and depends on information about surface layout defined by binocular disparity (He & Nakayama, 1994).

5.3   Neural Implementation of Edge Detection and Scene Segmentation

Neurons in the earliest cortical visual area, V1, respond preferentially to a particular orientation of luminance contrast and respond to stimuli in a restricted part of visual space that extends from 1° to 2° (Hubel & Wiesel, 1968). This area is called the classical receptive field (cRF), and its size is the result of input from neurons in lower tier areas; see figure 5.1B, connections running from the lateral geniculate nucleus (LGN) to V1. That is, it is purely determined by means of feedforward connections (Lamme & Roelfsema, 2000). The cRF is "tuned" to particular features; that is, it only responds to stimuli that meet particular requirements. There is also an area beyond the cRF in which stimuli do not elicit a response on their own but can modulate a cRF-driven response (Allman et al., 1985; Blakemore & Tobin, 1972). This is called the surround receptive field (sRF). The sRF concept is important for understanding the neural basis of edge detection and scene segmentation, since it represents the first stage in which a neuron responds toward the constellation in which a feature is presented.

   It could be argued that scene segmentation and edge detection are also examples of sRF effects. However, we believe it is important to differentiate between studies that deal with the responses of a neuron toward the direct context in which stimuli are presented, on the one hand, and studies in which the perceptual judgment of an animal is measured with regard to at least scene segmentation, on the other. We will therefore first discuss some important findings from research into sRF effects. After this, we will compare two different types of scene segmentation and edge detection models, the hierarchical model and the recurrent model.

5.4   sRF Effects in V1

The total size of the receptive field in V1 (cRF + sRF) is reported to be at least 2–5 times larger than the cRF (Maffei et al., 1976; Li & Li, 1994). When a stimulus is presented into the cRF of a neuron in one eye, and a context is presented into the sRF of the other eye, the sRF effects do not disappear (dichoptic presentation). Thus, sRF properties are not determined by means of pure feedforward processing (DeAngelis et al., 1994) but are cortical in origin. This means that either horizontal connections originating from cortical columns in the surroundings of the cell (see figure 5.1B, connections running within V1), input from higher tier areas (see figure 5.1B, connections running from V2 to V1), and potentially input from lower tier visual areas that have been modified by feedback connections are responsible for. the size of the sRF (Salin & Bullier, 1995).

The most typical type of sRF effect is response suppression. Approximately 72% of monkey V1 cells show this behavior when a central grating is presented that is successively increased in diameter (Walker et al., 2000; Sengpiel et al., 1997). A similar pattern is observed when a line element is presented in the cRF and randomly oriented line elements are presented in the sRF (Landy & Bergen, 1991). However, compared with this latter situation, the firing rate of the neuron will be higher if the line element is surrounded by line elements with an orthogonal orientation to that of the center stimulus (Knierim & VanEssen, 1992). Also, when a line element, presented in the cRF, is flanked by line elements that are collinear, the response may be enhanced instead of suppressed (Kapadia et al., 1995). The behavior of these neurons correlates with the anatomical structure and physiological properties of the horizontal connections, that is, long range projections that originate from pyramidal cells, between cortical columns in early visual cortex. Specifically, horizontal connections preferentially link orientation columns with a similar orientation tuning (Malach et al., 1993; Das & Gilbert, 1999), and these connections between similarly oriented cells are even stronger when these cells have receptive fields along a collinear axis (Schmidt et al., 1997). Behaviorally, these increases in firing rate coincide with an increase in the sensitivity of humans and monkeys to detect these stimuli (Kapadia et al., 1995). It is important to note that these effects are related to the direct context of the cRF.

5.5   The Hierarchical View of Edge Detection and Scene Segmentation

The most simple and elegant neural model of edge detection and scene segmentation perceives these processes as being implemented by a series of hierarchical processing steps that are effected by hierarchically organized brain areas, going from V1 via V2 and V4 to higher cortical areas such as the inferotemporal cortex (Livingstone & Hubel, 1988; DeYoe & Van Essen, 1988). In this model early visual areas, with their tuning for elementary shapes and small cRFs, are involved in edge detection, while higher visual areas, with their more specific tuning characteristics and larger cRFs, are involved in scene segmentation. Such a model is hierarchical in the sense that the properties of the sRF are seen as a result of the contribution of horizontal connections within a cortical area, and as to reflect the integration of information from downstream areas into a "higher" level representation.

Empirical support for the role of V1 in edge detection comes from the studies described in the section on sRF effects in V1, in particular the effects of line elements with an orthogonal orientation in the sRF of a receptive field. A more complex level of representation, border ownership, seems to be represented in areas V2 and V4 (and to a lesser extent V1). More than 50% of the neurons in areas V2 and V4, and probably area V3, signal border ownership (Zhou et al., 2000; Baumann et al., 1997), and indicate whether a particular edge belongs to a figure. This border ownership is signaled 10–25 ms after the response onset, and the sRF related to this effect appears to be at least 20° (Zhou et al., 2000). Finally, studies with functional magnetic resonance imaging (fMRI) have indicated that areas V1, V2, and V3 are involved in the processing of motion boundaries (Reppas et al., 1997).

The region of space over which information has to be analyzed to achieve scene segmentation is typically much larger than the cRF of a neuron in V1 or V2. Areas in higher tier regions do have cRF sizes that are large enough to encapsulate the region of a particular surface. These areas also show an increase in the complexity of the tuning. For instance, neurons in V4 are tuned to elementary shapes (Desimone & Schein, 1987; Gallant et al., 1996; Pasupathy & Connor, 2002a), making them well suited for the integration of edge-like information from lower tier areas. Also, it has been shown that areas V3, V4, temporal occipital cortex (TEO), and V3a (Kastner et al., 2000) respond to texture-defined surfaces compared to homogeneous textures.

In summary, the hierarchical model of edge detection and scene segmentation is both simple and elegant. It conforms to the main features of the visual system (increase in cRF size, increase in the specificity of the tuning of the cRF) and is supported by a great number of studies. It portrays V1 as an area involved in feature detection, V1 and potentially V2 and V3 as areas involved in edge detection, and areas V3, V3a, V4, and TEO as areas involved in scene segmentation.

5.6   The Recurrent Processing View on Scene Segmentation

The notion of hierarchal processing in edge detection and scene segmentation is strongly challenged by findings that show sRF effects in V1 with a relatively large delay (30–70 ms) after response onset (Rossi et al., 2001) and/or sRF effects at a large (more than 3°) spatial distance from the cRF (Lamme, 1995; Zipser et al., 1996; Bair et al., 2003; Lee et al., 1998; Marcus & Van Essen, 2002).

For example, Lamme (1995) found that a V1 neuron responds more strongly when its cRF is on the inside of the figure presented in figure 5.1A than when it is stimulated by identical background elements, even though its cRF is smaller than the figure. One result from this study is presented in figure 5.2A. In the top row of this figure the single-unit response from a neuron in V1 is shown, obtained by presenting a texture with homogeneously oriented line elements. The black circle in the adjacent texture represents the cRF of this neuron. After approximately 80 ms, the

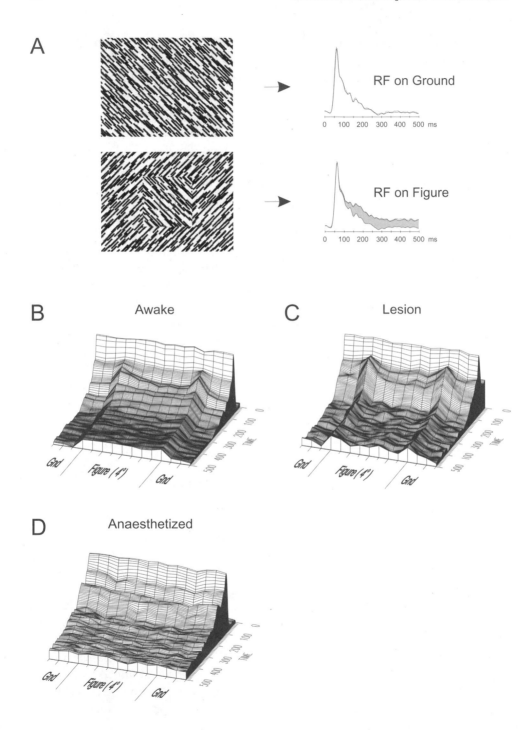

response of this neuron is influenced by the global context in which the line elements within the receptive field of the neuron are presented. For instance, neurons with their receptive field on the boundary between figure and ground show an increase in firing rate at this interval (Lamme et al., 1999). Subsequently, neurons within the boundaries show an increase in firing rate (compared to the condition in which only a homogeneous texture is presented) that starts after ~100ms. This is shown in figure 5.2B, in which the activity evoked by a figure texture is plotted over time for different positions of the cRF relative to the figure and the figure–ground boundary. Zipser et al. (1996) found that modulation, as measured in the center of a figure, is large for smaller figures and declines as figures grow larger. No significant modulation was found for figures larger than 10° (see also Lamme, 1995). More important, these studies also showed that an asymmetry, also visible in figure 5.2B, of modulation across the figure–ground boundary, was present in area V1. As soon as the cRF is outside the figure, the sRF modulation is absent.[1]

These findings implicate the involvement of recurrent or feedback processing (Salin & Bullier, 1995; Lamme & Roelfsema, 2000), that is to say, the influence of higher tier areas on lower tier areas in scene segmentation (for instance, the connections going from V2 to area V1 in figure 5.1B). This inference can be made for three different reasons: the first based on the anatomical layout of the visual system and the conduction speed of different types of neurons, the second based on findings from lesion studies, and the third based on the close connection in some reported studies on scene segmentation between measured neuronal activity and the perceptual interpretation of the scene.

5.6.1 Speed of Processing in the Visual System

Feedforward and feedback corticocortical connections conduct information at an extremely high speed of approximately 2 to 3.5m/s (Girard et al., 2001; Bullier, 2001), activating neurons in area V1 between 35 and 72ms and neurons in the frontal eye field between 43 and 91ms. Given that the synaptic relays add only an additional 5

Figure 5.2
General phenomology of contextual modulation. (A) The responses of a neuron in V1 (single unit, smoothed) when the classical receptive field (cRF) falls on a texture with homogeneously oriented line elements (top) and additional activity (bottom right, in gray) that can be measured when the line elements that fall in the cRF are part of a figure. (B) The neural activity (z-axis, smoothed spiking activity) evoked by a figure texture plotted over time (more horizontal axis) and across a line circumcising a figure (more vertical axis). Measured in V1 of a macaque monkey. Notice that the neurons start to fire vigorously after 40ms (visual response); 40ms later it is possible to see a difference in activity between neurons with their cRF on the edge and other neurons. After this, it becomes possible to see "filling in" in the area between the boundaries. (C) When the peristriate areas are removed, isolating V1 and V2 from the rest of the brain, activity related to the filling in disappears, while the activity related to edge detection remains visible. (D) When a monkey is brought under anesthesia (sensory + motor), activity related to edge detection and scene segmentation disappears. Gnd, ground.

to 20 ms to the relay time per synaptic cleft (Nowak & Bullier, 1997; Azouz & Gray, 1999) and that there are long distance corticocortical projections from, for instance, V1 to MT (Felleman & Van Essen, 1991), it is no surprise that all visually responsive areas in the macaque cortex are activated approximately 115 ms after stimulus onset (Lamme & Roelfsema, 2000), including regions in motor and frontal cortex.

This rapid speed of the corticocortical projections contrasts with the lower conduction velocity of horizontal connections that are on the order of 0.1 to 0.33 m/s (Girard et al., 2001; Grinvald et al., 1994; Bringuier et al., 1999). This 10-fold difference in conduction speed is caused by a difference in myelination and diameter between horizontal and interareal corticocortical connections (Bullier, 2001). Because of the relatively low conduction speed of horizontal connections and the high magnification factor in the fovea (horizontal connections span only about 0.6° of visual space [Dow et al., 1981] in the region of cortex representing the fovea), information can be spread by means of these connections at a rate of approximately 100 ms per degree of visual space (Bullier, 2001). However, contextual effects of scene elements at a distance up to 3–10° influence the measured spiking activity 100 ms after stimulus presentation (Marcus & VanEssen, 2002; Rossi et al., 2001; Zipser et al., 1996).

That is to say, while horizontal connections can explain sRF effects at a short spatial scale and appear to be important for the integration and segregation of short-range contour segments, they are probably too slow to explain the large field sRF effects reported in a number of studies (Bair et al., 2003; Lamme, 1995; Zipser et al., 1996; Marcus & VanEssen, 2002).

5.6.2 Lesion Studies

The involvement of recurrent connections has been indicated by lesion studies, showing the contribution of higher areas in figure–ground signals in V1 (Hupe et al., 1998; Lamme et al., 1998a). A lesion that removed the connections between areas V1 and V2, on the one hand, and the rest of the brain, on the other hand, resulted in a disappearance of the surface-related signal in area V1 but not of the boundary-related signal in V1. Results from this study (Lamme et al., 1998a) are illustrated in figure 5.2C (figure 5.2B represents activity from the same monkey before the lesion). Activity is still evoked at the boundary between figure and ground but is no longer present for the surface elements of the figure. This indicates that edge detection is completed within area V1 and V2 but subsequent surface segregation signals depend on feedback from higher areas. Likewise, Hupe et al. (1998) showed, by using reversible inactivation of area MT, that feedback connections serve to amplify the response of neurons in area V1 and enhance suppression evoked by the background (Hupe et al., 1998; Hupe et al., 2001).

5.6.3   Correlation Between Neuronal Activity in V1 and Perceptual Interpretation

While classical receptive field tuning properties in early visual areas are hardly different when animals are anesthetized or awake (Schiller et al., 1976; Lamme et al., 1998b), the sRF effects related to scene segmentation can only be recorded in the awake animal (see figure 5.2B). When a monkey is under anesthesia by isoflurane (see figure 5.2D), the sRF effects disappear entirely (Lamme et al., 1998b). Also, it has been shown that when monkeys do not detect figures in a saccade detection task, the sRF effects are strongly reduced or absent (Super et al., 2001). The correlation between neuronal activity in V1 and perceptual interpretation is further strengthened by a study that shows that masking the stimulus in such a way that a monkey is not capable of detecting the stimulus anymore coincides with an abolishment of the sRF effects (Lamme et al., 2002). Results from this experiment are depicted in figure 5.3. When a figure is masked by a stimulus that follows the presentation of a figure immediately (16 ms), the monkey is incapable of detecting this figure. With an increase in time between the presentation of the figure and the presentation of the mask, the capability of the monkey to detect the figure also increases (see figure 5.3A) and the size of the sRF effect (see figure 5.3B) that can be measured at these different masking intervals correlates with the reported visibility of the monkey. Finally, when the figure stimulus is followed by a blank screen mask, the figure is much easier to detect (see figure 5.3C). The sRF effect again correlates with the visibility of the stimulus, and this indicates that the effect presented in figure 5.3B is a result not of the presentation duration of the figure stimulus but of the perceived presence of the figure.

Since the large majority of horizontal connections do not have the speed or the extent to explain sRF effects at the spatial and temporal scale reported and these sRF effects are absent or influenced by recurrent top-down processing, we feel confident in concluding that some sRF effects, especially those related to scene segmentation, are related to recurrent processing between lower and higher tier areas. The source of this feedback projection is probably not area V2 but most likely extrastriate cortex or, potentially, areas in the temporal lobe (Roelfsema et al., 2002).

5.7   Separating Scene Segmentation and Edge Detection in Humans

Event-related potential (ERP) studies with human subjects have revealed that when the evoked response, obtained by presenting homogeneous textures, is subtracted from the response obtained by presenting figure textures (such as the one in figure 5.1A), a signal with peak latencies between 140 and 219 ms in occipital channels

A   Behavior for Pattern and Blank Masks

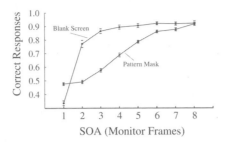

B   Contextual Modulation, Pattern Mask

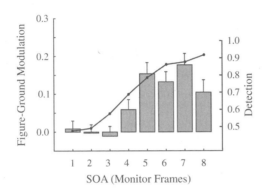

C   Contextual Modulation, Blank Screen

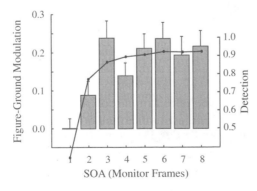

Figure 5.3
Contextual modulation while the perceivability of the stimulus is manipulated. (*A*) Performance of a monkey when a stimulus is followed by a pattern mask or a blank screen. (*B*) Contextual modulation when a pattern mask is presented after the figure texture. (*C*) Contextual modulation when a blank screen is presented. SOA, stimulus onset asynchrony.

remains (Bach & Meigen, 1992; Lamme et al., 1992). The systematic manipulation of the visibility of the figure has indicated that the latter part of this response, around 200 ms, is more related to scene segmentation, while the earlier part of this response, around 150 ms, appears to be more related to edge detection (Caputo & Casco, 1999). These ERP findings indicate that edge detection appears to precede scene segmentation in time but also illustrate one of the central problems of edge detection and scene segmentation research in humans: how to separate activity induced by the edge from activity induced by the surface.

We are currently working on this problem in our lab and are running experiments with stimuli similar to the ones presented in figure 5.4A. The goal of these studies

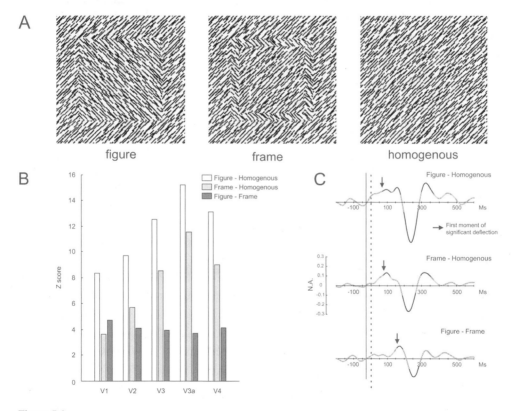

Figure 5.4
EEG and fMRI data measured in humans evoked by stimuli in which the amount of figure and edge was manipulated. (*A*) Example of a figure texture (left), frame texture (middle) and homogenous texture (right). (*B*) *Z* scores (vertical axis) for different fMRI contrasts in different early visual cortical areas. A generalized linear model was fitted to signals obtained by averaging over all voxels in a particular cortical area (horizontal axis). (*C*) Evoked subtraction responses of channel PO3 for all relevant comparisons (normalized activity on vertical, time in ms on horizontal).

is to differentiate between edge detection and scene segmentation and to try to separate sRF and cRF effects in human subjects; we will next describe one of these experiments in more detail, since this work has not been published.

5.8 Edge Detection and Scene Segmentation in Human Subjects

We recorded electroencephalogram (EEG) and fMRI data in human subjects viewing stimuli that were constructed so as to make it possible to differentiate between texture boundary detection and scene segmentation. We presented three types of textures in this experiment: textures with "solid" square figures (figure 5.4A, left), textures with frame figures (figure 5.4A, middle), and textures with homogeneously oriented textures (figure 5.4A, right). From the responses to these textures, we calculated subtracted EEG activity or fMRI contrasts that we here refer to as Fig–Hom (figure texture induced activity vs. homogeneous texture induced activity), Frame–Hom (figure texture induced activity vs. homogeneous texture induced activity), and Fig-Frame (figure texture induced activity vs. frame texture induced activity). The contribution from mechanisms involved in boundary formation or local texture contrast should be at least as large in the Frame–Hom contrast as in the Fig–Hom contrast, as the texture frames have the same size as the texture figures and could be considered to contain "more" edge. The amount of surface, however, is larger in the Fig–Hom contrast. If early visual processing is limited to boundary detection, the Frame–Hom activity should be higher than or equal to the Fig–Hom activity. If, on the other hand, a substantial part of the activity in occipital areas is related to surface formation, Fig–Hom signals should be largest.

The results from this experiment support the latter hypothesis (see figures 5.4B and 5.4C). Both the Fig–Hom and Frame–Hom EEG difference signals (see figure 5.4C) are characterized by a small but significant positive deflection starting at around 100 ms, followed by a large negative deflection starting at ~200 ms. The difference between these two signals is significant at a latency of about 155 ms, where the Fig–Hom signal is more positive than the Frame–Hom signal, and continues until about 300 ms, where the Fig–Hom signal is more negative than the Frame–Hom signal. Boundary detection therefore seems to precede surface segregation (in concurrence with Caputo & Casco, 1999).

The results of the fMRI contrasts of Fig–Hom, Frame–Hom, and Fig–Frame are depicted in figure 5.4B. The contrast Fig–Hom yielded a significant response in all cortical areas (at least $p < .0001$). This significance was highest for areas V3a and V4.

When we compare the significance of activation in the contrast Frame–Hom over cortical areas, it becomes clear that, going from V1 via V2 to V3, there is an increase in significance. This could indicate that edge detection is processed in a hierarchical fashion. An opposite pattern is present in the contrast Fig–Frame. Here, V1 shows a higher activation than V2 or V3, at least in terms of relative activation compared to Frame–Hom activity.

Therefore, the temporal order of events is not reflected in a hierarchical process at the cortical level: It is not the case that boundary detection predominates at low-level areas, while surface segregation signals predominate at higher areas. Rather, the reverse seems to hold. Boundary detection signals are stronger in higher areas than in lower areas; surface segregation signals are at least equally distributed over visual areas, and may even be strongest in V1. Therefore, the temporal order of events is not reflected in a hierarchical process at the cortical level; that is, boundary detection *does not* predominated at low-level areas, and surface segregation signals *do not* predominate at higher-level areas.

5.9 Conclusions

Neurons in V1 respond to particular orientation of luminance contrast (Hubel & Wiesel, 1968), and it is believed that this activity reflects the detection of simple features in a scene (see figure 5.5, top panel). Edge detection could be implicated by means of hierarchical processing, where horizontal connections in area V1 are involved in boundary detection at proximal distances and relay this information via feedforward connections to higher tier areas with larger receptive fields, where this process is repeated at a more distal scale (see figure 5.5, middle panel); Roelfsema et al., 2002).

However, there is strong evidence that, while edge detection might occur in a hierarchical fashion, this is not the case for scene segmentation. Instead, scene segmentation–related activity in V1 involves recurrent processing (see figure 5.5, bottom panel) from cortical areas beyond V2 (Lamme et al., 1998a), and we would like to distinguish this "contextual modulation" from normal sRF effects for the following reasons:

• This activity is absent in monkeys when the monkey is sensory anesthetized, while other sRF effects generally remain.

• This activity is a reflection of the interpretation (Zipser et al., 1996) of a scene, while most sRF effects are a reflection of the anatomical layout of the horizontal connections (Kapadia et al., 1999).

• This activity is absent when the surface organization is masked (Lamme et al., 2002) or not perceived (Super et al., 2001).

Feature detection

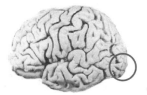 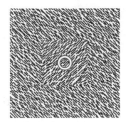

40-70 ms V1

Boundary formation

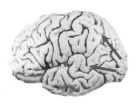 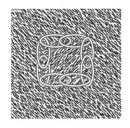

Feedforward sweep
75-95ms, V1, V2, V3, V4 etc

Surface formation

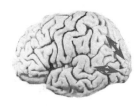 

Recurrent processing
< 90 ms, V1 and V2, V3, V4

Figure 5.5
Schematic overview of our current model of edge detection and scene segmentation. Feature detection between 40 and 70 ms involving mainly V1 (top); boundary formation, by means of a feedforward sweep from V1, via V2 to higher cortical areas between 75 and 95 ms (middle); scene segmentation, involving recurrent processing between higher and lower visual areas (bottom).

In short, contextual modulation appears to reflect widespread cortico-cortical inter-actions related to perceptual organization (Lamme & Roelfsema, 2000) and the phenomenal experience of the visual scene (Lamme et al., 2000).

Notes

1. Two other studies found a similar size tuning, but with an earlier cutoff, showing no modulation for figures larger than 5° (Marcus & Van Essen, 2002) or 3° (Rossi et al., 2001). However, these studies did not investigate whether an asymmetry across the figure–ground boundary was present or absent; there-fore, it is hard to interpret these studies in terms of figure–ground segmentation, since figure–ground seg-regation in terms of neural processing must coincide with an asymmetry in the neural response toward the figure, on the one hand, and the background, on the other.

6 Consciousness Absent and Present: A Neurophysiological Exploration of Masking

Edmund T. Rolls

6.1 Overview

Backward masking was used to investigate the amount of neuronal activity that occurs in the macaque inferior temporal visual cortex when faces can just be identified. It is shown that the effect of the pattern mask is to interrupt neuronal activity in the inferior temporal visual cortex. This reduces the number of action potentials that occur to a given stimulus, and it decreases even more the information that is available about which stimulus was shown because the variance of the spike counts is increased. When the onset of the mask follows the onset of the test stimulus by 20 ms, each neuron fires for approximately 30 ms, provides on average 0.1 bits of information (see figure 5 of Rolls et al., 1999, which shows cumulated information values), and human observers perform at a level approximately 50% better than chance in forced-choice psychophysics yet say that they are guessing and frequently report that they are unable to consciously see the face and identify which face it is. At a longer stimulus onset asynchrony (SOA) of 40 ms, the neurons fire for approximately 50 ms, the amount of information carried by a single neuron is 0.14 bits, and human observers are much more likely to report conscious identification of which face was shown. The results quantify both the amount of neuronal firing and information that are present when stimuli can be discriminated but not reported on consciously and the additional amount of neuronal firing and information that are required for human observers to consciously identify the faces. It is suggested that the threshold for conscious visual perception may be set to be higher than the level at which small but significant information is present in neuronal firing, so that the systems in the brain that implement the type of information processing involved in conscious thoughts are not interrupted by small signals that could be noise in sensory pathways.

The results also show that there is insufficient time for top-down processing from higher cortical areas (such as the inferior temporal visual cortex) to lower order cortical areas (such as V1) to be a requirement for conscious visual perception

Simultaneous recordings from populations of neurons in the macaque inferior temporal visual cortex also show that most of the information about which stimulus was shown is available in the number of spikes (or firing rate) of each neuron and not from stimulus-dependent synchrony, so that it is unlikely that stimulus-dependent synchrony (of which oscillations could be a degenerate form) is an essential aspect of conscious visual perception in humans.

6.2 Introduction

Damage to the primary (striate) visual cortex can result in blindsight, in which patients report that they do not see stimuli consciously yet, when making forced choices, can discriminate some properties of the stimuli such as motion, position, some aspects of form, and even face expression (Weiskrantz et al., 1974; Weiskrantz, 1997, 1998; Stoerig & Cowey, 1997; de Gelder et al., 1999). In normal human subjects, *backward masking* of visual stimuli, in which another visual stimulus closely follows the short presentation of a test stimulus, reduces the visual perception of the test visual stimulus, and this paradigm has been widely used in psychophysics (Humphreys & Bruce, 1989). In this chapter I consider how much information is present in neuronal firing in the part of the visual system that represents faces and objects, the inferior temporal visual cortex (Rolls & Deco, 2002), when human subjects can discriminate in forced choice, but cannot consciously perceive, face identity. I also consider the implications that the neurophysiological findings have for consciousness.

The representation of faces and objects is in the inferior temporal visual cortex as shown by evidence that position, size, and even (for some neurons) view-invariant representations of objects and faces are provided by neurons in the inferior temporal visual cortex (Rolls, 2000a; Rolls & Deco, 2002); that this is the last stage of unimodal visual processing in primates; and that lesions of what may be a homologous region in humans, the fusiform gyrus face and object areas (Ishai et al.,1999; Kanwisher et al., 1997), produce face and object identification deficits in the absence of low-level impairments of visual processing such as visual acuity (Rolls & Deco, 2002; Farah et al., 1995a; Farah et al., 1995b; Farah, 2004). The inferior temporal visual cortex is therefore an appropriate stage of processing at which to relate quantitative aspects of neuronal processing to the visual perception of faces and objects. We have therefore studied the quantitative relationship between neuronal activity in the macaque inferior temporal visual cortex and visual perception (Rolls & Deco, 2002), and in this article I focus on the relation between inferior temporal visual cortex and conscious visual perception, using the results from combined neurophysiological studies on the inferior temporal visual cortex and perceptual studies in humans with the paradigm of backward masking of visual stimuli

(Rolls et al., 1994; Rolls & Tovée, 1994; Rolls et al., 1999). A subsequent study by Kovacs et al. (1995) using a similar backward masking paradigm combined with primate electrophysiology confirmed the results.

6.3 Neurophysiology of the Backward Masking of Visual Stimuli

Rolls and Tovée (1994) and Rolls et al. (1994) measured the responses of single neurons in the macaque inferior temporal visual cortex during backward visual masking. Neurons that were selective for faces, using distributed encoding (Rolls & Tovée, 1995; Rolls et al., 1997; Treves et al., 1999; Rolls & Deco, 2002), were tested in a visual fixation task conducted as shown in figure 6.1. The visual fixation task was used to ensure that the monkey looked at the visual stimuli.

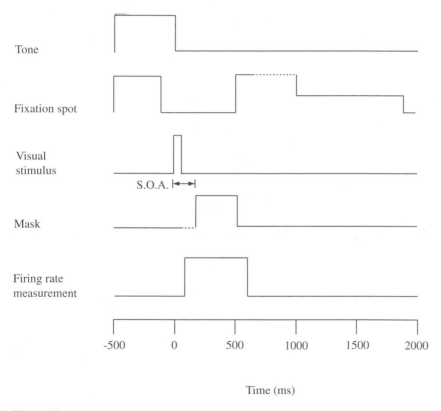

Time (ms)

Figure 6.1
The timing used in the backward masking visual fixation blink task. The stimulus onset asynchrony (SOA) is the time between the onset of the visual test stimulus and the onset of the pattern mask stimulus. The test stimulus duration was 16 ms. (After Rolls et al., 1994)

The methods used have been described by Rolls and Tovée (1994) and Rolls et al. (1994), and a few salient points follow. As shown in figure 6.1, at –100 ms, the fixation spot was blinked off so that there was no stimulus on the screen in the 100-ms period immediately preceding the test image. The screen in this period, and at all other times including the interstimulus interval and the interval between the test image and the mask, was set at the mean luminance of the test images and the mask, so that pattern discrimination with equally intense test and mask stimuli was investigated (see Bruce & Green, 1989). At 0 ms, the 500-ms warning cue tone was switched off and the test visual image was switched on for one 16-ms frame of a raster display image. The monitor had a persistence of less than 3 ms, so that no part of the test image was present at the start of the next frame. SOA (time between the onset of the test stimulus and the onset of the mask) values of 20, 40, 60, 100, or 1000 ms (chosen in a random sequence by the computer) were used. The duration of the masking stimulus was 300 ms. The stimuli were static visual stimuli subtending 8° in the visual field presented on a video monitor at a distance of 1.0 m. Faces were used as test stimuli. The usual masking stimulus (to which the neuron being analyzed did not respond) was made up of letters of the alphabet {N, O}, as illustrated in Rolls et al. (1994). The masking pattern consisted of overlapping letters; this masking pattern was used because it is similar to the mask used in the previous psychophysical experiments (see Rolls et al., 1994). (In some cases the masking stimulus was a face stimulus that was ineffective for the neuron being recorded.)

Figure 6.2 shows examples of the effects of backward masking on the responses of a single inferior temporal cortex neuron in peristimulus rastergram and time histogram form. The top rastergram/spike density histogram pair shows the responses of the neuron to a single frame of the test stimulus (an effective face stimulus for that neuron). Relative to the prestimulus rate, there was an increase in the firing produced with a latency of approximately 75 ms, and this firing lasted for 200–300 ms, that is, for much longer than the 16-ms presentation of the target stimulus. In the next pairs down, the effects of introducing a noneffective face as the masking stimulus with different SOAs are shown. It is shown that the effect of the mask is to limit the duration of the firing produced by the target stimulus. Very similar masking was obtained with the standard N–O pattern mask. Similar experiments were repeated on 42 different cells (Rolls et al., 1994; Rolls & Tovée, 1995), and in all cases the temporal aspects of the masking were similar to those shown in figure 6.2.

One important conclusion that can be drawn from these results is that the effect of a backward masking stimulus on cortical visual information processing is to limit the duration of neuronal responses by interrupting neuronal firing. The neuronal firing of inferior temporal cortex neurons often persisted for 200–300 ms after a

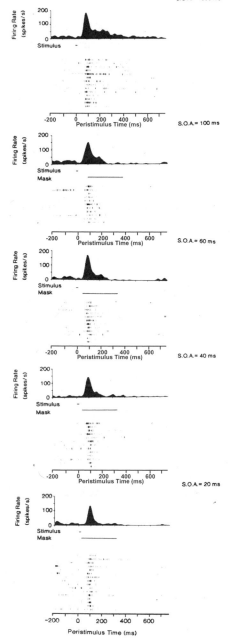

Figure 6.2
Peristimulus rastergrams and smoothed peristimulus spike density histograms based on responses in 8–16 trials to the test face alone (top raster–histogram pair) and to the test face followed by a masking stimulus (which was a face that was ineffective in activating the cell) with different stimulus onset asynchrony (SOA) values. (The SOA is the delay between the onset of the test stimulus and the onset of the mask stimulus.) The mask alone did not produce firing in the cell. The target stimulus was shown for 16 ms starting at time 0. (The top trace shows the response to the target stimulus alone, in that with this 1,000-ms SOA, the mask stimulus was delayed until well after the end of the recording period shown.) (After Rolls & Tovée, 1994)

16-ms presentation of a stimulus. With a 20-ms SOA, the neuronal firing was typically limited to 30 ms. With a 40-ms SOA, the neuronal firing was typically limited
to 50 ms. This persistence of cortical neuronal firing when a masking stimulus is not
present is probably related to cortical recurrent collateral connections that could
implement an autoassociative network with attractor and short-term-memory properties (see Rolls & Treves, 1998; Rolls & Deco, 2002), because such continuing poststimulus neuronal firing is not observed in the lateral geniculate nucleus (K. Martin,
personal communication).

6.4 Information Available in Inferior Temporal Cortex Visual Neurons During Backward Masking

To fully understand quantitatively the responses of inferior temporal cortex neurons
at the threshold for visual perception, Rolls et al. (1997) applied information theoretic methods (see Shannon, 1948; Rolls & Treves, 1998; Rolls & Deco, 2002) to the
analysis of the neurophysiological data with backward masking obtained by Rolls
et al. (1994) and Rolls and Tovée (1994). One advantage of this analysis is that it
shows how well the neurons discriminate between the stimuli under different conditions by taking into account not only the number of spikes but also the variability from trial to trial in the number of spikes. Another advantage of this analysis is
that it provides information about the extent to which the neurons discriminate
between stimuli in bits, which can then be directly compared with evidence about
discriminability obtained using different measures, such as human psychophysical
performance. The analysis quantifies what can be determined about which of the set
of faces was presented from a single trial of neuronal firing.

As a preliminary to the information theoretic analysis, the effect of the SOA on
the neuronal responses, averaged across the population of 15 neurons for which a
sufficient number of trials was available, is shown in figure 6.3. The responses for
the most (max) and the least (min) effective stimuli are shown for the period 0–
200 ms with respect to stimulus onset. There was little effect (not significant) of the
mask on the responses to the least effective stimulus in the set, for which the number
of spikes was close to the spontaneous activity.

The transmitted information carried by neuronal firing rates about the stimuli was
computed with the use of techniques that have been described previously (e.g., Rolls
et al., 1997; Rolls & Treves, 1998; Rolls & Deco, 2002) and have been used previously to analyze the responses of inferior temporal cortex neurons (Optican &
Richmond, 1987; Gawne & Richmond, 1993; Tovée et al., 1993; Tovée & Rolls, 1995;
Rolls et al., 1997). In brief, the general procedure was as follows (Rolls et al., 1999).
The response r of a neuron to the presentation of a particular stimulus s was

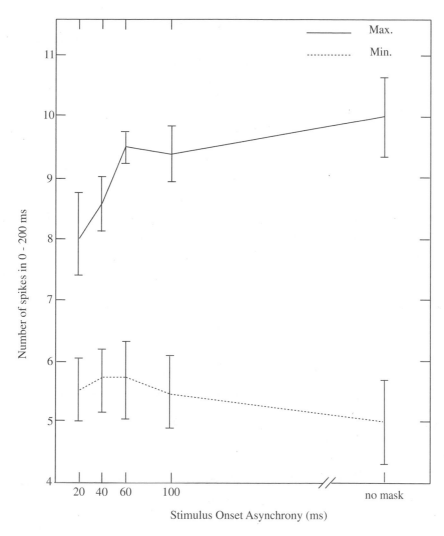

Figure 6.3
The mean (±*SEM*) across cells of the number of spikes produced by the most effective stimulus (Max.) and the least effective stimulus (Min.) as a function of stimulus onset asynchrony. (After Rolls et al., 1999)

computed by measuring the firing rate of the neuron in a fixed time window after the stimulus presentation. The firing rates were then quantized (separated) into a smaller number of bins d than there were trials for each stimulus. After this response quantization, the experimental joint stimulus–response probability table $P(s, r)$ was computed from the data (where $P(r)$ and $P(s)$ are the experimental probability of occurrence of responses and of stimuli, respectively), and the information $I(S, R)$ transmitted by the neurons averaged across the stimuli was calculated by using the Shannon formula (Shannon, 1948; Rolls & Deco, 2002):

$$I(S,R) = \sum_{s,r} P(s,r) \log_2 \frac{P(s,r)}{P(s)P(r)}. \tag{6.1}$$

The finite sampling correction of Panzeri and Treves (1996) was then subtracted to obtain estimates unbiased for the limited sampling. This procedure yields the information available in the firing rates about the stimulus.

Figure 6.4 shows the average across the cells of the cumulated information available in a 200-ms period from stimulus onset from the responses of the 15 neurons as a function of the SOA. This emphasizes how as the SOA is reduced toward 20 ms the information does reduce rapidly but shows that nevertheless at an SOA of 20 ms there is still considerable information about which stimulus was shown. One-way analysis of variance (ANOVA) indicated that the reduction of the information at different SOAs was highly significant at $p < .001$. It was notable that the information reduced much more than the number of spikes on each trial as the SOA was shortened. The explanation for this is that at short SOAs the neuronal responses become noisy, as shown by Rolls et al. (1999). This underscores the value of measuring the information available and not only the number of spikes (Rolls et al., 1999).

6.5 Human Psychophysical Performance with the Same Set of Stimuli

Rolls et al. (1994) performed human psychophysical experiments with the same set of stimuli and with the same apparatus as used for the neurophysiological experiments so that the neuronal responses could be closely related to the identification that was possible of which face was shown. The monitor provided maximum and minimum luminance of 6 and 0.13 footlamberts, respectively, and was adjusted internally for linearity, within an error of no more than 3%.

Five different faces were used as stimuli. All the faces were well-known to each of the eight observers used in the experiment. In the forced-choice paradigm, the observers specified whether the face was normal or rearranged, and they identified whose face they thought had been presented. The observers were instructed that

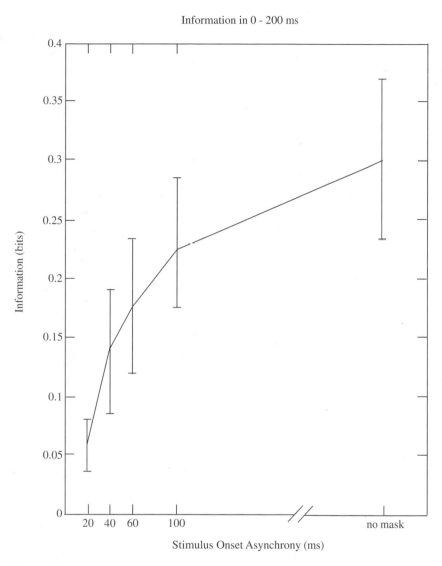

Figure 6.4
The mean (±*SEM*) across the cells of the cumulated information available in a 200-ms period from stimulus onset from the responses of the cells as a function of the stimulus onset asynchrony. (After Rolls et al., 1999)

even if they were unsure of their judgment, they were to respond with their best guess. The data were corrected for guessing to aid in the comparison between classification and identification. This correction was arranged such that chance performance would be shown as 0% correct on the graphs, and perfect performance as 100% correct.

The mean proportion of correct responses for the identification task (and for the classification of normal vs. rearranged) are shown in figure 6.5. The proportion correct data were submitted to an arcsin transformation (to normalize the data), and a repeated measures ANOVA was performed. This analysis showed statistically significant effects of SOA, $F(4, 28) = 61.52, p < .0001$.

Forced-choice discrimination of face identity was thus better than chance at an SOA of 20 ms. However, at this SOA, the subjects were not conscious of seeing the face, or of the identity of the face, and felt that their guessing about which face had been shown was not correct. The subjects did know that something had changed on the screen (and this was not just brightness, as this was constant throughout a trial). Sometimes the subjects had some conscious feeling that a part of a face (such as a mouth) had been shown. However, the subjects were not conscious of seeing a whole face or of seeing the face of a particular person. At an SOA of 40 ms, the subjects' forced-choice performance of face identification was close to 100% (see figure 6.6), and at this SOA, the subjects became much more consciously aware of the identity of which face had been shown (Rolls et al., 1994).

6.6   Comparison of Neuronal Data With the Identification and with the Conscious Perception of Visual Stimuli

The neurophysiological data (Rolls et al., 1994; Rolls & Tovée, 1994), and the results of the information theoretic analysis (Rolls et al., 1999), can now be compared directly with the effects of backward masking in human observers, studied with the same apparatus and with the same stimuli (Rolls et al., 1994). For the human observers, identification of which face from a set of six had been seen was 50% correct (with 0% correct corresponding to chance performance) with an SOA of 20 ms, and 97% correct with an SOA of 40 ms (Rolls et al., 1994). Comparing the human performance purely with the changes in firing rate under the same stimulus conditions suggested that when it is just possible to identify which face has been seen, neurons in a given cortical area may be responding for only approximately 30 ms (Rolls & Tovée, 1994; Rolls et al., 1994). The implication is that 30 ms is enough time for a neuron to perform sufficient computation to enable its output to be used for identification. The results based on an analysis of the information encoded in the spike trains at different SOAs support this hypothesis by showing that a

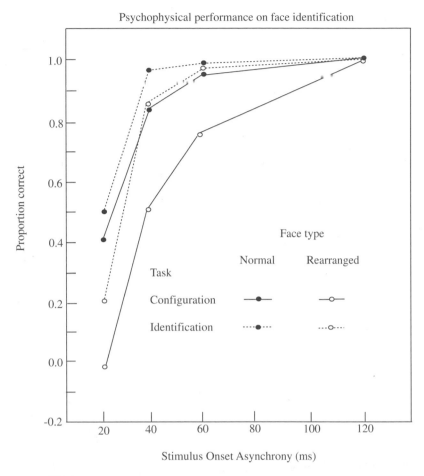

Figure 6.5
Psychophysical performance of humans with the same stimuli as used in the neurophysiological experiments described here. The subjects were shown "normal" faces or faces with the parts "rearranged" and were asked to state which of five faces had been shown ("Identification"), and whether the face shown was in the normal or rearranged ("Configuration"). The plots show the proportion correct on the tasks of classification of spatial configuration (i.e., whether the face features were normal or rearranged), and of determination of the identity of the faces for faces in the normal or rearranged spatial configuration of face features, as a function of stimulus onset asynchrony. The data have been corrected for guessing. The means of the proportions correct are shown. The test stimulus was presented for 16 ms. (After Rolls et al., 1994)

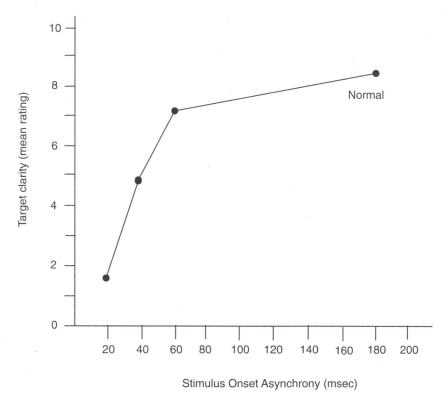

Figure 6.6
Rating of the subjective clarity of faces as a function of stimulus onset asynchrony (SOA). The mean of
the magnitude estimation ratings is shown. The clarity of the face, when presented without being followed by a masking stimulus, was assigned the number 10. If the observer was not able to see the features of the face, that was to be considered 0. The observers assigned a number from 0 to 10 to represent
the perceived subjective clarity of the face. The effect of SOA was statistically significant at $p < .001$.
(After Rolls et al., 1994)

significant proportion of information is available in these few spikes (see figure 6.4),
with, on average, 0.1 bits available from each neuron at an SOA of 20 ms (see figure
5 of Rolls et al., 1999, which shows cumulated information values). Thus, when subjects feel that they are guessing and are not conscious of seeing whose face has been
shown, macaque inferior temporal cortex neurons provide small but significant
amounts of information about which face has been shown. When the SOA was
increased to 40 ms, the inferior temporal cortex neurons responded for approximately 50 ms and encoded approximately 0.14 bits of information (for cumulated
information for the subset of face-selective neurons tested, see Rolls et al., 1999,
figure 5). At this SOA, not only was face identification 97% correct but the subjects
were much more likely to be able to report consciously seeing a face and/or whose

face had been shown. One way in which the conscious perception of the faces was measured quantitatively was by asking subjects to rate the clarity of the faces. This was a subjective assessment and therefore reflected conscious processing, and it was made using magnitude estimation. It is shown in figure 6.6 that the subjective clarity of the stimuli was low at the 20-ms SOA, was higher at the 40-ms SOA, and was almost complete by the 60-ms SOA.

It is suggested that the threshold for conscious visual perception may be set to be higher than the level at which small but significant sensory information is present, so that the systems in the brain that implement the type of information processing involved in conscious thoughts are not interrupted by small signals that could be noise in sensory pathways. Consideration of the nature of this processing, and the reason why it may be useful to not interrupt it unless there is a definite signal that may require the use of the type of processing that can be performed by the conscious processing system, is left to later in this chapter because the issues raised necessarily involve hypotheses that are not easy to test.

6.7 The Speed of Visual Processing Within a Cortical Visual Area Shows That Top-Down Processes Are Not Essential for Conscious Visual Perception

The results of the information analysis (Rolls et al., 1999) emphasize that very considerable information about which stimulus was shown is available in a short epoch of, for example, 50 ms of neuronal firing. This confirms the findings of Tovée et al. (1993), Tovée and Rolls (1995), and Heller et al. (1995) and facilitates the rapid readout of information from the inferior temporal visual cortex and the use of whatever information is available in the limited period of firing under backward masking conditions. It was notable that the information in the no-mask condition did outlast the end of the stimulus by as much as 200–300 ms, indicating some short-term memory trace property of the neuronal circuitry. This continuing activity could be useful in the learning of invariant representations of objects (Rolls, 1992; Wallis & Rolls, 1997; Rolls, 2000a; Rolls & Deco, 2002). The results also show that even at the shortest SOA of 20 ms, the information available was on average 0.1 bits (see figure 5 of Rolls et al., 1999, for cumulated information values). This compares to 0.3 bits with the 16-ms stimulus shown without the mask (Rolls et al., 1999, figure 5). It also compares to a typical value for such neurons of 0.35–0.5 bits with a 500-ms stimulus presentation (Tovée & Rolls, 1995; Rolls et al., 1997). The results thus show that considerable information (33% of that available without a mask, and approximately 22% of that with a 500-ms stimulus presentation) is available from neuronal responses even under backward masking conditions that allow the neurons to have their main response in 30 ms. Also, we note that the information available from a

16-ms unmasked stimulus (0.3 bits) is a large proportion (approximately 65%–75%) of that available from a 500-ms stimulus.

These results provide evidence on how rapid the processing of visual information is in a cortical area and provide a fundamental constraint for understanding how cortical information processing operates (see Rolls & Treves, 1998; Rolls & Deco, 2002). One direct implication of the 30-ms firing with the 20-ms SOA is that this is sufficient time both for a cortical area to perform its computation and for the information to be read out from a cortical area, given that psychophysical performance is 50% correct at this SOA. Another implication is that the recognition of visual stimuli can be performed using feedforward processing in the multistage hierarchically organized ventral visual system comprising at least V1–V2–V4–inferotemporal visual cortex, in that the typical shortest neuronal response latencies in macaque V1 are approximately 40 ms and increase by approximately 15–17 ms per stage to produce a value of approximately 90 ms in the inferior temporal visual cortex (Rolls & Deco, 2002; Oram & Perrett, 1992; Dinse & Kruger, 1994; Raiguel et al., 1989; Vogels & Orban, 1994; Nowak & Bullier, 1997). (The fact that considerable information is available in short epochs,—e.g., of 20 ms—of the firing of neurons provides part of the underlying basis for this rapid sequential activation of connected visual cortical areas; Tovée & Rolls, 1995; Rolls & Deco, 2002.) Given these timings, it would not be possible in the 20-ms SOA condition for inferior temporal cortex neuronal responses to feed back to influence V1 neuronal responses to the test stimulus before the mask stimulus produced its effects on the V1 neurons. As an example, in the 20-ms SOA condition with 30 ms of firing, the V1 neurons would stop responding to the stimulus at $40 + 30 = 70$ ms but would not be influenced by backprojected information from the inferior temporal cortex until $90 + (3$ stages $\times 15$ ms per stage$) = 135$ ms. This shows that at least some recognition of visual stimuli is possible without top-down backprojection effects from the inferior temporal visual cortex to early cortical processing areas.

The processing time allowed for each cortical area to perform useful computation and for the information to be read out to the next stage of cortical processing is on the order of 15–17 ms as shown by the neuronal response latency increases from cortical area to cortical area noted above (see further Rolls & Deco, 2002) and less than 30 ms as shown by the duration of the firing in the 20-ms SOA condition when face identification was 50% better than chance. This is sufficient for recurrent collaterals to operate by feedback within a cortical area to allow them to implement attractor-based processing, as shown by analyses of the speed of settling of such attractor or autoassociation networks, provided that they are implemented with neurons with continuous dynamics (as implemented in models by integrate-and-fire neurons) and with spontaneous firing (Treves, 1993; Battaglia & Treves, 1998; Rolls & Treves, 1998; Rolls & Deco, 2002). Indeed, the dynamics of a four-layer hierar-

chical network with an architecture like that of the ventral visual system are sufficiently rapid to allow recurrent feedback attractor operations to contribute usefully
to information processing in the system (Panzeri et al., 2001; Rolls & Deco, 2002;
contrast with Thorpe et al., 1996).

The inferior temporal visual cortex is an appropriate stage to analyze the identification of objects and faces, and to link to face identification in humans, because
the inferior temporal visual cortex contains an invariant representation of faces and
objects (Booth & Rolls, 1998; Rolls, 2000a; Rolls & Deco, 2002), and damage to
corresponding areas in humans may produce face and object agnosias (Farah et al.,
1995a; Farah et al., 1995b; Farah, 2004).

The quantitative information theoretic analyses of neuronal encoding referred to
in this chapter entailed measurement of the information represented by neuronal
firing in short time windows (of, e.g., 20 ms) starting as soon as the neuron starts to
respond, which for the macaque inferior temporal visual cortex is 80–100 ms after
stimulus onset (Tovée & Rolls, 1995; Rolls & Deco, 2002). There is considerable
information in this time period, and the number of spikes given typical firing rates
of visual cortical neurons (up to approximately 100 spikes/s) is likely to be 0, 1, or
2. This number of spikes through a single synapse of a postsynaptic neuron would
produce a graded current injection that would be integrated over 10–20 ms because
of the synaptic and postsynaptic dendrite time constants involved (Rolls & Deco,
2002). This is the biophysical basis for the relevance of a period of perhaps 20 ms
for spikes on incoming synapses to have their effect on the postsynaptic neuron.
The postsynaptic neuron would integrate (i.e., sum) the injected currents across the
whole vector of synaptic inputs in approximately this time period (Rolls & Deco,
2002). This shows that the number of spikes in the first 20 ms or so of firing after a
stimulus is presented is very relevant to decoding what the stimulus is (Rolls &
Deco, 2002; Franco et al., 2004). However, it would require much extra implausible
machinery to suppose that the postsynaptic neuron is somehow able to work out
the order in which spikes arrive on its different synapses, and thus reflect the time
of arrival of each spike on each of its synapses, and use this order information to
encode which stimulus has been presented (van Rullen et al., 2005).

The same information theoretic analyses show that from the earliest spikes of the
anterior inferior temporal cortex neurons described here after they have started to
respond (at approximately 80 ms after stimulus onset), the neuronal response is specific to the stimulus, and it is only on more posterior parts of the inferior temporal
visual cortex that neurons may have an earlier short period of firing (of perhaps
20 ms) that is not selective for a particular stimulus. The neurons described by Sugase
et al. (1999) thus behaved like more posterior inferior temporal cortex neurons, not
like typical anterior inferior temporal cortex neurons. This evidence thus suggests
that in the anterior inferior temporal cortex, recurrent processing that may sharpen

up representations is not evident in early nonspecific firing (cf. Hochstein & Ahissar, 2002; Lamme & Roelfsma, 2000; Rensink, 2000).

6.8   A Higher Threshold for Conscious Visual Perception Than for Identification

The quantitative analyses of neuronal activity in an area of the ventral visual system involved in face and object identification described here, which show that significant neuronal processing can occur that is sufficient to support forced choice but implicit (unconscious) discrimination in the absence of conscious awareness of the identity of the face, are of interest in relation to studies of blindsight (Weiskrantz et al., 1974; Weiskrantz, 1997, 1998; Stoerig & Cowey, 1997; de Gelder et al., 1999). The issue in blindsight is that conscious reports that a stimulus has been seen cannot usually be made, and yet some forced-choice performance is possible with respect to, for example, the motion, position, and some aspects of the form of the visual stimuli. It has been argued that the results in blindsight are not due simply to reduced visual processing, because some aspects of visual processing are less impaired than others (Weiskrantz, 1997, 1998, 2001; Azzopardi & Cowey, 1997). It has been suggested that some of the visual capacities that do remain in blindsight reflect processing via visual pathways that are alternatives to the V1 processing stream (Weiskrantz, 1997, 1998, 2001). If some of those pathways are normally involved in implicit processing, this may help to give an account of why some implicit (unconscious) performance is possible in blindsight patients. Further, it has been suggested that ventral visual stream processing is especially involved in consciousness, because it is information about objects and faces that has to enter a system to plan actions (Milner & Goodale, 1995; Rolls & Deco, 2002); and the planning of actions that involves the operation and correction of flexible one-time multiple-step plans may be closely related to conscious processing (Rolls, 1999; Rolls & Deco, 2002). In contrast, dorsal stream visual processing may be more closely related to executing an action on an object once the action has been selected, and the details of this action execution can take place implicitly (unconsciously) (Milner & Goodale, 1995; Rolls & Deco, 2002), perhaps because they do not require multiple-step syntactic planning (Rolls, 1999).

   The implication of this discussion is that in blindsight the dissociations between implicit and explicit processing may arise because different visual pathways, some involved in implicit and others in explicit processing, are differentially damaged. In contrast, in the experiments described here, the dissociation between implicit and explicit processing appears to arise from allowing differential processing (short, information-poor vs. longer) in the same visual processing stream and even area, the inferior temporal visual cortex. Thus, the implications of the dissociations described here, and their underlying neuronal basis, may be particularly relevant in a different way to understanding visual information processing and consciousness.

One of the implications of blindsight thus seems to be that some visual pathways are more involved in implicit processing, and other pathways in explicit processing. In contrast, the results described here suggest that short and information-poor signals in a sensory system involved in conscious processing do not reach consciousness and do not interrupt ongoing conscious processing or engage conscious processing. The findings described here thus provide interesting and direct evidence that there may be a threshold for activity in a sensory stream that must be exceeded in order to lead to consciousness, even when that activity is sufficient for some types of visual processing such as visual identification at levels well above chance in an implicit mode. The latter implicit mode processing can be revealed by forced-choice tests and by direct measurements of neuronal responses. (Complementary evidence at the purely psychophysical level using backward masking has been obtained by Marcel, 1983a, 1983b, and discussed by Weiskrantz, 1998, 2001.) Possible reasons for this relatively high threshold for consciousness are considered next.

It is now suggested that the threshold for conscious visual perception may be set to be higher than the level at which small but significant sensory information is present. This functionality may exist so that the systems in the brain that implement the type of information processing involved in conscious thoughts is not interrupted by small signals that could be noise in sensory pathways. These small signals may nevertheless be useful for some implicit (nonconscious) functions (which are interpreted as guesses) and may be reflected in the better than chance recognition performance at short SOAs even without conscious awareness.

6.9   What Is the Nature of the Information Processing That Is Linked Essentially to Consciousness?

The exact nature of the information processing that is linked essentially to consciousness is the subject for great debate. My own theory is that phenomenal consciousness is the state that occurs when one is thinking about one's own syntactic (or more generally linguistic) thoughts (Rolls, 1997, 1999, 2000b). In that the theory is premised on thoughts about thoughts, it is a higher order thought (HOT) theory of consciousness (see also Rosenthal, 1990, 1993), and in that the theory is about linguistic thoughts, I have termed it a HOLT theory of consciousness (Rolls, 1999, 2000b). It may also be called a HOST theory, as the higher order thoughts are about syntactic thoughts (Rolls, 2004). The computational argument I offer to specify why the higher order thoughts are computationally useful if they are syntactic is as follows. If a multistep plan involves a number of different symbols, and requires the relations (e.g., the conditional relations) between the symbols to be specified correctly in each step of the plan, then some form of syntax is needed, for otherwise the symbols would not be bound together correctly in each step of the plan. If the plan produces an incorrect outcome, then a process that can reflect on and evaluate each step of the plan, and determine which may be the incorrect step, is a way to solve the credit assignment problem (Rolls, 1999). It is argued that it is implausible that such HOST processes would occur without having a feeling like something to be the system that implements these processes, especially when the thoughts are grounded in the world (Rolls, 1999). This is only a plausibility argument. It should be noted that the higher order thoughts are linguistic in the sense that they require syntax, but not necessarily, of course, human verbal language. However, to the extent that some form of syntactic processing is closely related to consciousness, it is likely that a serial and time-consuming process is needed (with serial processing used to limit the binding problem to whatever syntax the brain can implement). Given the serial nature of this process, and its use for implementing long-term and/or multistep planning, it is suggested that it may be useful not to interrupt it unless the processing systems that can perform nonsyntactic implicit processing to detect stimuli or stimulus change have sufficiently strong evidence that the signal is strong, and is of a type that may be behaviorally significant, such as a moving spot on the horizon or an emotional expression change on a face.

6.10   Is Temporal Synchrony Linked to Conscious Processing?

Some have suggested that oscillations in the brain may be related to consciousness (Crick & Koch, 1990). It is difficult to see what useful purpose oscillations per se could perform for neural information processing, apart from perhaps resetting a population of neurons to low activity so that they can restart some attractor process (see, e.g., Rolls & Treves, 1998), or acting as a reference phase to allow neurons to provide some additional information by virtue of the time that they fire with respect to the reference waveform (Huxter et al., 2003). Neither putative function seems to be closely related to consciousness. Stimulus-dependent neuronal synchrony of subsets of neurons might be useful for grouping together subsets of neurons, though probably not for binding the spatial relations between the features represented by each neuron (Rolls & Deco, 2002, section 13.7). Singer and colleagues—see, e.g., Singer, 1999, 2000—had proposed that synchronous firing between a subset of neurons representing a set of features that are part of the same stimulus might indicate that they should be bound together and not bound to other features.) However, some form of grouping might facilitate paying attention to one input relative to another, and such an effect might conceivably be related to consciousness. It is therefore useful to assess to what extent stimulus-dependent synchrony of groups of neurons does convey information additional to that provided by the spike counts (that is, firing rates) in a short period about which stimulus was shown. Although Singer and colleagues, and others, (e.g., Singer, 1999, 2000) have examples of experiments in which stimulus-dependent synchrony is present, there has been very little quantification of the relative contributions of the spike counts and stimulus-dependent synchrony effects, and whether they are independent contributions, by an information theoretic measure that provides the only metric by which their relative contributions can be quantitatively assessed (Rolls & Deco, 2002). We have therefore performed such comparisons for the inferior temporal visual cortex as described next.

Using a second-order expansion of the Shannon information equation (Panzeri et al., 1999), we found for small sets (2–5) of simultaneously recorded inferior temporal cortex neurons that, on average, more than 96% of the total information available about which of 20 stimuli was shown was available in the spike counts, with stimulus-dependent correlations between the firings of different neurons thus adding very little independent information (Rolls et al., 2003, 2004). To enable more neurons and more spikes from each neuron to be considered, and the contribution of stimulus-dependent neuronal synchrony to be more directly assessed, we developed a new decoding method for the information measurements (Franco et al., 2004) and found that, again, the spike counts contributed 93%–99% of the information about which of two stimuli had been seen under natural vision conditions with a complex background, leaving only a minor independent contribution, on average, across experiments with 2–5 simultaneously recorded neurons of stimulus-dependent synchrony to the total information (Aggelopoulos et al., 2005). In the investigation of Aggelopoulos et al. (2005), the monkey had to choose and touch one of two objects shown just above or below the center of a screen in order to obtain fruit juice. The positions of the rewarded and punished object were randomized from trial to trial. In this task, the monkey had to segment the two objects from the background, and from each other, and then, after object recognition, reach to touch the object that was associated with reward. This is an interesting situation in which to test neural encoding, for the visual system is operating under natural visual conditions in which, to the extent that this is required with natural vision, features must be segmented from the background, and bound together only if the features are part of the same object.

These investigations thus show that the encoding of information in terms of stimulus-dependent synchrony does not appear to be a major contributor to the information available in the inferior temporal visual cortex about what is being seen in the world. Of course, it would be useful to see this quantitative methodology applied to other visual cortical areas, but the evidence at present does not suggest that grouping or binding by temporal synchrony is likely to be a major contributor to the encoding of what objects we see. Instead, it is proposed that the spatial binding of features occurs in a feature hierarchy network at an early stage of cortical visual processing (e.g., V2 and V4) by forming neurons that respond only to a combination of a few features in the correct spatial relation to each other. These feature combination neurons are then an adequate basis for invariant object recognition performed by higher stages in the hierarchy, in which the relative spatial positions of the features remains important but the neuronal responses are invariant with respect to the global position, size, and so forth of the whole object (Rolls & Deco, 2002; Elliffe et al., 2002).

Acknowledgments

This research was supported by Medical Research Council Programme Grant PG9826105. The author wishes to acknowledge the excellent contributions of many scientific colleagues to the work described here, including P. Azzopardi, D. G. Purcell, S. Panzeri, A. L. Stewart, A. Treves, and M. J. Tovée.

III VISUAL MASKING AND THE DYNAMICS OF VISION

7 Computational Models of Visual Masking

Gregory Francis and Yang Seok Cho

7.1 Introduction

Backward visual masking refers to impaired performance on some judgment of a target stimulus when it is followed by a mask. Both the target and the mask stimuli are usually very brief (often less than 50 ms), and the target is chosen such that if it is presented by itself, it is easy for observers to perform whatever judgment is required. However, presentation of a mask stimulus, even 100 ms after the target has been turned off, can make the observer's judgment exceedingly difficult. In some cases, observers report not seeing the target at all. Backward masking is a fundamental tool in cognitive psychology and vision research, where it is used to limit the amount of information processing (see recent reviews by Breitmeyer and Öğmen, 2000; Enns & Di Lollo, 2000). Backward masking is also used to investigate aspects of various types of mental diseases (e.g., Braff & Saccuzzo, 1981; Green et al., 1994a; Slaghuis & Bakker, 1995).

Often the properties of the target and mask stimuli are held fixed, and the stimulus onset asynchrony (SOA), the time between the target onset and the mask onset, is varied. The resulting set of data is called a *masking function*. One particularly interesting characteristic of backward masking is that the masking function is sometimes U-shaped. For short SOAs, the target is clearly seen, and the required task fairly easy to perform. For middle-duration SOAs (often less than 100 ms), the target is harder to see and the task difficult to perform. For long SOAs, the task performance is again quite good, perhaps because the target is partially processed before the mask appears.

U-shaped masking functions are not always observed, however. In some cases the strongest masking occurs when the target and mask are presented at the same time (SOA = 0), and masking effects grow weaker as the SOA between the target and mask increases. In such situations a monotonic-shaped masking function is found. This chapter explores quantitative theories of the appearance of U-shaped and monotonic-shaped masking functions. There are a variety of computational models that account for the existence of both U-shaped and monotonic-shaped masking functions (Weisstein, 1972; Bridgeman, 1971, 1978; Anbar & Anbar, 1982; Francis, 1997, 2003a). Francis (2000) showed that all but one of these, which was subsequently analyzed further in Francis (2003a), have a common behavioral property that is responsible for the appearance of a U-shaped masking function. This property is called *mask blocking*. The next section discusses a simple system that uses mask blocking and describes how it produces U-shaped or monotonic-shaped masking functions under different conditions. This analysis then suggests an experiment that tests the entire class of models that use mask blocking and also tests some alternative explanations of the shape of masking functions.

7.2 Analysis of Simplified Mask Blocking

Most of the current quantitative models produce a U-shaped masking function with a common computational approach called *mask blocking*. An analysis of mask blocking in the individual quantitative models can be found in Francis (2000). Rather than describe each of the individual models, this discussion will explore a simple system that uses mask blocking.

To make things concrete, consider a system that generates initial responses $X_T(t)$ and $X_M(t)$, respectively, for the target and mask. These are single-value variables that characterize some aspect of the visual system's response to the stimuli.

$$\frac{dX_T}{dt} = -AX_T + I_T(t) \tag{7.1}$$

and

$$\frac{dX_M}{dt} = -AX_M + I_M(t). \tag{7.2}$$

As is common in writing differential equations, the dependence of X_T and X_M on time is implied but not written. The terms $I_T(t)$ and $I_M(t)$ indicate input from the target and mask stimuli, respectively. Without any input, each variable will decay to a value zero at a rate set by parameter A. The values of these variables do not correspond to perceptual awareness of the stimuli. Instead, these equations contribute to a visual response function (VRF), $v(t)$ that takes excitatory activity from the target response and inhibitory activity from the mask response. A key property of the inhibition is that it is only present if the mask signal is stronger than the target signal. It is in this way that mask blocking occurs; a strong target signal can block the inhibitory effect of the mask:

$$\frac{dv}{dt} = -Av + X_T - [X_M - X_T]^+ \tag{7.3}$$

The term $-[X_M - X_T]^+$ in equation 7.3 describes the interaction of the target and mask. The notation $[\,]^+$ represents a rectification function, so that if the term inside the brackets is not positive, then the function returns the value zero. If the term inside the brackets is positive, the function returns the value unchanged. Thus, the term $-[X_M - X_T]^+$ will be negative if X_M is larger than X_T and will be zero otherwise. Hence, masking occurs when X_M is bigger than X_T. This implements mask blocking because if the target response, X_T, is bigger than the mask response, X_M, the mask has no influence on the target VRF.

The value of the target VRF does not correspond to perceptual awareness of the target stimulus. The percept is assumed to be computed from the value of the target VRF by an integration over time:

$$P = \int_0^T [v(t) - G]^+ \, dt, \tag{7.4}$$

where G is a threshold parameter, the value zero as the lower limit of the integral indicates the onset of the target, and T is some upper limit of time for the integral. This form of the integral treats as zero any values of $v(t)$ that are below the threshold value. The values of P should be related to experimental data on masking, and changes in the value of P should correspond to changes in the behavioral measure of masking.

In the simulations described below the parameters were set as $A = 0.1$ and $G = 0.1$, and T was chosen so that the integral in equation 7.4 included all nonzero terms. The input for the target was defined as

$$I_T(t) = \begin{cases} 10 & \text{for } 0 \le t < 10 \\ 0 & \text{otherwise,} \end{cases} \tag{7.5}$$

so that it turned on at time zero and off at time 10. The input for the mask was

$$I_M(t) = \begin{cases} I_M & \text{for } \tau_l \le t < \tau_l + 10 \\ 0 & \text{otherwise,} \end{cases} \tag{7.6}$$

so that it turned on at SOA equal τ_l and turned off 10 time units later. The value of I_M is the intensity of the mask. In figures 7.1a–b, $I_M = 5$, and in figures 7.1c–d, $I_M = 20$.

Mask blocking refers to a situation where signals generated by the target block mask-generated inhibition. In the present system this is implemented by a rectified

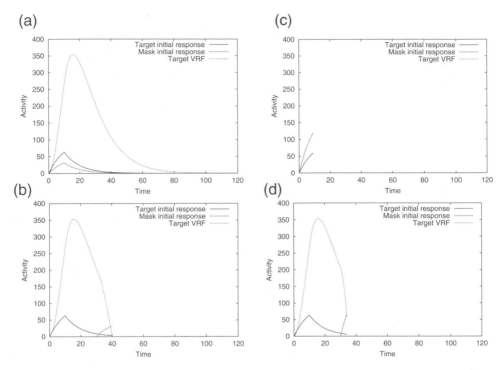

Figure 7.1
Simulations of a system that uses mask-blocking to generate a U-shaped masking function. (*a*)–(*b*) A weak mask at stimulus onset asynchronies (SOAs) of 0 and 30 ms. (*c*)–(*d*) A strong mask at SOAs of 0 and 30 ms. Each simulation stops after offset of the stimuli when the target visual response function (VRF) becomes negative (not shown)

subtraction in equation 7.4. However, quite similar behavior can be implemented using other computations (e.g., division of the mask inhibitory signal by the target signal).

The effect of strong mask blocking is indicated in figure 7.1a. In this situation, the target and the mask stimuli start and end at the same time (SOA = 0). The mask input is weaker than the target input, so the mask response is always below the target response. As a result, the mask has no effect on the target VRF; the integral of the target VRF is equivalent to the case in which the mask is not present at all. The strong target signal blocks the mask from producing any masking.

Weaker mask blocking, and thus stronger masking, is indicated in figure 7.1b. Here, the mask onset follows the target onset by an SOA of 30 time units. As a result of this time delay, the rising part of the mask response overlaps a fading part of the target response. When the mask response is larger than the target response, it begins to send an inhibitory signal that quickly drives the target VRF below zero. The area under the target VRF in this case is smaller than for figure 7.1a. Thus, increasing the SOA between the target and mask stimuli results in stronger masking. This release from mask blocking is what produces the downward sloping part of a U-shaped masking function. For much longer SOAs, the mask will have less influence on the target VRF because it arrives too late. This effect produces the upward slope of a U-shaped masking function.

A system that includes mask blocking will produce a U-shaped masking function if the mask is weak enough that it cannot produce much masking for short SOAs but can produce some masking when the target response has faded during medium SOAs. For longer SOAs, the later arrival of the mask will always free the target VRF from any masking that might have occurred over medium or short SOAs.

The same system can produce a monotonically increasing masking function if the mask is strong. Figure 7.1c–d shows simulation plots for a strong mask signal (twice the intensity of the target). In figure 7.1c, with SOA = 0, the mask response is stronger than the target response at all times, so the target VRF immediately receives strong inhibition and never rises above zero. In figure 7.1d, the mask is delayed by SOA = 30, and the target VRF is not inhibited until the mask's response is larger than the (fading) target response.

Thus, for a strong mask, mask blocking does not occur and the masking function will be monotonic as SOA varies. Such a system predicts U-shaped masking functions should appear for relatively weak masks and monotonic-shaped masking functions should appear for relatively strong masks. For the system and parameters of the present simulations, the masking functions are shown in figure 7.2 and demonstrate this property. An online version of this system has been created following the methods described in Francis (2003b). It is available online at http://www.psych.purdue.edu/~gfrancis/Publications/BackwardMasking/.

Many quantitative models create a U-shaped masking function with a version of masking blocking (Francis, 2000). Although the models differ substantially in terms of mechanistic implementation, equations, parameters, and physiological interpretations, further analysis of the models reveals that they all follow the same pattern of behavior as the simple mask-blocking system described above. Francis and Herzog (2004) showed through computer simulation that when the mask is weak, each model produces a U-shaped masking function, and when the mask is stronger, each model produces a monotonic-shaped masking function. The definition of weak and strong varies across the models, but the overall behavior of the models is the same. This relationship between the strength of the mask and the shape of the masking function is a fundamental aspect of any system that uses mask blocking and so is a robust property of these models. The relationship will not disappear with changes in the model parameters.

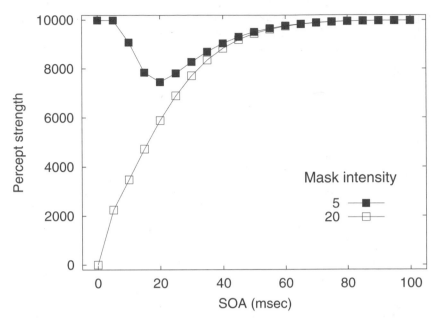

Figure 7.2
Masking functions for the mask-blocking system. The monotonic masking function occurs for the high-intensity mask, while the U-shaped masking function occurs for the low-intensity mask. A property of these systems is that, at each stimulus onset asynchrony (SOA), a monotonic masking function must lie below a U-shaped masking function.

Consistent with the properties of mask-blocking systems, Kolers (1962) noted that monotonic-shaped masking functions appeared for high-energy masks and U-shaped masking functions appeared for masks that were similar in energy to the target. Subsequent work has shown that this observation holds for a variety of mask types, including pattern masks that have contours overlapping the target (e.g., Hellige et al., 1979; Spencer & Shuntich, 1970; Turvey, 1973), metacontrast masks that do not overlap the target (e.g., Schiller, 1965; Weisstein, 1972), and masks consisting of a homogeneous field or disk that covers the target (e.g., Stewart & Purcell, 1974).

A fundamental characteristic of a system that uses mask blocking is that the shape of the masking function is related to the *strength* of the target and the mask signals. In a mask-blocking system, the intensity and spatial properties of the target and mask stimuli are converted into response strengths and such strengths determine the shape of the masking function. Thus, all mask-blocking systems make a common prediction: For a fixed target, task, and SOA, any kind of masking situation that produces a U-shaped masking function must have weaker masking than any kind of masking situation that produces a monotonic-shaped masking function.

7.3   Other Explanations

It may be worthwhile to compare the predicted relationship between mask strength and masking function shape against other explanations of masking function shapes:

1. *Target property.* Weisstein (1972) noted that U-shaped masking functions appeared when the target and mask had roughly the same intensity but that decreasing the target intensity led to monotonic-shaped masking functions. More generally, one could hypothesize that the shape of the masking function is solely related to the target stimulus, with some target stimuli producing U-shaped masking functions and other target stimuli producing monotonic-shaped masking functions.

2. *Type of mask.* Several researchers have noted (e.g., Enns & Di Lollo, 2000) that some types of masks seem to produce U-shaped masking functions and other types of masks tend to produce monotonic-shaped masking functions. For example, noise masks, pattern masks, and light masks often produce monotonic-shaped masking functions, while metacontrast masks (where the mask shape does not spatially overlap with the target shape) tend to produce U-shaped masking functions.

3. *Level of masking.* Turvey (1973) suggested that monotonic-shaped masking functions indicated low-level (e.g., retinal) masking, while U-shaped masking functions indicated high-level (e.g., cortical) masking.

4. *Source of mask inhibition.* Breitmeyer and Ganz (1976) and Breitmeyer (1984) proposed that U-shaped masking functions appeared because of differential delays in sustained and transient streams of the visual system. Strongest masking occurred when the transient inhibition of the mask overlapped with the sustained information of the target. Since the transient system was faster than the sustained system, the ideal overlap occurred when the mask followed the target. However, monotonic-shaped masking functions could occur if the mask had a strong enough sustained signal to allow for sustained-on-sustained inhibition. It follows that in this theory monotonic-shaped masking functions should correspond to stronger masking than U-shaped masking functions because the monotonic-shaped masking functions are the result of additional inhibition. The quantitative model of Purushothaman et al. (2000) uses this approach to explain various masking effects.

5. *Type of masking effect.* Some researchers (e.g., Eriksen, 1966; Haber, 1969) have proposed that there are at least two different masking effects: integration and interruption. *Integration masking* occurs when the target and mask temporally integrate and the target becomes difficult to process. Such masking produces monotonic-shaped masking functions because integration is less likely to occur as the target and mask are separated in time. *Interruption masking* occurs when the mask

interrupts the processing of the information about the target. Such masking has been hypothesized to produce U-shaped masking functions.

6. *Integration effects.* A different interpretation of the effect of integration has been proposed by Navon and Purcell (1981) and Reeves (1982). They proposed that integration of the target and mask's would sometimes still allow the target properties to be judged well. In this view, the decrease in target visibility/identifiability as SOA increases is the result of the target and mask's being less likely to integrate into a single percept. Thus, contrary to the previous explanation, U-shaped masking functions would be evidence of integration at short SOAs, while monotonic-shaped masking functions would indicate that such integration either had no effect, had a deleterious effect, or did not occur at all.

Clearly, these alternative explanations are conceptually quite different from the strength-based explanation that makes up the explanation for all models that are based on mask blocking. The next section describes an experiment that tests the prediction of the mask-blocking systems and simultaneously turns out to investigate many of the alternative explanations as well.

7.4   Experiment 1: Backward Masking

We investigated the relationship between U-shaped and monotonic-shaped masking functions with an experiment that varied the properties of the target and the mask stimuli. Figure 7.3 schematizes the target and mask stimuli (in reverse contrast). The target frame consisted of four elements (one target and three distractors) arranged on the corners of a virtual square measuring 12.06° on each side. There were two types of target frames: sparse and filled. The sparse distractor stimuli consisted of five dots arranged with four dots on the corners of a 0.92° by 0.92° square and an additional dot in the middle. The sparse target stimulus was similar, but was constricted horizontally to make a vertical rectangle (0.57° by 0.92°). The filled stimuli were similar, except an outline square and rectangle were drawn for the distractor and target stimuli, respectively, and there was no central dot. The target frame was displayed for one frame of the 60 Hz monitor (approximately 17 ms).

Around each target and distractor stimulus a mask stimulus was drawn that was either sparse or filled. The sparse masks were four dots drawn on the corners of a 1.43° by 1.43° square. The filled mask was an outline square (thickness of 0.17°) of the same size. The mask stimuli were shown for two refresh frames of the monitor (approximately 34 ms). Both target and mask stimuli were drawn in white (225 cd/m^2) on a black (0.6 cd/m^2) background in a room with standard overhead lighting. Luminance measurements are for white or black fields that completely covered the measurement area of a light meter.

Target stimuli   Mask stimuli

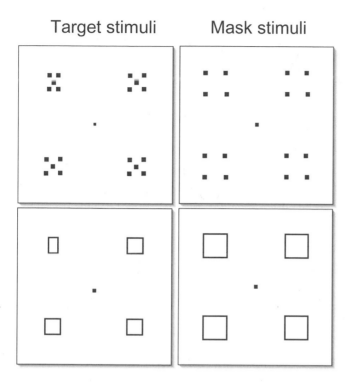

Figure 7.3
The target and mask stimul; used in the backward masking experiment (in reverse contrast). Each target type was paired with each mask type separately.

The observer's task was to report the location of the (virtual) rectangle in the target frame. Each of the four target–mask combinations was constant for a given session. The experiment consisted of 12 sessions, each with a 20-trial practice block and three 90-trial experimental blocks. Each block included five SOAs (0, 17, 34, 51, and 68 ms) between the target and the mask. Two observers participated. One observer was the second author and the other was naive to the purpose of the experiment.

The choice of stimuli were derived from an earlier study (Cho & Francis, 2003) that compared masking functions with a sparse mask and an outline mask. That study found that a sparse mask produced a monotonic-shaped masking function while the outline mask produced a U-shaped masking function. The current study additionally varied the properties of the target stimuli.

7.4.1   Results

The key question to be resolved is whether the shape of the masking functions is related to properties of the target, the mask, or target–mask combinations. Figure 7.4a–d plots masking functions for the different conditions for each observer. There are substantial overall differences between the observers, which is consistent with earlier studies (e.g., Weisstein & Growney, 1969); nevertheless, both observers show a similar pattern of results.

Figure 7.4a–b plots the masking functions for the sparse (dot) target and distractors. The curve with the filled elements is for the sparse (four-dot) mask, and the curve with the open elements is for the filled (outline square) mask. For both observers, the sparse mask produced a U-shaped masking function and the filled mask produced a monotonic-shaped masking function.

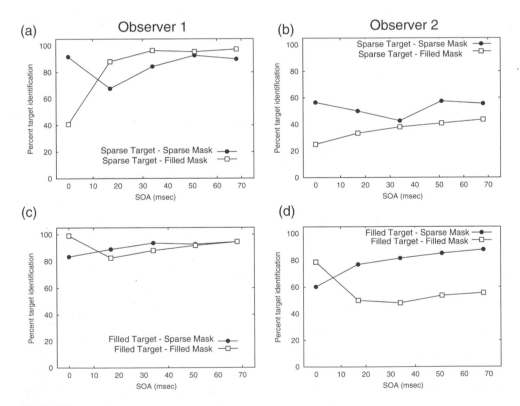

Figure 7.4
Results from experiment 1 for two observers. (*a*)–(*b*) Masking functions for the sparse target and both types of masks. (*c*)–(*d*) Masking functions for the filled target and both types of masks. SOA, stimulus onset asynchrony.

Figure 7.4c–d plots the masking functions for the filled (outline square) target and distractors. The curve with the filled elements is for the sparse (four-dot) mask, and the curve with the open elements is for the filled (outline square) mask. For both the observers, the sparse mask produced a monotonic-shaped masking function and the filled mask produced a U-shaped masking function.

7.4.2   Discussion

The experimental data do not agree with the prediction of the mask-blocking systems. Moreover, the data are also incompatible with many alternative explanations of the appearance of U-shaped and monotonic-shaped masking functions.

With regard to the mask-blocking systems, the models that use mask blocking predict that, with a fixed target and task, at each SOA a monotonic-shaped masking function should always lie below a U-shaped masking function. This is violated for both observers (see Figure 7.4a, c, and d) where the monotonic-shaped masking function is sometimes above the U-shaped masking function. The one case consistent with the prediction (see Figure 7.4b) does little to obviate the conclusion that the models are invalid because the prediction is that the relationship between masking strength and masking function shape must *always* hold. The existence of a counterexample is enough to negate the prediction. Moreover, the frequency of the violation of the prediction suggests that the violation does not involve a particularly unusual circumstance. This conclusion agrees with and extends the experimental findings of Francis and Herzog (2004).

As noted above, the data are also incompatible with some of the alternative explanations of the appearance of U-shaped and monotonic-shaped masking functions. For much the same reasons that the mask-blocking systems are rejected, the transient–sustained source of inhibition explanation is rejected because monotonic masking functions sometimes produce weaker masking than U-shaped masking functions.

The data are incompatible with the idea that masking function shape is related solely to the properties of the target. A sparse/filled target can produce either a monotonic-shaped masking function or a U-shaped masking function, depending on the type of mask that is used. Likewise, the data are incompatible with the idea that the masking function shape is related solely to the properties of the mask. A sparse/filled mask can produce either a monotonic-shaped masking function or a U-shaped masking function, depending on the type of target that is used.

The data also challenge the level-of-masking hypothesis. Whenever there is a monotonic-shaped masking function, this hypothesis would hold that low-level masking effects were occurring. However, if strong low-level inhibition exists for a given mask, it is difficult to explain how changing the target stimulus would somehow make such low-level inhibition ineffective (which would be necessary to produce a U-shaped masking function).

It should be emphasized that this result does not mean that none of the explanations ever apply to backward masking effects. It is possible that they do apply under some conditions. The data do allow us to conclude that none of these explanations apply to the particular conditions of this experiment, and so these explanations do not provide a *complete* description of backward masking.

Thus for the conditions of this experiment, the only remaining viable explanations involve integration and interruption masking. There are two such explanations. One is based on the hypothesis that temporal integration of the target and the mask produces a type of masking by camouflaging the target. Such camouflage can produce masking at the shortest SOAs and thus a monotonic-shaped masking function. The other explanation suggests that temporal integration of the target and the mask does not produce strong masking but leads to visibility of some features of the target at short SOAs. In this explanation integration of the target and mask corresponds to a U-shaped masking function.

We prefer a generalization of these two proposals. When the target and the mask temporally integrate, we imagine that the unified percept can sometimes render the target more difficult to identify and sometimes render the target easier to identify. Thus, we hypothesize that performance on the masking task at the shortest SOAs, which determines whether a U-shaped or monotonic-shaped masking function is found, is related to the ability of the observer to perform the experimental task on the integrated target and mask combination. We tested this hypothesis in a second experiment.

7.5   Experiment 2: Visual Search

To validate the hypothesis that performance on the masking experiment at the shortest SOAs is related to the temporal integration of the target and mask stimuli, we conducted a visual search experiment with similar stimuli. The four possible combinations of target and mask stimuli were used to make a set of displays for a visual search experiment. Figure 7.5 shows (in reverse contrast) samples of the displays for each target–mask combination. In addition, displays were created that did not include a target but instead consisted of four distractor elements. The observer's task was to judge as quickly as possible whether or not a target element was present. On each trial one of the displays appeared and remained visible until the observer made a target-present or target-absent response by pressing the appropriate key on a keyboard. Reaction time was recorded, and incorrect responses were

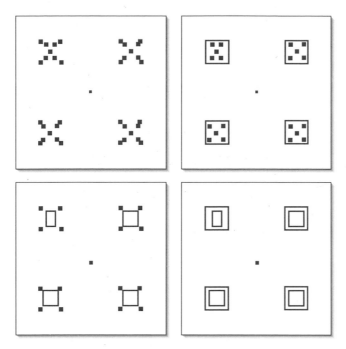

Figure 7.5
Sample displays for experiment 2 (in reverse contrast). The displays are the same as for the backward masking experiment, except the target and mask are superimposed.

discarded from further analysis. The same observers as in experiment 1 participated in experiment 2.

If performance at the shortest SOAs in the backward masking experiment was determined by the temporally integrated percept of the target and mask stimuli, one would expect that reaction times would be longest for those target–mask combinations that produced monotonic-shaped masking functions and shortest for those target–mask combinations that produced U-shaped masking functions. On the other hand, if the difference in masking function shape was due to some other form of interaction between the target and mask, then there seems to be no reason to think that performance on the visual search task would be related to performance on the backward masking task.

7.5.1 Results

Figure 7.6 plots the percentage correct identifications of the target for SOA = 0 in the masking experiment against the reaction time in the visual search experiment. The individual points are for the different target–mask combinations. The points lie

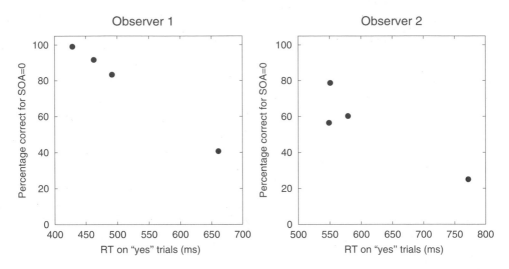

Figure 7.6
Comparison of target identification in the backward masking task and reaction time (RT) in the visual search task for different target–mask combinations. SOA, stimulus onset asynchrony.

nearly on a straight line, which indicates that the two variables are closely related. The correlation between reaction time and percentage correct was −.99 for observer 1 and −.91 for observer 2. Both of these correlations are statistically significant ($p < .005$ for observer 1 and $p < .05$ for observer 2).

7.5.2   Discussion

The data from the visual search experiment are correlated with the data from the backward masking experiment at the shortest SOA. This result is consistent with the hypothesis that performance on the backward masking experiment is determined by the ability of the observer to extract information about the target when it temporally integrates with the mask.

7.6   Conclusions

An analysis of quantitative models of backward masking based on mask blocking led to a prediction regarding how variation in the properties of the mask might change the shape of the masking function. An experiment to test this prediction demonstrated that it was not valid. This is a significant finding because these models have successfully explained a large variety of data on backward masking. The failure of the prediction to hold also suggests that the key limitation of these models is that the interactions between the target and mask representations are fundamentally strength based. It is this characteristic that leads to the prediction that monotonic-shaped masking functions should correspond to stronger masking than U-shaped masking functions.

Indeed, other computational models that do not use the mask-blocking approach turn out to face similar problems with this set of data. The model of Purushothaman et al. (2000) does not use mask blocking computations, but it still makes the same flawed prediction regarding masking function shape. A quite different model proposed by Francis (2000, 2003a) also does not use mask blocking but also makes the same flawed prediction. Finally, if parameters are set appropriately, a quantitative model of reentrant processing proposed by Di Lollo et al. (2000) can also produce a U-shaped masking function (Francis, 2003b). However, with the parameters used so far, the model makes the same prediction regarding masking strength and masking function shape as the other models. This model has not undergone a full analysis, though, so there may be parameter sets that produce a different pattern of results.

The experimental result is particularly interesting because the various quantitative models of backward masking have been characterized as being fundamentally different from each other. Some of the models involve recurrent or reentrant feedback, while other models have a strictly feedforward flow of information. Some of the models are based on complicated neural network architectures, while other models are described with a single differential equation. Some of the models are hypothesized to work at an object-level description of stimuli, while other models are hypothesized to describe low-level interactions involving lateral inhibition. Despite these substantial differences, all of the models make essentially the same prediction about the shape of the masking function and the overall strength of masking, and all of the models are wrong for essentially the same reason.

The experimental data simultaneously cause us to reject a variety of other explanations for the differences between U-shaped and monotonic-shaped masking functions. The only alternative that seems to remain viable is to consider the role integration of the target and the mask might have at the shortest SOAs. We explored this possibility with a second experiment that provides an independent measure of the ease of identifying the target when the target and the mask stimuli produce a combined percept. The percentage of correct identification at the shortest SOA in experiment 1 correlates with reaction time in experiment 2, which suggests that whether one obtains a U-shaped or a monotonic-shaped masking function depends on whether integration of the target and mask at the shortest SOAs leads to easy visibility of the target or camouflage of the target, respectively.

What remains unclear is whether the role of integration accounts for the shape of the masking function in every situation, or whether other mechanisms (such as mask blocking) sometimes also apply. A goal of future research will be to identify experiments that can test between these quite different methods of producing a U-shaped backward masking function.

Acknowledgments

Gregory Francis and Yang Seok Cho were supported by National Science Foundation Grant 0108905.

8 A Reentrant View of Visual Masking, Object Substitution, and Response Priming

James T. Enns, Alejandro Lleras, and Vince Di Lollo

When a mask follows a briefly presented target, there are several consequences. The one that has historically received the most attention is a reduction in the visibility of the target. This is the conventional definition of *masking*. Yet, another equally important consequence is that errors in target identification are biased toward the identity of the mask rather than being randomly distributed among the target alternatives. This is evidence of *object substitution*. Finally, when the target is a signal to make a speeded action, this action can be influenced by a prime stimulus that is not even visible to the participant. This is known as masked *response priming*. In this chapter we review evidence concerning all three of these consequences of viewing rapid visual sequences. We argue that these consequences are difficult to understand, either individually or together, as the consequence of strictly feedforward processing in the visual brain. In contrast, when these results are considered from the perspective of reentrant visual circuitry, they are easier to understand and to relate to one another. Moreover, predictions derived from a reentrant view of the brain lead to unexpected and novel results that are confirmed when tested against psychophysical data.

Most theories of vision hold to the view that from the time the eye first encounters a scene to the time that conscious perception occurs the scene has been coded at several levels in the visual system. Moreover, most theories propose some form of interaction between the anatomically lower levels of processing involved in registering details of the scene (e.g., retina, lateral geniculate nucleus, area V1) and the anatomically higher levels involved in the meaningful categorization and conscious experience of the scene (e.g., extrastriate cortical regions including the temporal cortex). Some theorists have even referred to this as the distinction between "seeing" and "understanding," or between stimulus driven and conceptually driven processing (Broadbent, 1958; Hebb, 1949; Helmholtz, 1866/1962; Hochberg, 1968; Neisser, 1967).

But how do these two levels of visual processing interact? On one option, the influence is unidirectional, meaning that lower levels of processing feed their results

forward to the higher levels, where the resulting processes are increasingly
abstracted away from the original image (Hubel, 1988; Pylyshyn, 2003). The proposed benefit of such abstraction is that it permits perception to concern itself with
the invariant or intrinsic attributes of the objects in the scene (i.e., their true color,
their actual size) rather than with the momentary or superficial attributes of the
image (i.e., the luminance and wavelength characteristics of light at the eye, their
retinal extent).

However, on another option, the influences between levels of processing are
bidirectional, such that processing consists of iterative exchanges of neural signals
among levels (Damasio, 1994; Di Lollo et al., 2000; Grossberg, 1976a, 1976b,
Hochstein & Ahissar, 2002; Lamme & Roelfsema, 2000; Mumford, 1992; Zeki, 1993).
An initial wave of stimulation ascends rapidly through the system (feedforward
processing), followed by descending signals between levels (feedback processing or
reentry). Together, the ascending and descending pathways form an iterative-loop
system, aimed at noise reduction and hypothesis verification, thereby establishing
the most plausible perceptual interpretation of the incoming stimulus. Most notably,
in this view, the roles played by neurons at the lower levels differ considerably over
time, depending on whether they are participating in the signaling of information
about the first glance at a scene or whether they are participating in the iterative
checking of hypotheses about the scene generated by neurons at the higher levels.

In the research we have conducted over the past few years, we have been increasingly attracted to the reentrant position, largely because of the improved understanding that comes from adopting the iterative reentrant perspective. We have
found that when we try to incorporate the vast anatomical evidence for reentrant
communication in the brain (Bullier et al., 1988; Felleman & Van Essen, 1991;
Mignard & Malpeli, 1991; Zeki, 1993) into theories we use to account for psychophysical (behavioral) data, many of the apparent puzzles in these results can be
explained by adopting a reentrant stance. Yet this is not to claim that adopting this
approach comes without its own potential pitfalls and dangers. Constructing arguments about the structure of the brain on the basis of behavioral data is always an
uncertain business.

In what follows we will summarize our recent research in three different areas of
visual masking. In each section, we will first describe a feedforward account of a
phenomenon, that is, one premised on unidirectional flow of visual information from
lower to higher brain regions. We then describe experiments we have conducted
that have led us to the reentrant position. In a final section we identify several
emerging areas of research in which we hope to broaden the reentrant perspective
beyond the scope of visual masking and priming.

8.1 Metacontrast Masking: Thinking Outside the Box

Metacontrast masking has been defined as ". . . the reduction in visibility of one briefly presented stimulus, the target, by a spatially adjacent and temporally succeeding, briefly presented second stimulus, the mask" (Breitmeyer, 1984, p. 4). Masking is known to occur within a narrow band of temporal intervals. When the stimulus onset asynchrony (SOA) between the target and the mask is either very brief or very long, the target is clearly visible. At intermediate SOAs, however, perception of the target is impaired, leading to a U-shaped function of accuracy over SOA.

The main mechanism thought to be at work in metacontrast masking involves inhibitory interactions between neurons representing the contours of the target and the mask (Breitmeyer & Ganz, 1976; Macknik & Livingstone, 1998; Weisstein et al., 1975). For example, in the model of Breitmeyer and Ganz (1976) the key idea is that the onset of each stimulus initiates neural activity in two channels: a transient channel, which has short latency and responds optimally to low spatial frequencies of fast-changing stimuli, and a sustained channel, which has longer latency and is attuned to figural aspects of the stimulus such as details carried by higher spatial frequencies. Activity in the transient channel is said to inhibit concurrent activity in the sustained channel. Masking occurs when the faster acting signals triggered by the onset of the mask inhibit the activity of slower signals carrying information about the earlier target.

These "two-channel" theories are predicated on strict temporal and spatial relationships between the target and the mask. In the temporal domain, an optimal interval must elapse from the onset of the target to the onset of the mask: It is the onset of the mask that interferes with the processing of the earlier target. In the spatial domain, there are two main requirements: first, that the mask contain a substantial amount of contour and, second, that the contours of the mask be in close spatial proximity to the contours of the target (Breitmeyer, 1984; Growney et al., 1977).

8.1.1 Common Onset: A New Masking Paradigm

Research carried out over the past several years in our and other laboratories has revealed a new form of masking that is difficult to reconcile with either the temporal or the spatial requirements of the two-channel view. More important, the new form of masking is not predictable from a strictly feedforward model of visual information processing. Here, we give only a brief introduction to this new form of masking in order to give the reader an indication of what needs to be explained. Interested readers can experience this masking effect firsthand through demonstrations on the Internet (http://www.interchange.ubc.ca/enzo/).

In a typical experiment (Di Lollo et al., 2000), the display sequence consisted of an initial brief pattern containing from 1 to 16 rings, each with a gap in one of four cardinal orientations. One of the rings (the target) was singled out by four small surrounding dots that acted as both cue and mask (figure 8.1a). The display continued without interruption to a second frame that contained only the same four small dots for durations varying from zero to several hundred milliseconds. Observers reported the orientation of the target's gap. A critical aspect of the display was that the target and the four dots appeared *simultaneously* in frame 1. We have referred to this temporal contingency as the *common-onset masking paradigm* (Di Lollo et al., 2000).

The results, illustrated by the segmented lines in figure 8.1b, revealed little or no masking when the display contained only one potential target or when the mask

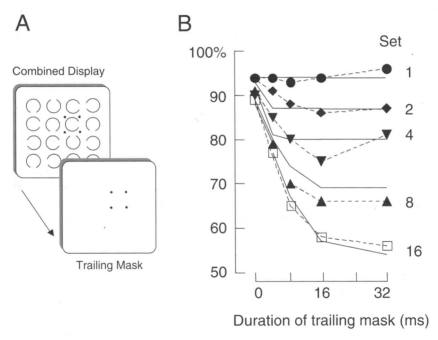

Figure 8.1
(*A*) Schematic diagram of the display sequence in common-onset masking. The sequence began with a display containing between 1 and 16 rings, one of which (the target) was singled out by four surrounding dots. The sequence continued without interruption with a display of the same four dots for durations between 0 and 320 ms. (*B*) Target identification accuracy in a four-dot masking study (Di Lollo et al., 2000). No masking occurs when attention can be rapidly deployed to the location of the target, as occurs when set size is equal to one. Accuracy is also affected little by increments in set size, provided that the four-dot mask terminates with the target display. Pronounced masking occurs, however, as both set size and mask duration are increased. According to the reentrant hypothesis, this occurs because the representation of the unattended target has been replaced by the mask representation before target identification could be completed.

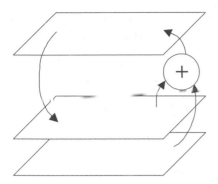

Figure 8.2
A computational model for object substitution (Di Lollo et al., 2000). A large number of three-layered modules, such as the one shown here, are arrayed over the visual field. Stimuli from the visual field arrive at the input layer (bottom), where the receptive fields are small, the features coded are simple, and activation decays rapidly unless maintained by continued external input. The contents of the input layer are summed with the current contents of the working space (middle) and sent to the pattern layer (top), where the receptive fields are much larger and code for more complex patterns.

terminated at the same time as the target display, regardless of the number of potential targets. In contrast, pronounced masking occurred provided that both of two conditions were met: first, that the initial display contain multiple potential targets and, second, that the mask remain on view beyond the termination of the target display.

Unidirectional inhibitory models cannot account for masking obtained with the common-onset paradigm because those models were explicitly designed to explain why masking had never been found when the target and the mask were presented simultaneously (Alpern, 1953; Breitmeyer & Ganz, 1976; Matin, 1975; Weisstein et al., 1975). In light of the results in figure 8.1b, we can now assert that masking with common onset had never been obtained in earlier studies because the target and the mask not only started together but also ended together. This temporal contingency corresponds to the condition in which the duration of the trailing mask was equal to zero, where no masking was obtained. Strong masking developed, however, as the duration of the trailing mask was increased, provided that the display contained a sufficient number of potential targets (figure 8.1b). Thus, the critical factor in metacontrast masking is not whether the target and the mask have a common onset but whether the mask remains on display beyond the offset of the target. A recent study has even shown that the critical variable is really the temporal factor of mask duration and not simply the additional stimulus energy that comes from prolonging a visual stimulus (intensity × time; Di Lollo et al., 2004).

A second reason why inhibitory models cannot account for the results in figure 8.1b is that the four-dot mask used in that experiment do not have a sufficient amount of contour to generate the required amount of inhibition. As noted above, the strength of classical metacontrast masking is known to decrease markedly as the amount of contour in the mask is reduced (Breitmeyer, 1984).

8.1.2   Object Substitution: A New Understanding of Masking

We believe that an account of common-onset masking with a four-dot mask can be developed in the broader context of how the visual system handles rapidly occurring sequential stimuli. In keeping with reentrant thinking, we suppose that conscious perception of a stimulus emerges from neural activity triggered not only by feedforward signals but also by iterative exchanges between cortical regions connected by reentrant pathways. On the first cycle, the input from the initial display is encoded at a low level within the system and then proceeds to higher levels where tentative cognitive representations are produced. These representations are in need of confirmation because they may be incomplete and ill defined or, equivalently, the ascending signals might activate more than one representation at the higher level. This creates an ambiguity for perception that can be resolved by comparing the high-level codes with the initial pattern of activity at the lower level. Reentrant pathways enable such a comparison.

We assume that, on the second and later iterations, the high-level representation reenters the lower level and is compared to what is currently there. If the image on the screen has not changed, a match is found and processing continues. If the screen has been blanked after the initial display, there is nothing on the screen to compete with the decaying initial stimulus representation. Thus, for a short time a match can still be found with this decaying trace. If, however, the reentrant information does not match the current information at the lower level (i.e., if the input has changed), then a new tentative representation emerges and processing continues as for a new stimulus.

We propose that common-onset masking occurs when the initial display (target plus mask) is replaced on the screen by a different configuration (mask alone) before the required processing iterations have taken place for the target to be identified. Thus, the emerging percept of the compound image (target plus mask) is replaced in consciousness with the percept of the mask alone. It is as though the visual system treats the trailing configuration as an updated replacement of the earlier one (Kolers, 1972).

Implicit in this description is a general account of backward masking in which a process of perceptual updating plays a critical role. It is our view that this type of masking occurs when the emerging representation of a target is replaced by the emerging representation of a trailing mask as the visual pattern or object occupying a given spatial location. We refer to this process as masking by *object substitution*.

8.1.3   CMOS: A Computational Model for Object Substitution

We have incorporated these theoretical ideas in a computational model of masking by object substitution, CMOS, in short (Di Lollo et al., 2000). CMOS belongs to a class of models known as *closed-loop controllers* that are common in several areas of industry and robotics (e.g., Carpenter & Grossberg, 1987). In their most general form, these models describe a process in which some form of input is collected and coded before being sent on to an output device. However, the output device, in addition to generating an output signal, sends a copy of that signal back to the input device. This leads to another round of coding to facilitate the comparison of this feedback signal with the current signals entering the input device. In this way, the output signal is influenced in an ongoing way by both current input and information already processed.

The central assumption in the CMOS model is that visual perceptions emerge from the activity of three-layered modules such as illustrated in figure 8.2, arrayed throughout the visual field. Each module can be conceptualized as a circuit involving the connections between cortical area V1 and a topographically related region in an extrastriate visual area. The output of each module is a representation of the spatial pattern within its receptive field.

Here, we give the reader only a general idea of how the model operates (details are given in Di Lollo et al., 2000). The onset of a visual stimulus triggers the first of several cycles of activity in the three layers illustrated in figure 8.2. The activity in the pattern layer is then fed back to the working space by means of a simple overwriting operation. As part of this transfer, pattern information is translated back to the pixel-like codes of the input layer, permitting a direct comparison. This comparison is necessary for resolving ambiguities and for achieving fine spatial registration between the reentrant code and the ongoing activity at the lower level.

Masking is produced in this model by the fact that the contents of the input layer change dynamically with new visual input. The contents of the pattern layer change more slowly because its input is a weighted sum of what is currently in the input layer and what was in the working space on the previous iteration. This produces a degree of inertia in response to changes in input that is an unavoidable consequence of reentrant processing. If the visual input changes during this critical period of inertia, masking will ensue. We refer to this process as *object substitution* because the emerging representation of a target in the pattern layer is replaced by the emerging representation of the mask as the visual pattern or object occupying a given spatial location.

The continuous lines in figure 8.1b illustrate simulations from a formal implementation of CMOS. The model curves provide a remarkably good fit to the empirical data. Notably, the simulation captures the two fundamental factors that mediate object-substitution masking: Attention must be distributed over multiple potential targets, and the mask must continue to be visible during the period in which the iterations between higher level pattern representations and lower level contour representations are likely to occur.

Several recent investigations have confirmed the occurrence of object-substitution masking under a variety of conditions and have explored its limits (e.g., Giesbrecht et al., 2003; Jiang & Chun, 2001a, 2001b; Lleras & Moore, 2003; Neill et al., 2002; Tata, 2002). Especially revealing is an investigation by Woodman and Luck (2003a), who recorded event-related potentials to explore dissociations among attention, perception, and conscious awareness during object-substitution masking. They found that the target is identified by the visual system even when it is masked and, therefore, cannot be reported accurately. Under these conditions, however, the target triggers a shift of attention so that, by the time attention is deployed, only the mask remains visible, leading to impaired accuracy of target identification. These findings buttress the interpretation that object-substitution masking is critically dependent on reentrant processing.

8.2   Object Substitution as a General Theory of Masking?

Although object substitution theory does a reasonably good job of accounting for masking in the common onset paradigm, and even metacontrast-like masking involving four small dots, a critic might legitimately wonder whether this theory can account for masking obtained in conventional paradigms, including metacontrast involving snugly fitting surrounding contours and pattern masking involving overlapping shapes and visual noise. According to the reentry hypothesis, there is no difference in principle between masking with common onset and many aspects of classical metacontrast and pattern masking. All forms of backward masking should be subject to the influences of object substitution, in that the emerging representation of a temporally leading target will be replaced in consciousness by that of the mask if it follows the target closely in time and appears before target identification is complete. However, it is also possible that there will be differences in each form of masking with, for example, metacontrast masking producing specific types of contour interactions that are not shared by pattern masking or masking by four dots.

The approach taken to this question in a recent study (Enns, 2004) involved a systematic comparison of the effects of the four-dot mask with the "classic" masks used in metacontrast, noise, and pattern masking. To accomplish this, a simple letter identification task and identical target–mask sequences were used to compare six different masking stimuli as illustrated in figure 8.3. The distribution of attention was

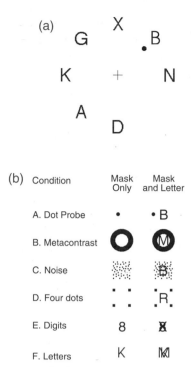

Figure 8.3
Example target display in the comparison of masks (Enns, 2004). The cross at the center indicates the fixation point; the black dot indicates the target letter to be reported, in this case the letter *B* (top). The target letter was preceded by, presented concurrently with, or followed by, one of these masks (bottom)

manipulated by varying the potential number of targets randomly among one, four, and seven items. The temporal relation between target and mask was varied from −150 ms (mask before target) to +600 ms (target before mask). In experiment 1 the mask itself acted as the target "probe," indicating to the observer which letter was to be identified. This meant that for all the positive temporal intervals, the letter to be identified was only indicated after the mask had been presented, preventing spatial attention from focusing on the target prior to the arrival of the mask. In subsequent experiments a spatial cue was placed near the target location, either simultaneously with the target display (experiment 2) or 100 ms prior to its arrival (experiment 3).

Three critical predictions were derived from the reentrant view. First, under ditions of spatially distributed attention (experiment 1, where the mask was also the target probe), the reentrant hypothesis predicts that all forms of backward masking should have, at a first approximation, an equal effect on target accuracy. This prediction derives directly from the idea that the contents of the mask will replace those of the target if the target has not been identified prior to its replacement on the screen by the mask. Second, the differences among masking effects should be greatest when the target and mask are in close spatiotemporal proximity and are therefore temporally integrated with one another (all three experiments). Under these conditions, the problems of target identification will not concern those of object substitution. Rather, they will involve problems of camouflage, in the case of noise and pattern masking, and local contour interactions, in the case of metacontrast masking. Third, backward masking will be minimized when attention can be prefocused on the spatial location of the target (experiment 3). This prediction follows directly from the idea that if target identification can be completed before only the mask remains on view, object substitution will not occur.

Target identification accuracy in experiment 1 (figure 8.4) showed that all backward masks had very similar effects, provided that attention was distributed (display size = 7). The primary consequence of each of these masks under distributed attention conditions was to reduce target accuracy to the level obtained in the baseline (dot probe) condition but to do so within a target–mask interval of 50 ms to 150 ms rather than the 600 ms that is required when no backward mask replaced the spatial location occupied by the target.

However, there were two notable exceptions to this general trend of equal backward masking for all mask types. One concerned the four-dot mask. Unlike the other four masks, which had their maximum influence at an interval of 50 ms and beyond, the four-dot mask had its full effect only at intervals of 150 ms and longer. This suggests that although backward masks are equal in their effects at intervals of 100 ms or more, they contain important differences in their effects at shorter intervals, as per the second prediction we derived from the reentry theory for this paradigm. This deviation from the general trend is therefore in keeping with the proposal that masking has at least two distinct ways to influence target identification: an early or fast-acting component associated with object formation and a later or slower acting component associated with object substitution.

A second deviation from the general pattern was seen in two of the mask types, digits and letters, which reduced target accuracy much more severely than the simple decay of information that occurs without a backward mask (dot probe condition). Although this appears superficially to be a violation of the prediction derived from reentry, a closer look reveals that the specific errors made in these two cases are actually consistent with it. Recall that the theory states that if only the mask remains on view prior to the complete identification of the target, processing will become focused on the mask. This means that if the mask itself activates target-relevant features or properties, these features may come to control the observer's response. This is exactly what happened. An examination of the responses made when targets were

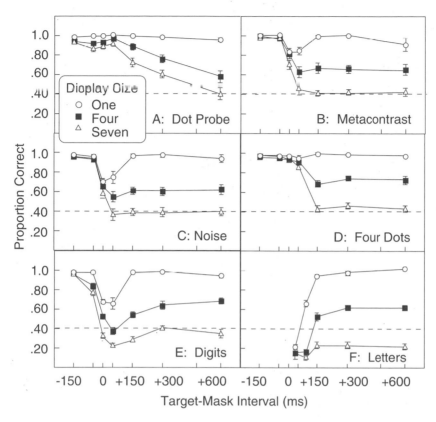

Figure 8.4
Target identification accuracy when the mask is the probe (Enns, 2004). (*A*) Dot probe baseline, (*B*) metacontrast, (*C*) noise, (*D*) four dots, (*E*) digits, and (*F*) letters. Dashed line indicates baseline accuracy on display size = 7, with a postdisplay dot probe and no mask.

incorrectly identified indicated that many of them were related to the target-relevant features in the mask rather than being random. For digit masks this meant that, for example, the digit 4 led to target responses that were visually similar to the digit (e.g., *A*); for letter masks, the identity of the mask was often incorrectly reported as the target letter. In both cases the mask seemed to be replacing the target as the object of conscious report by the observer.

Target identification accuracy in experiment 3 (figure 8.5) showed that all forms of backward masking have minimal effects if spatial attention can be focused on the target location prior to the target–mask sequence. This prediction derives from the idea that object substitution will not occur if the target shape can be identified prior to the time that the mask shape, remaining alone on view, will become the focus of the identification processes. However, as in experiment 1, substantial masking was

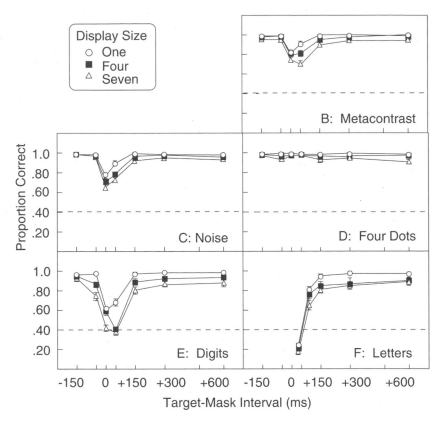

Figure 8.5
Target identification accuracy with a spatial precue (Enns, 2004). (*B*) Metacontrast, (*C*) noise, (*D*) four dots, (*E*) digits, and (*F*) letters. Dashed line indicates baseline accuracy with a postdisplay dot probe and no mask. (*A*) is omitted for ease of comparison with figure 8.4.

observed for all masks other than the four dots in the range of intervals between −50 ms and +50 ms. Strong masking occurred even when there was only a single display item and when a spatial precue indicated with 100% certainty where this item would appear. In this range of intervals, the focus of spatial attention had little influence on target identification. This attention-insensitive aspect of masking is consistent with the idea that temporal integration and local contour interaction are influenced relatively little by the distribution of spatial attention.

This comparison of the effects of spatial attention (display size and spatial cuing) on various types of visual masks (metacontrast, random noise, four dots, and patterns) provides strong support for the idea, derived from the object substitution theory of masking, that there are two distinct visual masking processes at work in a typical masking paradigm.

The first process is active in the range of target–mask intervals of 0–100 ms. It interferes with object formation, and at least in the case of pattern masking, this seems to be through the mechanism of temporal integration. Although it is the formal task of the observer to identify the target object (letter), when targets and masks are presented in close temporal proximity, the first "object" formed by the visual system is actually a composite of the target and mask patterns. For some masks, such as the four dots, such a composite object interferes little if at all with the task of identifying the target letter. However, for other masks, such as the random dots, digits and letters, the fusion of target and mask slows down target identification. For this early process, the effects of the mask are essentially those of "camouflage," which must be removed or segmented before the target can be identified.

This temporally early masking process is influenced very little by whether spatial attention is widely distributed, equally ready to select any one of eight different possible target locations, or whether it is already narrowly focused on only a single display location. This can be seen by comparing target accuracy for the smallest set size in both experiments (display size = 1 in figures 8.4 and 8.5). The data points for each masking condition are almost all identical when this comparison is made, illustrating the point that the object formation process is uninfluenced by the spatial focus of attention and that it is over by the time 150 ms has elapsed between the presentation of target and mask.

The second process, masking by object substitution, is critically dependent on the existence of a temporal delay between target presentation (a physical event initiating visual processing) and target identification (a mental achievement). This is evident in three critical features of the data. First, when attention was widely distributed at the onset of the target display, there was no backward masking in effect for a single display item beyond a target–mask interval of 100 ms (see figure 8.4). This held true whether the mask was a metacontrast frame, random noise, or even a competing shape such as another letter. This means that aside from the expected masking effects during object formation, there were no additional masking effects that arose from a delay in selecting the correct display item for perceptual report. Second, the four-dot mask yielded no evidence of any masking during the object formation stage, either when attention was distributed (see figure 8.4), or when attention could be focused earlier on the target location (see figure 8.5). Evidently, four dots pose no significant "camouflage" problems for target identification. Finally, the absence of all backward masking effects for target–mask intervals of 150 ms and more when the target location was cued in advance (see figure 8.5) is consistent with object substitution masking depending critically on a delay between display presentation and the identification of a specific item in that display.

Taken together, these results suggest that a mask will interfere with target identification only when each of two conditions is satisfied: (1) The mask must be presented prior to the completion of target identification, and (2) a temporally integrated target–mask composite must interfere with target identification. Masks that fail to satisfy both of these conditions will be ineffective. This was the case for the common-onset four-dot mask that terminated with the target (in section 8.1 of this chapter and in the present experiments at target–mask intervals of 0 ms). These stimulus sequences satisfy condition 1 but not condition 2. The converse was the case for experiments described in the present section with digit and letter masks presented 150 ms or more following a precued target letter. These tests satisfied condition 2 but not condition 1. In summary, the reentrant hypothesis leads to a unification of the principles for many different kinds of masking that have not been anticipated previously when researchers have taken a unidirectional approach to theorizing about visual masking.

8.3   A Cautionary Tale of Mask-Dependent Response Priming

Backward masking has been used in myriad studies to date, and much is known about the relevant factors involved (Breitmeyer & Öğmen, 2000; Enns & Di Lollo, 2000). Yet its most frequent use by vision researchers has not been to better understand why it occurs. Instead, it has been used most often as a tool of convenience to reduce the visibility of a stimulus. But its use as such a tool is premised on masking's being understood as a strictly feedforward process, one in which the mask simply interrupts the processing of the target. In this view, which has become quite standard, processing of the target has simply been abandoned upon presentation of the mask, in favor of processing of the mask.

For example, research in visual priming often uses a backward mask to reduce the visibility of a stimulus referred to as the *prime*. In a typical *masked priming* procedure, a prime shape is first presented briefly, followed by presentation of a mask shape that renders the prime very low in visibility, and then these shapes are followed by a target shape that remains on view and must be responded to rapidly. The goal of this procedure is to determine whether and how the advance information conveyed by the prime influences the processing of the later occurring target. Within a feedforward view of visual processing, it therefore seems reasonable to assume that the chief determinant of priming is the prime shape. The mask shape only indirectly influences target processing by weakening or strengthening the information carried by the prime shape. In what follows, we will show how misguided such an assumption can be and how the concept of object updating through reentrant processing can shed light on a type of masked priming that is often claimed to index the inherently "inhibitory" nature of visual unconscious processing.

The negative compatibility effect (NCE) was first described by Eimer and Schlaghecken (1998) and has since been the subject of much research (Eimer & Schlaghecken, 2001, 2002; Eimer et al., 2002; Klapp & Hinkley, 2002; Lleras & Enns, 2004; Schlaghecken & Eimer, 2001, 2002; Verleger et al., 2004). In a typical experiment, a brief prime is first presented (a double arrow pointing either right or left), followed by presentation of a mask (typically, a pattern mask composed of superimposed right- and left-pointing double arrows), which is then followed by a target (a double arrow pointing either right or left). The participants' task is to indicate as rapidly as possible in which direction (right or left) the target arrow is pointing. NCE refers to the counterintuitive finding that participants are reliably faster to respond to the target when prime and target point in opposite directions (incompatible trials) than when prime and target point in the same direction (compatible trials).

Most interpretations of the NCE have relied on feedforward models of perception, where the role of the mask is confined to reducing or even eliminating perceptual awareness of the prime (Eimer & Schlaghecken, 2002; Klapp & Hinkley, 2002). These authors have claimed that when perceptual awareness of the prime is limited, the prime is processed by unconscious mechanisms that are intrinsically inhibitory in nature. From this perspective, the NCE arises because a low visibility prime activates the unconscious inhibitory processes associated with it, causing the response to an identical visible target to be inhibited relative to a target corresponding to the opposite response.

In a recent paper, we called these unconscious inhibition theories of the NCE into question (Lleras & Enns, 2004). We began by noting that most previous studies had used pattern masks composed of the superimposition of both possible primes. In those studies where different masks were used, the masks still contained what we referred to as "task-relevant features" (i.e., arrowlike features pointing right and left) rather than task-irrelevant features (Klapp & Hinkley, 2002; Schlaghecken & Eimer, 2002). To test what role these kinds of masks may have played in producing the NCE, we conducted a series of experiments in which masks containing task-relevant features and task-irrelevant features were compared. Figure 8.6 shows a summary of the priming effects observed under both conditions. As can readily be seen, relevant masks systematically produced negative priming effects (replicating previous studies on the NCE), whereas irrelevant masks systematically yielded positive priming effects.

These results directly refute unconscious inhibition theories of the NCE because in such accounts "a mask is a mask is a mask." That is, the type of mask used should not affect the direction of the priming effect, provided that it reduces the visibility

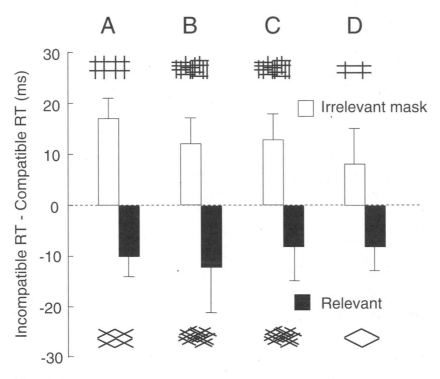

Figure 8.6
Mean priming effects—incompatible reaction time (RT) minus compatible RT—as a function of prime type (Lleras & Enns, 2004). Primes and targets were double-headed arrows. Primes were presented for 15 ms, 1.5° above or below fixation. Masks were presented for 120 ms at both possible prime locations. Targets were presented at fixation 100 ms after the mask's offset. The prime–mask interval was 45 ms in conditions (A) and (B), 15 ms in condition (C) and 90 ms in condition (D). (A) and (B) represent priming data for which prime visibility was higher on irrelevant-mask trials than on relevant-mask trials: For irrelevant and relevant masks, respectively, (A), 87% and 72%; (B), 88% and 74%. (C) and (D) show data for which prime visibility was equal on irrelevant-mask trials and on relevant-mask trials: For irrelevant and relevant masks, respectively, (C), 58% and 66%; (D) 94% and 89%). Examples of the masks used in each condition are shown next to the corresponding bar.

of the prime sufficiently to activate the unconscious inhibitory processes associated with the subsequent target. Only prime visibility should determine priming magnitude, with low levels of visibility yielding an NCE and high levels of visibility a positive priming effect. However, this was not what we found. We found that completely opposite priming effects could be obtained at equal levels of high or low prime visibility. What determined the direction of the priming in both cases was whether the mask contained task-relevant (negative priming) or task-irrelevant features (positive priming).

Unconscious inhibition theory falls far short of explaining these data. What we proposed instead was based on the concept of object updating, as presented in the preceding sections. At the core of this proposal is the possibility, derived from our previous studies of masking by object substitution, that the prime and mask may be interpreted by the visual system as changes in the same object over time. As a result, the prime–mask stimulus sequence is susceptible to the normal processes of object updating, and a single object representation may represent both stimuli as one object changing over time. When the prime (say, a left arrow) first appears, an object representation is established and attributes of the prime are encoded and associated with it. Notably, if task-relevant attributes are encoded, these attributes will start priming their associated response (a left response, in this example). When the mask (say, a juxtaposition of left and right arrows) appears afterward, the same object representation is updated with information from the mask. Because some of the attributes of the mask are already represented in this object representation (those corresponding to the left arrow embedded within the mask and also present in the prime), updating will primarily involve those "novel" features that are present in the mask but are absent from the prime (those corresponding to the right-arrow features embedded in the mask).

In accordance with previous literature on masked priming, we therefore proposed that priming is determined by the most recent set of task-relevant features encoded at the object level of representation, provided that strong links already exist between those features and their corresponding response (see Neumann, 1990; Scharlau & Ansorge, 2003). This assumption, in combination with object updating, is sufficient to account for the NCE observed with relevant masks as well as for the positive priming observed with irrelevant masks. On relevant-mask trials, the most recent set of task relevant features detected prior to target onset are those present in the mask and absent from the prime, therefore creating an opposite-to-prime facilitation. This opposite-to-prime facilitation results in faster responses to the target when the prime is opposite in shape (because the novel features in the mask point in the same direction as the target) and to slower responses to the target when the prime is identical (the novel features in the mask now point in a direction opposite to the target). Although the observed priming effect may superficially appear to be negative with respect to the prime, it actually corresponds to a positive priming effect induced by the novel task-relevant features in the mask. In sum, the observed priming effect reflects the influence not of the prime alone but of the prime–mask bundle on response selection. Correspondingly, on irrelevant-mask trials, the most recent set of task-relevant features encoded prior to target onset are those present in the prime (the mask has none of these features). Thus, the observed priming effect truly reflects the positive influence of the prime on response selection to the target.

We showed that this object updating account could even be applied to masks that did not contain exact replicas of the primes but merely contained similar features in spatially noncorresponding locations to those in the target (Lleras & Enns, 2004). We also tested this account in an experiment in which the roles of the prime and mask were reversed. For example, in one experiment either the superimposed set of double arrows (task relevant) or the double pound sign (task irrelevant) were used as a prime and the double-headed arrows were used as a mask. Although neither of these primes could now bias a particular response, the priming observed from the masks was influenced by these response-neutral primes. Task-relevant primes led to more priming than task-irrelevant primes, consistent with the prime–mask sequence contributing jointly to the priming effects on the target.

Standard feedforward accounts of masking would predict no influence of the prime type in this experiment. Priming ought to be determined solely by the mask–target sequence, which was identical in both types of trials. However, the object updating account predicts that more priming ought to be observed in the relevant prime condition than in the irrelevant prime condition. This follows because if prime and mask are associated with the same object representation in the relevant prime condition, the processing of the task-relevant priming features will begin at the onset of the prime. This is slightly earlier in time than in the irrelevant prime condition. Thus, by the time the "mask" appears in the relevant prime condition, any further updating of the priming features in the mask can only add strength to the representation that has already begun to be formed. In contrast, in the irrelevant prime condition, the object updating process could only begin to represent the target-relevant information at the onset of the mask. The results were consistent with these predictions: Task-relevant primes resulted in a significantly larger priming effect than task-irrelevant primes.

In sum, these experiments help to demonstrate that (1) the behavioral consequences of masking should always be examined directly rather than simply being assumed; (2) object updating is a powerful concept that can be applied to studies of unconscious processing of stimuli that are reduced in visibility, as well as to studies of response priming to objects with strongly associated response tendencies; and (3) the object updating concept produces testable predictions and can help to explain some behavioral phenomena with a simpler set of assumptions than those needed when standard feedforward theories of perception are applied.

8.4   The Future of Reentrant Theorizing

In the preceding sections of this chapter we have summarized the consequences of our reentrant theorizing in the realm of masking and masked priming. However, we are growing more confident every day that the reentrant hypothesis does not apply only to this restricted set of laboratory phenomena. Even in everyday vision, it is our view that the perception we are able to accomplish in a momentary glance is influenced by the perception we have of the larger schema of the scene that we have recently formed or have simply assumed to be true. The processes of perception in a glance will automatically evoke hypotheses about what lies beyond that glance, leading to a bias in where the next glance will be placed. In turn, having the expectation of particular schema will lead to the testing of specific hypotheses in subsequent glances. In other words, vision is almost always influenced as much by what lies in the mind as what lies before the eyes of the observer. Here, we will briefly point to two examples of phenomena illustrating the point that these recursive aspects of vision are as relevant in everyday visual functioning as they are in visual masking and priming.

8.4.1 Beyond the Limits of the Attentional Blink

Everyone who watches television is aware that not all the images that flash before our eyes are processed to an equal level of comprehension and awareness. Rather, we are aware that the cost of attending to a specific image in detail is a loss in comprehension of the images that follow, at least for a brief period of time. In the laboratory, this phenomenon is known as the *attentional blink*, and it is measured by inserting two visual targets into a stream of visual distractors that are displayed in rapid serial visual presentation. When the lag between the two targets is varied systematically in steps of 100 ms or so, the first target can be identified very accurately, but at the cost of a severe reduction in second-target accuracy. This is the attentional blink. It is commonly largest when the intertarget lag is short, and it diminishes gradually as the lag is increased to 500 ms or more.

The standard feedforward theoretical account of the attentional blink proposes some form of limited attentional resource that is allocated to the leading target at the expense of the trailing target. We have recently proposed an alternative account based not on depletion of a limited resource but on a temporary loss of perceptual control over the processes of perception in a glance (Di Lollo et al., 2005). The main idea is that processing of initial items in the visual stream is governed by a hypothesis-testing mechanism that is configured to pass target items and exclude nontarget items. This "input filter" is maintained by reentrant signals from a central processor that can perform only one function at a time. As soon as the central processor has detected an item from the target set and has begun to identify it, the maintenance signals for this initial monitoring task are discontinued, and the input filter comes under exogenous control by the next item in the visual stream. Therefore, if the next item belongs to the same category as the first target, the filter's configuration remains unaltered, and the item can be processed efficiently. If, however, the next item belongs to a different category from the first target, it will take longer to process than a same-category stimulus because it does not match the configuration of the input filter. This delay makes the trailing item vulnerable to masking by the next item in the stream. In addition, the configuration of the input filter will be altered, so that even ensuing items belonging to the same category as the first target will not be processed efficiently.

This reentrant account of the perception of rapid visual sequences makes the bold prediction that no attentional blink will occur if two or even three items from the target class are presented in succession. This is in sharp contrast to the standard theories that predict a decrease in accuracy for targets that follow the first in rapid succession. Although some of these theories try to accommodate the result that up to one additional target may occasionally sneak through the "sluggish attentional window" used to process the first target, none of the theories predict that up to three targets in a row will be processed efficiently. Yet this is exactly what the data show.

We conducted a series of experiments comparing report accuracy for items in a visual stream with three successive targets (which was uniformly high) versus two targets separated by a single distractor (resulting in the attentional blink for the second target; Di Lollo et al., 2005). The pattern of results revealed that it was the appearance of the distractor, during the period when the participant was identifying the first target, that inadvertently caused the input filter to become reset to the distractor class of items. Thus, the cognitive limit measured in the attentional blink is not one of a failure to be able to identify multiple items appearing in succession but is instead a failure to be able to control the hypotheses that are currently being tested in the information seen in a glance.

8.4.2 Using Memory to Resume an Interrupted Search

Think of the last time you drove or walked down a busy commercial street while searching for a friend whom you had arranged to meet. You did not know exactly where you would find your friend, so you alternated between searching for faces in the crowd and paying attention to the traffic around you. We have recently begun to examine the ability of participants engaged in visual a search to resume the search after a forced interruption (Lleras et al., under review). In contrast to some theories that have regarded visual search as being largely amnesic—on the grounds that observers have little memory for previously inspected locations and that a secondary visual memory task does not interfere with search—we have found that young adults are unusually good at resuming a search after it has been interrupted. This is seen in their exceptionally rapid response times to displays that they have viewed only once very briefly.

Having begun a search that is interrupted, searchers are often able to resume their task at a rate comparable to the speed with which they can respond to a target in the absence of any distracting items. In other words, they no longer need to search among the candidate items; they merely need to test the hypothesis they formed in their initial glance at the display on the second presentation of the same display. We have confirmed that the hypothesis being tested is linked to a particular location in the display and that perturbations of display items that are not near this location do not impair the rapid resumption of the search.

These results are consistent with our general view that visual perception consists of a recursive sequence of hypothesis generation and hypothesis testing. In a single glance at a scene, hypotheses about it must first be generated before they can be tested (confirmed or rejected). Hypotheses based on an initial glance can be tested very rapidly in a second glance, simply because the initial generation step has already been accomplished. On this account, only a limited portion of a scene—namely, that involving the hypothesis—has to be remembered during the interruption. This is a very different conceptualization of the "memorial processes" involved in visual search than has typically been assumed. Rather than memory consisting of some "finished product" of perception (something like a photograph) at the end of a long chain of neural events, memory in visual search seems to consist instead of a rough map of where detailed processing has already been completed and what one expects to find at the next location to be examined (Hochberg, 1968).

9 Dynamics of Perceptual Epochs Probed by Dissociation Phenomena in Masking

Haluk Öğmen, Bruno G. Breitmeyer, and Harold E. Bedell

9.1 Introduction

Visual masking can be defined as a reduction in the visibility of one stimulus, called the *target*, due to the presence of another stimulus, called the *mask*. Typically, the target and the mask are presented briefly and their relative onset asynchrony (stimulus onset asynchrony; SOA) is varied systematically. This paradigm can be viewed as one in which the temporal dynamics of target's neural processing is measured by using the mask as a "measuring probe." As the SOA varies, the mask exerts its effect during different phases of target's processing, thereby providing information on how the target's processing unfolds in time. In order to interpret these measurements, one needs to understand the nature of interactions between processes devoted to the target and those devoted to the mask. Extensive studies on visual masking have shown that masking is not a unitary phenomenon and that the mask can exert its effect on the processing of the target at various loci from the retina to the cortex (Bachmann, 1994; Breitmeyer, 1984; Breitmeyer & Öğmen, 2000). Different stimulus configurations engage different neural levels at varying degrees: For example, if the mask consists of a light field (masking by light), the main interference on the processing of the target occurs at the retinal level. When the mask is presented dichoptically, the interference occurs at cortical levels. Therefore, a systematic use of masking paradigms can reveal *the stages* of information processing along with their dynamics.

Because target–mask interactions are distributed and often highly nonlinear, it is difficult to produce precise predictions from qualitative, descriptive models of masking. The use of masking paradigms to probe neural dynamics is facilitated by computational models. These models can incorporate various stages of target–mask interactions as informed by neurophysiological and neuroanatomical studies. In this chapter, we will discuss such a model. We provide in the Appendix an outline of how basic aspects of neural processing are incorporated in our computational model. This model stemmed from a theory in which dynamical constraints of visual information processing and the neurophysiological structure of the primate visual system were used as guiding functional and structural principles, respectively. As a result, the model provides a link between function and structure within the framework of visual information-processing dynamics.

We start the chapter by discussing some general functional constraints in real-time information processing and argue that these constraints lead to a fundamental trade-off between the ability to achieve perceptual synthesis through feedback (reentrant) mechanisms and the ability to maintain sensitivity to changes in the stimulus. We then review a theory of retinocortical dynamics that offers a solution to this problem by using a sustained–transient dual-channel structure. The dual-channel structure of the theory is mapped to parvo- and magnocellular pathways in the primate visual system. According to the theory, under normal viewing conditions the dynamics of the visual system undergoes a succession of brief epochs, each lasting about a few hundred milliseconds. Therefore, understanding the "first-half-second" dynamics of visual processing is key to understanding the general dynamics of vision. The theory suggests that the initiation and the maintenance of perceptual epochs are carried out by a competition between sustained and transient systems. Dissociation paradigms offer a powerful technique to investigate dual-channel structures. We discuss dissociation phenomena in masking and suggest that these phenomena provide a window into the dynamics of visual processing in feed-forward and feedback modes across parallel pathways.

9.2   Functional Constraints in Real-Time Information Processing

9.2.1   Feedback and Modularity

Feedback and modularity are two of the most fundamental concepts in systems engineering. In the case of feedback, re-injecting the output (or a function of the output) back at the input level allows the system to autonomously keep track of its state and correct in real time undesirable deviations from its pre-established performance characteristics. This makes the system more robust to both internal and external noise compared to feedforward systems. Another important use of feedback, which is often encountered as loop structures in computer programs, is the resource efficiency that it provides through iterative adjustment of processing according to the prevailing context.

Assume that there are n different inputs producing m different outputs. This mapping can be implemented by a *single* mechanism. However, in general such an approach will not be fault tolerant, for a change in a small part of the system can have wide-ranging effects in overall performance. Moreover, a single mechanism is not easily amenable to modifications, for example, as required by adaptation. In engineering, typically a *modular* approach is preferred, for it allows easier and more robust design and modification. It is also a method of choice when the design problem has trade-offs that cannot be met by a single system. A modular approach in biology is attractive from the points of view of genetics, development, and adaptation. In problems in which the input and output spaces are well-defined and well delimited, one can usually divide the problem into a reasonable number of relatively simple modules. However, in a natural environment, an object's appearance can vary drastically as a function of lighting conditions and the overall spatiotemporal configuration of the scene. This problem is compounded further by the mapping of the three-dimensional space on two-dimensional retinas. Therefore, the input space in visual perception is, in general, ill defined and ill delimited. As a result, theories based on feedforward modular approaches (e.g., Marr, 1982) led to a proliferation of narrowly specialized modules without a clear methodology whereby a coherent percept can be synthesized from the outputs of the modules. Given this fundamental limitation of feedforward approaches, a major effort in computational modeling has been the synthesis of feedback and nonlinear interactions within and across a relatively small number of modular neural systems (e.g., Grossberg, 1988).

9.2.2 Feedback and Stability

Feedback can be negative or positive; negative feedback has, in general, corrective action and, when properly designed, tends to stabilize the system. On the other hand, positive feedback has an amplificatory action. The large majority of engineering use of feedback has been negative feedback because of its stabilizing action. Positive feedback has been, in general, used in digital systems where signal saturation controls the self-reinforcing action of the feedback. However, because of saturation, the system loses its analogue representational and information-processing power. Another important requirement for the use of stabilizing feedback is that delays in the system should be modest: Delayed feedback, even when negative, typically leads to unstable oscillatory behavior.

The primate visual system exhibits extensive anatomical feedback, including significant excitatory connections. The functional role of these feedback connections is largely unknown. Information processing at different neural loci exhibits a broad range of latencies (e.g., Schmolesky et al., 1998). As mentioned before, in terms of information processing, feedback appears essential for many models; however, a plausible model has to address the *real-time stability* of the system in the presence of positive feedback and delays.

9.2.3 Trade-Off Between Stimulus Readout and Perceptual Synthesis in a Feedback System

Consider the schematic diagram in figure 9.1 depicting the interactions between feedforward and feedback signals. The feedforward signal delivers the *stimulus-dependent* activity through afferent pathways. The feedback signal processes this activity in order to transform it into *percept-dependent* activities. There is a trade-off in setting the gains of the feedforward and feedback signals. If the gain of the feedforward signal is much higher than the gain of the feedback signal, then stimulus-dependent activities will energize feedback loops. However, because the feedforward signal remains dominant, the generation and establishment of *percept-dependent activities* will be hampered. This will lead to a failure to attain a perceptual synthesis. On the other hand, if the gain of the feedback signal is much stronger than the gain of the feedforward signal, then perceptual synthesis will occur. However, the percept will be very insensitive to changes in the input. Assume, for example, that the input shape changes from a square to a triangle. Because afferent signals are relatively weak, the synthesis corresponding to the square will persist in the positive feedback loops and the percept will be either the continuation of the previous object (square) or a highly blurred version of the two objects (a combination of a square and a triangle).

9.3   A Solution: Temporal Multiplexing of Conflicting Tendencies

We proposed a retinocortical dynamics theory that offers a solution to this trade-off by multiplexing in time the conflicting tendencies, namely, the need for strong feedforward signals (for a reliable readout of the input and for energizing the feed-

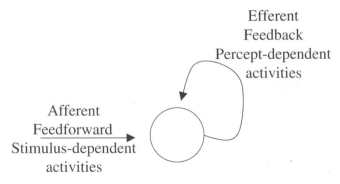

Figure 9.1
Interactions between stimulus-dependent feedforward (afferent) signals and percept-dependent feedback (functionally efferent) signals.

back loops) versus the need for a strong feedback signal to establish activities that underlie perceptual synthesis (Öğmen, 1993). According to this theory, the real-time dynamics of visual processes unfolds in three phases: (1) a "feedforward dominant" phase where strong afferent signals travel to higher cortical areas allowing the readout of the input and energizing the feedback loops; (2) a "feedback dominant" phase during which the afferent signal decays to a lower plateau value and the feedback, or reentrant, signals establish perceptual synthesis; and (3) a "reset phase" that is initiated when inputs change; during the reset phase the feedback signals receive a fast and transient inhibition so as to allow the dominance of the afferent signals (feedforward dominant mode) that deliver the new input. By limiting the real-time dynamics of the system to a succession of transient epochs, this scheme also has the advantage of avoiding asymptotic unstable behavior that can emerge in nonlinear positive feedback systems.

How can these phases be regulated in real time? We propose that the input is delivered to the feedback system by two parallel complementary pathways. A pathway with a relatively fast and transient response gets activated when changes occur in the input. The activity of this pathway is assumed to inhibit (reset) the reverberating activity in the feedback loop. A second pathway, with relatively slow and sustained response, delivers the input to the feedback system. Moreover, we assume that this input is nonmonotonic, overshooting to a peak first and then decaying to a lower plateau. The initial peak response corresponds to the feedforward dominant phase. The decay of the activity to a lower plateau allows the feedback signals to dominate; therefore, it provides a transition from feedforward dominant to feedback dominant phase.

9.4. RECOD: A Neural Model for the Theory

9.4.1 The Dual-Channel Structure in RECOD

In this section, we outline the retinocortical dynamics (RECOD) model (Öğmen, 1993; Öğmen et al., 2003), which suggests how this theory can be realized in the visual system. Figure 9.2 shows the general structure of the model. The two ellipses at the bottom of the figure represent two populations of retinal ganglion cells; one with fast–phasic (transient) response and a second with slower–tonic (sustained) response (e.g., Gouras, 1969; De Monasterio, 1978; Croner & Kaplan, 1995). These two populations of retinal ganglion cells project to distinct layers of the lateral geniculate nucleus (LGN) and form two parallel afferent pathways (the magnocellular and the parvocellular) as shown in the figure. The properties of functionally identified transient and sustained channels in humans (Kulikowski & Tolhurst, 1973; Breitmeyer, 1975; Legge, 1978; Breitmeyer et al., 1981a; Breitmeyer, 1984) and

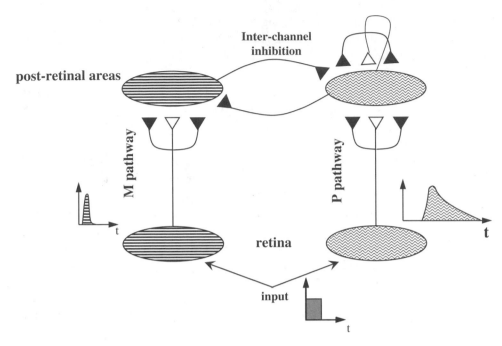

Figure 9.2
Schematic representation of the retinal cortical dynamics (RECOD) model. Filled and open triangular symbols depict inhibitory and excitatory synapses, respectively.

monkeys (Harwerth et al., 1980) parallel the properties of the magnocellular and the parvocellular pathways, respectively (Kremers, 1999), and we consider these pathways as neural correlates for the transient and sustained afferents in our model. Magnocellular and parvocellular projections to the cortex provide selective inputs to different visual areas subserving various functions such as the computation of motion, form, and brightness (Livingstone & Hubel, 1988). At the cortical level, these two pathways interact (Van Essen et al., 1992), but the loci and degree of their interactions are not fully established (e.g., Martin, 1992; Sincich & Horton, 2002). Neuroanatomical data indicate that the magnocellular afferents provide the *dominant* inputs to the dorsal ("where") pathway whereas parvocellular afferents provide the dominant inputs to the ventral ("what") pathway (Yabuta & Callaway, 1998). The model uses a lumped representation for the cortical targets of magnocellular and parvocellular pathways. The main cortical targets of the magnocellular pathway represent the areas in the dorsal pathway. The main cortical targets of the parvocellular pathway represent the areas in the ventral pathway (see the upper ellipses in figure 9.2).

9.4.2   Feedback in RECOD

The lumped representation for the areas involved in the computation of dynamic form and brightness contains recurrent connections to represent the extensive feedback observed between cortical areas as well as the feedback from cortex back to LGN (for a review, see Sherman & Guillery, 1996). In the model, these feedback connections provide the functionalities discussed in section 9.2.1. Consider the equation for the cells in the postretinal network driven by the parvocellular pathway. The activity of the ith cell, p_i, in this network is given by the equation

$$\frac{1}{\tau}\frac{dp_i}{dt} = -A_p p_i + (B_p - p_i)\{\Phi(p_i) + 2v_i(t-\eta)\} - p_i \left\{ \sum_{j=i-n_{pf};j\neq i}^{i+n_{pf}} \Phi(p_j) \right.$$
$$\left. + \sum_{j=i-n_p}^{i+n_p} H_{j-i}^{pi} v_j(t-\eta-\kappa_p) + \sum_{j=i-n_p}^{i+n_p} Q_{j-i}^{mp} m_j \right\}. \tag{9.1}$$

This equation is a variant of the Hodgkin–Huxley model, and a brief introduction to its neural basis can be found in the Appendix. The terms $\Phi(p_i) + 2v_i(t-\eta)$ and

$$\sum_{j=i-n_{pf};j\neq i}^{i+n_{pf}} \Phi(p_j) + \sum_{j=i-n_p}^{i+n_p} H_{j-i}^{pi} v_j(t-\eta-\kappa_p) + \sum_{j=i-n_p}^{i+n_p} Q_{j-i}^{mp} m_j$$

represent the excitatory and inhibitory inputs, respectively. The excitatory input has a feedforward component $2v_i(t-\eta)$ and a feedback component $\Phi(p_i)$. Similarly, the feedforward and feedback components of the inhibitory input are

$$\sum_{j=i-n_p}^{i+n_p} H_{j-i}^{pi} v_j(t-\eta-\kappa_p)$$

and

$$\sum_{j=i-n_{pf};j\neq i}^{i+n_{pf}} \Phi(p_j),$$

respectively. The summation operation indicates that inputs are pooled over space. The kernels H_k^{pi} and Q_k^{mp} determine the spatial extent of pooling. Parameter η represents the relative delay between the parvocellular and magnocellular signals. Parameter κ_p reflects the relative delay of the inhibitory signal with respect to the excitatory signal. Finally, the last component of the inhibitory input,

$$\sum_{j=i-n_p}^{i+n_p} Q_{j-i}^{mp} m_j,$$

represents interchannel transient-on-sustained inhibition, which is discussed in the next subsection.

This equation was developed to address specifically the encoding of edge blur. Because the extent and the spatial profile of edge blur can vary considerably in an image, the model was designed to include feedforward filters along with a flexible feedback mechanism. The nonlinear feedback function was defined as $\Phi(a) = 10a\{(a + 1)^2 - 1\}$, if $a < 0.05$ and $\Phi(a) = a(a + 0.975)$, otherwise. This particular form of feedback provides the network with the capability of flexible processing of edge blur (Öğmen, 1993).

9.4.3 Intra- and Interchannel Inhibition in RECOD

In the RECOD model, each channel, or pathway, possesses both positive and negative connectivity patterns. We will refer to the negative, that is, inhibitory, connections within each channel as *intrachannel* inhibition (Breitmeyer & Ganz, 1976; Breitmeyer, 1984). The aforementioned reset mechanism is implemented by inhibitory connections from the M (transient) pathway to the P (sustained) pathway. We will refer to this inhibition as *interchannel transient-on-sustained* inhibition (Breitmeyer & Ganz, 1976; Breitmeyer, 1984). As shown in figure 9.2, this inhibitory connection is accompanied by a reciprocal inhibitory connection, the *interchannel sustained-on-transient* inhibition. This is shown by the arrows between the upper ellipses in figure 9.2. This reciprocal inhibition creates a competition between the sustained and transient channels and allows the system to maintain a dynamic balance between figural synthesis and reset. As discussed before, the reset signal is required to allow the new afferent signal to reach the cortex in an effective manner. However, without a reciprocal inhibition, the system would be very sensitive to noise in the transient channel. Because figural synthesis requires time, without a reciprocal inhibition, noise would often reset the activity in the form channel, interfering with figural synthesis.

9.5 Other Reset Mechanisms

The importance of the trade-off between figural synthesis and reset has also been highlighted within the context of the boundary contour system (BCS) model (Francis et al., 1994). The BCS model includes positive feedback (Grossberg & Mingolla, 1985), and the analysis of the model showed that without a reset mechanism this feedback causes extensive persistence (Francis et al., 1994). In the BCS model, a competition between orientationally selective (cortical) mechanisms implements the reset. Francis and colleagues showed that this reset mechanism can form the basis of several visual illusions (Kim & Francis, 1998; Francis & Kim, 1999, 2001; Francis & Rothmayer, 2003).

Given that numerous cortical feedback circuits exist, it is highly likely that the nervous system uses multiple reset mechanisms. In the RECOD model, we used a reset mechanism that is *outside* of the feedback loops and *directly driven* by the external input. A static input can generate time-varying cortical activity, such as oscillatory potentials. The transient activity in the magnocellular pathway being closely related to the transients of the input (rather than intrinsic cortical time-varying activity), our reset mechanism is designed so that intrinsic cortical time-varying activity does not interfere with figural synthesis. On the other hand, a reset mechanism such as the one used in the BCS model can account for bistable percepts, that is, switches in perceptual organization in response to certain static stimuli.

9.6   Dynamic Competition Between Reset and Figural Synthesis and the Dissociation Phenomena in Masking

The balance between reset and persistence, discussed in the previous sections, is carried out through the reciprocal inhibition between parvo- and magno-driven cortical cells. In order to test this proposal, one can devise experiments where the stimulus configuration selectively biases the competition and, therefore, creates a dissociation between the functions carried out by the two parallel interacting systems. We will first discuss a dissociation between visibility and rapid spatial localization. According to our model, the qualia-rich visibility of a stimulus is based on the activities in the "form channel," that is, the channel that receives a parvo-dominant input. Rapid spatial localization is carried out by the "motion/temporal-change channel," that is, the channel that receives a magno-dominant input. We will then discuss a double dissociation between visibility and masking effectiveness in metacontrast. According to our model, these functions are carried out by the parvo- and magno-driven systems, respectively.

9.7   Dissociation Between Visibility and Spatial Localization

The visibility of a target stimulus can be strongly reduced when it is followed in time by a spatially nonoverlapping mask stimulus, a phenomenon known as *metacontrast* (Stigler, 1910, 1926; Fry, 1934; for reviews, see Breitmeyer, 1984; Bachmann, 1994; Breitmeyer & Öğmen, 2000). The nature of interactions between the target and the mask depends on several stimulus parameters, such as size, energy, eccentricity, and contour proximity. The *criterion content*, that is, the stimulus dimension(s) on which the observer bases his or her judgments, plays an important role in determining how target visibility depends on SOA (for reviews, see Kahneman, 1968; Breitmeyer, 1984, pp. 103–105). For example, for target and mask stimuli of equal energy, a

U-shaped ("type B") metacontrast function is obtained when the observers make judgments related to the target's surface properties (e.g., perceived brightness, contrast), contour properties (e.g., contour completeness, contour shape), or figural identity (e.g., letter recognition). U-shaped functions can be obtained using a variety of response tasks such as matching, magnitude estimation, and choice reaction times (RTs) as long as the criterion content required for the task falls into one of the aforementioned categories. However, when the observer's task is changed to reporting the presence or the spatial location of the target, instead of its visibility, the metacontrast mask has no effect on the observer's performance, as measured by simple/choice RTs or by response accuracy (e.g., Fehrer & Raab, 1962; Schiller & Smith, 1966). A "coarse localization" of the stimulus in time and/or in space is sufficient to accomplish this task. We will therefore make a distinction between task parameters and criterion content that require a *coarse* localization of the target (hereafter referred as *target localization*) and those that require surface, contour, and figural identification of the target (hereafter referred as *target visibility*).

The markedly different findings for the visibility versus localization of the target suggest that the processes that underlie the visibility of a stimulus can be dissociated from those that underlie the spatial localization of the same stimulus.

Several studies have provided evidence for the existence of two distinct neural pathways, a "what" pathway related to stimulus visibility/identity and a "where" pathway related to the spatial localization of the stimulus (Ungerleider & Mishkin, 1982; Ungerleider, 1985; Desimone & Ungerleider, 1989). Accordingly, one way to explain the dissociation between stimulus visibility and localization in visual masking is to postulate that the mask stimulus interferes with the target stimulus in the "what" pathway but not in the "where" pathway. This explanation would be consistent with the findings showing that figural aspects of stimuli such as size can be distorted at the perceptual level but not at the motor level (Milner & Goodale, 1995). On the other hand, as suggested in our model, it is also possible that the pathways processing the figural and the spatial localization information *interact* and that the dissociation observed in metacontrast is not a general property of neural processing. The top panel of figure 9.3 provides a schematic explanation according to our model for the dissociation between visibility and localization in metacontrast. The target stimulus is presented first and generates a fast transient and a slower sustained activity in the afferent transient and sustained pathways, respectively. The model postulates that the visibility of the target is correlated with the activities in postretinal areas receiving their main input from the sustained (parvocellular) pathway. Both sustained and transient activities carry information about the spatial location of the target. However, because of the shorter latency of the transient signals (Maunsell & Gibson, 1992; Nowak et al., 1985; Petersen et al., 1988; Schmolesky et al., 1998), the model postulates that the transient activities will play

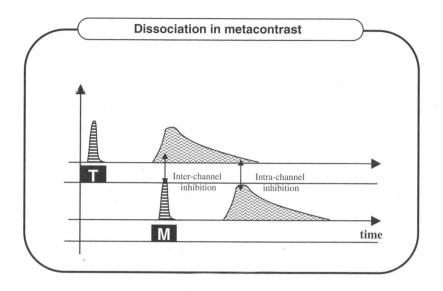

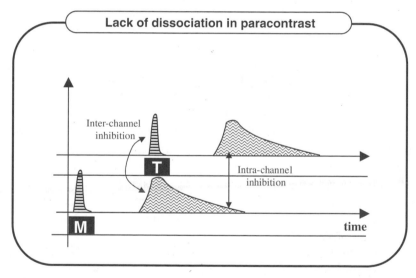

Figure 9.3
Depictions of model predictions for metacontrast (top panel) and paracontrast (lower panel).

a major role in target localization when the observer is asked to respond *as fast as possible*. In metacontrast, the mask is presented second and generates similar activities with a delay equal to the SOA. From the nature of the temporal overlap between the activities, one can see that both the intra- and interchannel inhibition will cause a suppression of activity in the sustained channel for the target. As a result, the visibility of the target is predicted to decrease. However, the transient activity generated by the target, and consequently the ability of the observer to report the presence or the location of the target, is predicted to remain intact. The bottom panel of figure 9.3 depicts the prediction of the model for paracontrast. In this case, both the transient and sustained activities generated by the target are inhibited. As a result, the model predicts that RTs should increase and the visibility of the target should decrease.

To test these predictions, we conducted two experiments (Öğmen et al., 2003). In a first experiment, we measured target visibility as a function of SOA for para- and metacontrast. The target stimulus consisted of a disk and the mask consisted of a ring that surrounded the target. Target and mask were presented in the right visual field, and a match stimulus of the same dimensions as the target was presented in the left visual field (see Öğmen et al., 2003, for details). The task of the observer was to indicate which of the two, the target or the match, appeared brighter. The luminance of the match stimulus was changed by a staircase procedure. Figure 9.4 shows the points of subjective equality between the perceived luminance of the match and the target stimuli as a function of SOA along with the model prediction. As expected, both para- and metacontrast show U-shaped functions with a smaller magnitude for para- than metacontrast. Peak metacontrast occurs at SOA = 50 ms. Peak paracontrast occurs in the −150-ms to −100-ms range.

Overall, the model predictions match the data well in terms of the location of the dips in the masking function. In the model, paracontrast masking at relatively large SOA magnitudes arises from a slow intrachannel *cortical* inhibition that was not included in the earlier versions of the dual-channel masking models. In our simulations, the relative delay of this intrachannel inhibition was 144 ms. The estimated delays for antagonistic interactions (center–surround) in the early visual pathways are at least an order of magnitude less than this value (e.g., Benardete & Kaplan, 1997). Therefore, this interaction is likely to occur at relatively higher levels. In our simulations, we used a *functional feedforward* signal to implement this inhibition (see Öğmen et al., 2003, and chapter 16 in this volume for a distinction between anatomical and functional feedback); however, a functional feedback signal is also possible. Additional experiments are needed to test these possibilities. Quantitatively, the model underestimates the magnitude of metacontrast and the span of masking at large SOA magnitudes. For computational simplicity, the simulations were based on a simplified (one-dimensional) version of the stimuli used in the

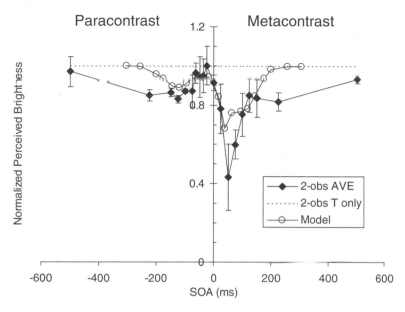

Figure 9.4
Filled symbols: Perceived brightness averaged (AVE) across two observers and normalized with respect to a condition where only the target (T) was presented (horizontal dashed line corresponding to the value 1) ±1 SEM. Open symbols: model predictions.

experiment. It is possible that the quantitative discrepancies between the model and the data are due to the failure in our model and simulations to represent adequately all stimulus parameters such as eccentricity, stimulus size, energy, and background level. These parameters are known to influence both the magnitude and the morphology of the masking functions (for a review, see Breitmeyer, 1984). Qualitatively, the model shows changes in stimulus visibility for both paracontrast and metacontrast and thus provides the necessary conditions to study the dissociation phenomenon. Our goal was to fit the model to the visibility data with a reasonable match so that quantitative predictions that provide a reasonable approximation for RT data could be obtained.

In a second experiment, we measured the spatial localization performance in para- and metacontrast. The stimulus was similar to the one used in the visibility experiment with the following main difference: The masks (rings) were presented on both sides of fixation, and, in each trial, the target was presented in a random manner either inside the left or inside the right ring. The task of the observer was to indicate as rapidly and as accurately as possible whether the target appeared to the left or to the right of fixation by pressing the left and right buttons of a joystick. In order to discount changes in RTs due to factors other than contour masking, we also had a control condition where the mask's contours were far from target's contours with highly reduced similarity between the two contours. This mask did not influence the visibility of the target at the eccentricity used in the experiment. The contour-masking-related RTs were computed by subtracting the RTs obtained in the control experiment from the RTs obtained in the main experiment (ΔRT). Figure 9.5 plots the change in RT due to contour masking as a function of SOA for two mask–target contrast ratios. The accuracy of responses was higher than 97% for all observers. For metacontrast, ΔRTs fluctuate around averages of −5.5 ms and 1.7 ms for mask–target energy ratios of 1 and 3, respectively. However, for paracontrast, ΔRTs depend strongly on SOA, peaking at SOA = −150 ms. The peak ΔRT values are 28.7 ms and 51.1 ms for mask–target ratios of 1 and 3, respectively.

Taken together, these results show that the dissociation between stimulus visibility and spatial localization does not hold in paracontrast. Figure 9.5 also shows the model prediction superimposed on the data. Both the data and the model show an inverse-U-shaped function for paracontrast and a relatively constant function for metacontrast.

Overall, we interpret the dissociation between visibility and spatial localization in metacontrast as evidence for parallel pathways subserving these functions and the failure of dissociation when the temporal order of stimuli is switched (i.e., paracontrast) as evidence that these parallel pathways interact.

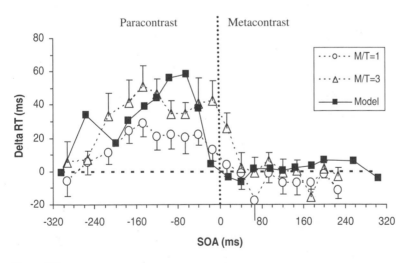

Figure 9.5
Change in reaction time (RT) due to contour masking as a function of stimulus onset asynchrony (SOA) for mask : target contrast ratios (M/T) of 1 and 3 (±1 *SEM*). Squares: model predictions.

9.8   Dissociation Between Visibility and Masking Effectiveness

According to our model, the main contributor to the U-shaped masking in metacontrast is transient-on-sustained inhibition. Therefore, the masking effectiveness of a mask stimulus can be correlated with the strength of its transient activity. On the other hand, the visibility of the mask stimulus is correlated with the strength of its sustained activity. Given that masking effectiveness and visibility are assumed to correlate with different neural processes, a dissociation between the two should be theoretically possible under appropriate experimental paradigms. *Target recovery* (also known as *target disinhibition*) is one such paradigm (e.g., Dember & Purcell, 1967). Breitmeyer et al. (1981b) used a stimulus configuration where the target (T) was a disk surrounded by a ring that served as the primary mask (M1), which in turn was surrounded by a second ring that served as a secondary mask (M2; see the inset in figure 9.6). They presented M1 at an SOA that produced a maximal metacontrast suppression of T. They systematically varied the T–M2 SOA and measured in separate experiments the visibility of T and the visibility of M1. They computed the *change* in visibility for T and M1 with respect to the baseline condition where

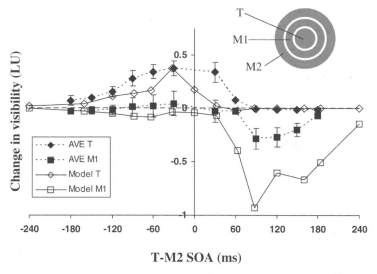

Figure 9.6
Changes in the visibility in log units (LU) of contrast for the target (T) and the primary mask (M1) as a function of the T-M2 stimulus onset asynchrony (SOA). Positive (negative) values indicate an increase (decrease) in visibility with respect to the condition where only T and M1 were displayed. Negative T-M2 SOA corresponds to the case where M2 was presented before T. The duration of each stimulus was 15 ms, and the T-M1 SOA was fixed at 45 ms. Filled symbols joined with dashed lines represent the data averaged (AVE) across the three observers in Breitmeyer et al. (1981). Open symbols joined by solid lines show the predictions of the model. The inset depicts the spatial configuration of the stimulus.

M2 was not presented. Their data show strong increases in the visibility of T without a concomitant change in the visibility of M1 for negative T–M2 SOAs (see figure 9.6). Because the increase in the visibility of T indicates a decrease in the masking effectiveness of M1, this finding shows a dissociation between the masking effectiveness of M1 and its visibility. For M2 presented after M1, an opposite effect is observed: While the visibility of M1 is strongly reduced, there is no change in its masking effectiveness.

Taken together, these results show a double dissociation between visibility and masking effectiveness. Figure 9.7 depicts schematically how our model can account for this double dissociation phenomenon: The top panel shows how M2 influences the transient activity of M1. When M2 precedes M1, the sustained activity of M2 inhibits the transient activity of M1. As M2 gets closer in time to M1, the transient activity of M2 also inhibits the transient activity of M1 (transient-on-transient inhibition). However, as the T–M2 SOA further increases, the sustained and transient activities of M2 no longer overlap with the transient activity of M1, and therefore changes in M1's masking effectiveness are restricted to mainly negative T–M2 SOAs. The influence of M2 on M1's visibility will be mainly due to the inhibition exerted by the transient activity of M2 on the sustained activity of M1. This occurs for positive T–M2 SOAs. Figure 9.6 shows the quantitative prediction of our model superimposed on the data. While the model overestimates the magnitude of the changes in M1's visibility, there is a good agreement in the timing of visibility changes, and more important, the existence of two SOA ranges yielding a double dissociation between visibility and masking effectiveness.

Overall, the double-dissociation phenomenon discussed in this section provides strong empirical support for the proposed dual-channel structure and the competition between these channels.

9.9   Other Models and the Double-Dissociation Phenomena

Francis (1997) simulated the BCS model and compared its predictions to Breitmeyer et al.'s (1981b) disinhibition data. Qualitatively, the introduction of the secondary mask led to the recovery of the target, in agreement with the data. However Francis (1997) noted that, in its current form, the model fails to explain the dissociation between the visibility and the masking effectiveness of the primary mask. Further studies are needed to establish whether other parameter values in the model can address this problem and the quantitative discrepancies between the model predictions and experimental data.

An alternative explanation of target recovery is the facilitatory effect by the preceding secondary mask on the target, either by acting as a cue or by activating a

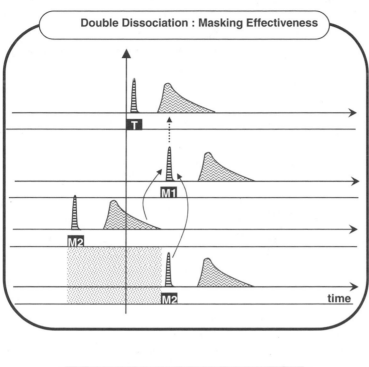

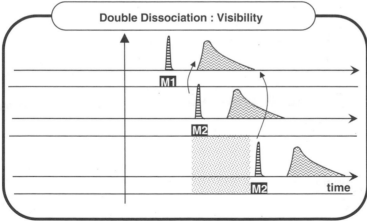

Figure 9.7
Double dissociation between visibility and masking effectiveness according to the retinocortical dynamics (RECOD) model. The top panel depicts how M2 modulates the masking effectiveness of the primary mask (M1). The top two traces of this panel show schematically the transient and sustained activities that are generated by the target (T) and M1 at the T-M1 stimulus onset asynchrony (SOA) that produces the optimal suppression of T's visibility. The masking effectiveness of M1 correlates with the strength of its transient activity, which suppresses the sustained activity of T (dashed arrow). The bottom two traces show the beginning and the end of the T-M2 SOA range where M2's sustained and transient activities inhibit M1's transient activity. The lower panel depicts the T-M2 SOA range wherein M2 modulates the visibility of M1.

nonspecific subcortical pathway, as postulated by the perceptual retouch model (Bachmann, 1984, 1994). However, such facilitatory effects should also act on the primary mask, M1, and, therefore, changes in M1's visibility should parallel target recovery curves for negative SOAs. This does not happen in the data. Moreover, in our recent experiments we found that in the absence of M1, that is, when only M2 and T are presented, T's visibility shows no change when M2 precedes T (Öğmen et al., 2004a). Hence, the facilitatory effect of M2 does not appear to be the basis of target recovery.

9.10   Conclusions

Under normal viewing conditions, our eyes shift from one fixation point to another, staying at each fixation locus for a few hundred milliseconds. During this short time interval, the object of interest is kept at a relatively fixed position at the fovea. Therefore, the operation of the visual system during normal viewing conditions can be viewed as a succession of short epochs. The theoretical framework presented in this chapter provides a functional rationale for why a succession of brief epochs is important for the visual system. It also provides a hypothesis for how the visual dynamics unfolds during each of these epochs. According to our approach, at the beginning of fixation, transient activity resets the previous activity in the form channel and a succession of feedforward- and feedback-dominant phases lead to a perceptual synthesis that occurs within a few hundred milliseconds (Öğmen, 1993). We suggested that a masking paradigm can be used as a way to probe the dynamics of these perceptual epochs. In particular, dissociation phenomena in masking were studied to analyze the dynamics of the competition between sustained and transient systems that regulates the initiation and maintenance of the epochs. Future research will address how interactions between motion and form systems are used to "fill in" between epochs so as to provide a phenomenal spatiotemporal continuity between perceptual epochs.

9.11   Appendix: Computational Basis of the RECOD Model

The computational structure of the model is built by specializing according to neurophysiological, neuroanatomical, and functional constraints a few canonical equations that describe basic aspects of neuronal dynamics. The first type of equation used in the model has the form of a generic Hodgkin–Huxley equation

$$C_m \frac{dV_m}{dt} = -(E_p + V_m)g_p + (E_d - V_m)g_d - (E_h + V_m)g_h, \tag{9.2}$$

where V_m represents the membrane potential, g_p, g_d, and g_h are the conductances for passive, depolarizing, and hyperpolarizing channels, respectively, with E_p, E_d, and E_h representing their Nernst potentials. C_m is the membrane capacitance. This equation has been used to characterize the dynamics of membrane patches and single cells, as well as networks of cells (reviewed by Grossberg, 1988; Koch & Segev, 1989). For simplicity, one can set $E_p = 0$ and use the symbols B, D, and A for E_d, E_h, and g_p, respectively, to obtain the generic form for the "multiplicative" or "shunting" equation (reviewed by Grossberg, 1988):

$$C_m \frac{dV_m}{dt} = -AV_m + (B - V_m)g_d - (D + V_m)g_h. \tag{9.3}$$

The depolarizing and hyperpolarizing conductances are used to represent the excitatory and inhibitory inputs, respectively.

The second type of equation is a simplified version of equation 9.2, called the "additive," "leaky-integrator" model, where the external inputs influence the activity of the cell not through conductance changes but directly as depolarizing and hyperpolarizing currents, yielding the form

$$C_m \frac{dV_m}{dt} = -AV_m + Excitatory Inputs - Inhibitory Inputs. \tag{9.4}$$

Mathematical analyses showed that, with appropriate connectivity patterns, shunting networks can automatically adjust their dynamic range to process small and large inputs (reviewed by Grossberg, 1988). Accordingly, we use shunting equations when we have interactions among a large number of neurons so that a given neuron can maintain its sensitivity to a small subset of its inputs without running into saturation when a large number of inputs become active. We use the simplified additive equations when the interactions involve few neurons.

Finally, a third type of equation is used to express biochemical reactions of the form

$$S + Z \xrightarrow{\gamma} Y \xrightarrow{\delta} X \xrightarrow{\alpha} S + Z,$$

where a biochemical agent, S, activated by the input, interacts with a transducing agent, Z (e.g., a neurotransmitter), to produce an "active complex," Y, that carries the signal to the next processing stage. This active complex decays to an inactive state, X, which in turn dissociates back into S and Z. It can be shown that (see the Appendix in Sarikaya et al., 1998), when the active state X decays very fast, the dynamics of this system can be written as

$$\frac{dz}{dt} = \alpha(\beta - z) - \gamma sz \tag{9.5}$$

with the output given by $y(t) = \dfrac{\gamma}{\delta} s(t)z(t)$, where s, z, and y represent the concentrations of S, Z, and Y, respectively, and γ, δ, and α denote rates of complex formation, decay to inactive state, and dissociation, respectively. This equation has been used in a variety of neural models, in particular to represent temporal adaptation, or the gain control property, occurring, for example, through synaptic depression (e.g., Grossberg, 1972; Carpenter & Grossberg, 1981; Öğmen & Gagne, 1990; Gaudiano, 1992; Öğmen, 1993; Abbott et al., 1997).

The detailed specialized equations of the model can be found in Öğmen et al. (2003). Here we will outline one example to show how the generic equations are specialized to represent neuronal networks in the model. Consider retinal cells with sustained activities. The retinal network is designed to capture the basic spatiotemporal properties of the retinal output without necessarily incorporating all details of the retinal circuitry. To the extent possible, parameters of the model reflect the physiologically measured parameters of the primate retina.

Functionally, we consider three important stages that shape the dynamics of the responses. The first functional stage is that of temporal adaptation, or gain control. When a step input is applied, the response of the sustained cells increases first to reach a peak and gradually decays to a lower plateau response. To achieve this adaptation we apply equation 9.5 as follows:

$$\frac{1}{\tau}\frac{dz_i}{dt} = \alpha(\beta - z_i) - \gamma(J + I_i)z_i, \tag{9.6}$$

where z_i represents the concentration of a transducing agent at the ith spatial location. J is a baseline input generating a dark current and I_i is the external input (luminance value) at the ith spatial position. Parameter τ is a constant that influences the overall time constant of the system.

Another important aspect of the retinal network is the spatial center–surround organization. To incorporate the center and surround of the receptive fields, signals from the first stage are convolved with the kernels G_k^{se} and G_k^{si}, which represent the excitatory center and the inhibitory surround of the receptive field. The kernels are Gaussian functions of the form $G_k^{se} = Amp_{se}\, e - (k^2/sd_{se}^2)$, and the parameters Amp_{se} and sd_{se} were selected according to the receptor spacing at the fovea (Coletta & Williams, 1987; Dacey, 1993) and the physiologically measured receptive field characteristics at the corresponding region of the primate retina (Croner & Kaplan, 1995). The membrane potential of the ith sustained cell, w_i, is described by using the Hodgin–Huxley (shunting) equation as follows:

$$\frac{1}{\tau}\frac{dw_i}{dt} = -A_s w_i + (B_s - w_i)\sum_{j=i-n_s}^{i+n_s} G_{j-i}^{se}\Psi(J_s + I_j)z_j - (D_s + w_i)\sum_{j=i-n_s}^{i+n_s} G_{j-i}^{si}\Psi(J_s + I_j)z_j, \tag{9.7}$$

where the center and surround convolution sums provide the excitatory and the inhibitory inputs. The input signal is processed by a second-order polynomial, $\Psi(.)$, whose coefficients were determined by fitting the contrast response of the model neurons to the physiological data from Kaplan and Shapley (1986).

Finally, to represent the output, that is, the spike activity, of the sustained retinal ganglion cells, we use a quadratic nonlinearity with threshold $\lambda([w_i - \Gamma_s]^+)^2$, where $[a]^+$ denotes the threshold, or half-wave rectification, function (i.e., $[a]^+ = a$ if $a > 0$, and $[a]^+ = 0$, otherwise). Parameters λ, and Γ_s represent the gain and the threshold level of this function, respectively.

Once the physiologically measured parameters are incorporated into the model, the equation can provide a good quantitative estimate for processes that can lead to masking. For example, a light mask will mainly exert its effect through equation (9.6), while a contour mask will have its retinal effect through the receptive field kernels in equation (9.7). Contributions of each of these components can be assessed quantitatively by analyzing the respective model processes.

Acknowledgments

This work was supported by National Institutes of Health Grant R01-MH49892 and National Science Foundation Grant BCS-0114533.

10 Backward Masking in Schizophrenia: Neuropsychological, Electrophysiological, and Functional Neuroimaging Findings

Jonathan K. Wynn and Michael F. Green

10.1 Introduction

Schizophrenia patients exhibit a wide range of neurocognitive and perceptual deficits. In particular, schizophrenia patients have great difficulty in processing visual stimuli that are presented in rapid succession. Visual backward masking has been used for more than 20 years in the study of these perceptual deficits to gain a better understanding of the early visual processing deficits commonly seen in schizophrenia. Studying backward masking deficits in schizophrenia has advantages over use of other visual processing paradigms in that we can gain a better understanding of the neural time course of schizophrenia patients' visual processing deficit. Commonly, backward masking deficits in schizophrenia appear as patients' requiring a longer interval between the target and the mask to correctly identify the target.

This chapter will discuss findings of visual backward masking deficits in schizophrenia patients over that past 15 years with a particular emphasis on our current research program. We will briefly discuss the background, history, and findings of visual backward masking deficits in schizophrenia using the research program from our laboratory as a way to illustrate key questions in the area. The remainder of the chapter will focus on our current research, which has taken advantage of recent theories of backward masking, as well as advances in electrophysiology and functional neuroimaging. In particular, we will discuss current research into gamma-range cortical oscillations and how they are related to schizophrenia deficits in visual backward masking. We will also present preliminary functional magnetic resonance imaging (fMRI) findings of visual backward masking in normal controls as a basis for our planned studies in schizophrenia patients. Finally, we will present findings elucidating the functional significance of a backward masking deficit in schizophrenia.

The success of our research program on schizophrenia is heavily dependent on the work of basic behavioral scientists working in the area of visual processing. Our explicit goal is to apply methodologies developed by basic researchers to gain a better understanding of the abnormal brain processes in schizophrenia patients. Our long-standing collaboration with Bruno Breitmeyer is a direct outgrowth of this programmatic approach to interdisciplinary research. This collaboration has led to the development and applications of novel methods to assess visual backward masking that have greatly increased our understanding of the early visual processing deficits seen in schizophrenia patients.

10.2 Backward Masking Deficits in Schizophrenia

Schizophrenia is marked by symptoms that range from hallucinations and delusions to flat affect and anergia (e.g., lack of energy). One of the core features of schizophrenia is an abnormality in information processing, especially when stimuli are presented in rapid succession (for a review, see Braff et al., 1992). Visual backward masking has been one informative paradigm for measuring early visual processing deficits in schizophrenia. Work over the years has shown that these deficits are central aspects of schizophrenia, rather than being due to psychotic symptoms or medications. Importantly, backward masking research in schizophrenia has been extended to study those at risk for schizophrenia (e.g., first-degree relatives).

Symptoms of schizophrenia can be categorized as positive (e.g., delusions, hallucinations, etc.) or negative (e.g., avolition, anhedonia, etc.; Andreasen & Olsen, 1982). Our initial masking studies in this area, where subjects were asked to report the identity of a letter positioned to the left or right of fixation, showed that masking deficits were more prominent in patients with negative symptoms, compared to those with positive symptoms (Green & Walker, 1984, 1986) and in comparison to normal control subjects. In addition, patients with negative symptoms needed a longer stimulus duration to see the target. This finding of a link between negative symptoms and visual masking has been replicated in several other laboratories (Butler et al., 2002; Cadenhead et al., 1997).

The masking deficits are clearly not a result of the psychoactive medications that patients take. A study of ours revealed substantial masking deficits in unmedicated patients in symptomatic remission compared to normal controls (Green et al., 1999). Several studies from other groups have shown that unmedicated patients show backward masking deficits just as large as, if not larger than, those in medicated patients compared to normal controls (Braff & Saccuzzo, 1982; Butler et al., 1996; Cadenhead et al., 1997).

A separate focus of research has been whether visual backward masking deficits are a trait characteristic of schizophrenia. If visual masking deficits are a trait feature of schizophrenia, then those who have a genetic predisposition to schizophrenia would be expected to show deficits compared to normal controls, even if they do not show any signs of psychiatric illness. Our laboratory published the first study to show that siblings of schizophrenia patients also exhibit backward masking deficits compared to normal controls (Green et al., 1997). A group of full siblings of schizophrenia patients who were screened for the absence of psychiatric disorders (including schizophrenia, schizotypal or paranoid personality disorder, bipolar disorder, or substance dependence) was compared with a group of normal control subjects. It was found that siblings showed backward masking deficits (i.e., target identification was significantly worse) relative to normal controls on the early component—that is, at stimulus onset asynchronies (SOAs) of 40 ms and less—of their masking functions, indicating that genetic vulnerability to schizophrenia leads to abnormalities in early sensory–perceptual processes. Studies from other laboratories generally support our findings in siblings of schizophrenia patients (Bedwell et al., 2003; Keri et al., 2001). Aside from the findings in siblings of patients, the observation that patients in remission also show deficits supports the idea that these deficits reflect a trait aspect of the illness (Green et al., 1999).

10.3   Mechanisms Underlying the Deficit

Our research program moved into questions of the specific mechanism involved with the deficits in schizophrenia. Namely, we were interested in whether schizophrenia patients showed a selective deficit in masking by integration, interruption, or both. Masking by integration results in a confusing, composite image of the target and mask, thus making accurate target identification difficult. Masking by interruption occurs when the mask interrupts or prevents later stage processing of the target. In a series of studies investigating the masking mechanism that was deficient in schizophrenia, we attempted to isolate the role of integration versus interruption neural pathways by altering the energy of the masks and to isolate the role of transient versus sustained changes by altering the clarity of the target (Green et al., 1994a, 1994b).

In this series of experiments, we attempted to limit the masking mechanism to interruption by using a low-energy mask. A high-energy masking condition presumably involved masking by both integration and interruption. Results showed that patients performed significantly worse compared to normal controls in both paradigms, and the magnitude of the deficits was comparable across conditions. The results of this experiment revealed the classic U-shaped curve in normal controls in the low-energy masking condition (e.g., masking by interruption). However, the patients showed deficits in this masking condition, in which masking by integration was greatly reduced: The patients' performance remained susceptible to masking by interruption for longer interstimulus intervals compared to normal controls.

We next examined in further detail the deficit in backward masking in schizophrenia by specifically examining the visual channels (i.e., transient and sustained) involved with masking by interruption (Green et al., 1994b). In the classic model of Breitmeyer and Ganz (1976), it was proposed that the transient onset of the mask interrupts sustained processing of the target. It may be the case in schizophrenia that patients have overactive transient channels, making them more susceptible to backward masking.

We attempted to determine the extent to which either the sustained channel or the transient channel contributes to schizophrenia patients' backward masking deficits by reducing the role of sustained channels. Most masking studies in schizophrenia at this time involved identification of a sharply focused target, a task heavily reliant on sustained channels. Whereas sustained cells are sensitive to high spatial frequency stimuli and are used in identification of stimuli, transient cells are sensitive to low-frequency (e.g., blurred) information and location of stimuli. Two conditions were used that took advantage of transient cells: In the first condition, a blurred target was presented at fixation in an identification task, and in the second condition, a sharply focused target was presented in a location task, where the target could appear at one of four locations away from fixation. The localization task theoretically reduced reliance on sustained channels even further than the identification task. In both conditions, schizophrenia patients exhibited a larger masking effect across SOAs than normal controls, whereby patients identified significantly fewer targets across all SOAs. These results showed that schizophrenia patients' deficit in backward masking is present even when the role of sustained channels is greatly limited. We hypothesized that schizophrenia patients have overactive transient (magnocellular) channels, which makes interruption of the target by the mask especially vulnerable.

To summarize, studies conducted in our lab point to an abnormality in the magnocellular system in schizophrenia patients. These results, as well as converging results from other studies of basic aspects of visual processing in schizophrenia (e.g., Butler et al., 2001; Doniger et al., 2002; Slaghuis & Bishop, 2001), show that abnormalities can be detected in low-level visual processes, such as detection of low-level frequency stimuli, that are linked to the functioning of the magnocellular pathway.

10.3.1   An Update of the Breitmeyer and Ganz Model

In a recent update to Breitmeyer and Ganz's (1976) model of backward masking, Öğmen (1993) proposed a model that incorporates retinal and postretinal activity in backward masking (see Breitmeyer & Öğmen, 2000, for a review). Dubbed *retinocortical dynamics* (RECOD), the model posits that recurrent, or feedback, transient inhibition occurs in both retinal and postretinal neurons.

The RECOD model predicts oscillations in the gamma range (30–70 Hz) in the sustained channels, and these oscillations should be observable in performance data. According to the RECOD model, transient inhibitory activity is more effective during synchronized firing of the postretinal neurons (Purushothaman et al., 2000). Strong masking occurs when transient activity generated by the mask temporally overlaps postretinal oscillatory activity generated by the target. Weak masking occurs when transient activity of the mask is not synchronous with the oscillatory firing of the target. As schizophrenia patients are known to exhibit gamma-range deficits in other areas such as auditory stimulation (Kwon et al., 1999), as assessed by electroencephalograph (EEG) recordings, we explored the possibility of whether their masking deficits may be due to abnormal gamma activity in masking.

10.4 Gamma Oscillations and Schizophrenia

10.4.1 Evidence of Gamma Deficits

It has been proposed that neural synchronization in the gamma range is important for information processing and feature binding (e.g., Tallon-Baudry et al., 1999), or how the brain integrates multisensory stimuli to form a coherent representation of an object processed in different areas of the cortex. It has also been suggested that abnormalities in synchronization may be present in schizophrenia patients (see Behrendt, 2003; Lee et al., 2003, for a review). The cognitive impairments seen in schizophrenia may be related to failures to integrate neural activity in both local and distributed networks. It has further been shown that gamma-aminobutyric acid (GABA) interneuronal interactions may be a possible mechanism underlying gamma synchronization (Traub et al., 1996; Whittington et al., 1995). GABAergic circuitry abnormalities have also been shown in schizophrenia patients (Grunze et al., 1996; McCarley et al., 1996). Partly for these reasons, there is a growing interest in gamma-range abnormalities in schizophrenia.

One of the first studies in this area examined whether schizophrenia patients exhibit normal gamma synchronization using an EEG entrainment to trains of auditory clicks (Kwon et al., 1999). While patients showed normal EEG synchronization to 20- and 30-Hz trains, they showed significantly less synchronization power and delayed synchronization to the 40-Hz train, which is in the gamma band. The investigators hypothesized that gamma abnormalities in schizophrenia may underlie abnormalities in perception and feature binding that may lead to reality distortions (i.e., hallucinations) and disorganized thought. Several recent studies, using various paradigms, have also shown abnormalities in schizophrenia patients to maintain gamma activity during auditory-oddball testing (Haig et al., 2000) and while viewing visual gestalts (Spencer et al., 2003).

Taken together, these results are suggestive of gamma-range abnormalities that exist in both early (evoked) and late (induced) gamma responses in schizophrenia, indicative of a failure to properly bind information to form percepts of stimuli as well as to process those stimuli. Considering the recent evidence that visual backward masking shows an oscillatory pattern in the gamma range, we decided to examine gamma activity, both psychophysical and physiological, during a backward masking task for schizophrenia patients and normal controls.

10.4.2   Gamma in Behavioral Data

Our first glimpse of oscillating performance came from a study that was not specifically designed to look for it. One of the studies mentioned above examined backward masking in unmedicated schizophrenia patients in psychotic remission (Green et al., 1999). Though not initially designed to examine cortical oscillations, results from this study revealed oscillations in normal controls that were suggestive of gamma activity. Moreover, schizophrenia patients failed to show these oscillations (figure 10.1).

In this study, each subject participated in three different masking conditions in a counterbalanced fashion. The first condition was a high-energy mask condition, which was expected to generate a monotonic masking function. The second condition was a low-energy mask condition, which was expected to generate a nonmonotonic U-shaped masking function. The final condition was a blurred target condition that reduced the reliance on sustained channels. For each condition, SOAs of 5, 10, 20, 40, 70, and 100 ms were used.

Schizophrenia patients showed deficits (i.e., significantly fewer correctly identified targets) across all three conditions compared to the normal controls, but there were also differences in the shapes of the functions. While patients showed U-shaped masking functions for all three conditions, normal controls showed a W-shaped (oscillating) masking function. Further analyses were then conducted between groups to assess the magnitude of the second-degree (U-shaped) and fourth-degree (W-shaped) shapes of the masking functions. Schizophrenia patients showed significant differences from normal controls on both the second- and fourth-degree polynomial function for each masking condition. To determine the exact nature of the group differences in the polynomial functions, within-group analyses were conducted. Controls showed a significant fourth-degree component on all three masking conditions, whereas the patients did not show any significant fourth-degree component for any of the masking conditions. The results show that only the normal controls exhibit oscillating masking functions whereas the lack of

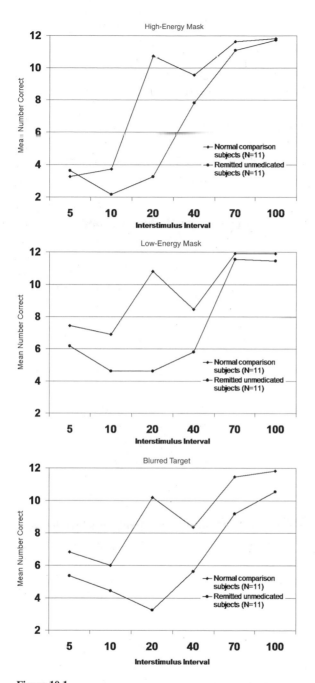

Figure 10.1
Visual masking performance of patients with schizophrenia in remission and normal control subjects. Three different masking conditions were used: top, target identification with a high-energy mask (20 ms for mask, 10 ms for target); middle, target identification with a low-energy mask (5 ms for mask, 10 ms for target); bottom, target identification with a blurred target (5 ms duration for mask, 20 ms for target). Targets were letters subtending 0.3° of visual angle presented at one of four locations that were 2.2° of visual angle from center of fixation. (From Green et al., 1999, *American Journal of Psychiatry*, 156, pp. 1367–1373, Copyright 1999, the American Psychiatric Association; http://ajp.psychiatryonline.org. Reprinted by permission)

an oscillating masking function in schizophrenia patients is consistent with abnormal gamma activity. In addition, the larger second-degree component of the masking function of the patients may reflect overactive transient channels, as suggested by our findings (Green et al., 1994b) and other independent laboratories (Schuck & Lee, 1989; Schwartz & Winstead, 1982). While the temporal resolution of the SOAs was not sufficient to adequately detect oscillations in the gamma range, the oscillations in the normal control data are at least consistent with gamma-range activity.

10.4.3 Reduced Gamma Oscillations During Masking: Behavioral and Electrophysiological Findings

To further explore the gamma deficits exhibited by schizophrenia patients, a large sample of patients and normal controls was recruited to examine their performance through nonlinear modeling (Green et al., 2003). Furthermore, a small subset of patients and controls underwent a masking procedure with simultaneous EEG recording to more directly measure their gamma responses.

Two masking conditions were chosen: an identification task (mainly reliant on sustained channels) and a location task (reliant on either transient or sustained channels). The two masking tasks were chosen because they both show maximum masking at an SOA near zero and lend themselves well to detrending and nonlinear modeling. The masking performance data were averaged for each SOA separately for the schizophrenia and normal comparison groups. The data were first detrended, to remove the upward slope. A two-stage model fitting was then performed on the residuals, following detrending, and analyzed with a four-parameter damped sine wave, which is the wave most consistent with the masking theory proposed by Purushothaman et al. (2000).

As expected, schizophrenia patients showed significant performance deficits in both masking tasks compared to normal controls for SOAs greater than zero. Normal controls had residuals that fit well with the damped sine wave for both masking functions, with frequencies of 30 Hz ($R^2 = .996$) for the location task and 35 Hz ($R^2 = .980$) for the identification task—that is, in the gamma range. However, for schizophrenia patients, no solution could be resolved using the damped sine wave, whereas a three-parameter undamped sine wave fit the patient data better with frequencies of 32.7 Hz for the location task and 14.9 Hz for the identification task (figure 10.2).

The second experiment directly measured gamma oscillations via simultaneously recording the EEG during the same target identification task as that in the first experiment. Event-related gamma activity was recorded during a target identification masking procedure across eight SOAs (12 trials at each SOA); unmasked trials were included in order to determine the specificity of the gamma findings to visual masking. Electrodes were positioned in the occipitoparietal area because of this region's relevance for visual processing during the masking task.

The results of this study are summarized in figure 10.3. All four sites were summed, and gamma amplitude was converted to z scores. Results revealed a trend in the Group × Epoch (i.e, evoked vs. induced) × Condition (masked vs. unmasked) interaction, $F(1, 13) = 3.42, p < .10$. Further exploration of this interaction revealed no significant group differences for activity elicited by unmasked targets. However, as can be seen in figure 10.3, normal controls showed significantly ($p < .05$) greater induced gamma activity (i.e., in the range of 200–400 ms) in the masking condition compared to schizophrenia patients, suggestive of normal feature binding and perceptual organization in normal controls (Tallon-Baudry & Bertrand, 1999).

The results from the behavioral data of the first experiment and the physiological data of the second experiment reveal that schizophrenia patients are unable to maintain normal gamma activity during a visual backward masking task. While the data strongly implicate gamma abnormalities in schizophrenia, they do not directly indicate that gamma abnormalities cause the backward masking deficits in schizophrenia. Masking deficits may be due to abnormalities in patients' transient channels, they may be partially due to abnormal gamma activity that is a characteristic of sustained channels (Purushothaman et al., 2000), or the gamma abnormalities may entirely explain the poor masking performance in schizophrenia patients. In current studies in our laboratory, we are attempting to distinguish between these alternatives in a larger sample by using a larger electrode array, examining gamma activity for each SOA, and examining correct and incorrect trials in both the unmasked and masked conditions.

10.5 fMRI Findings During Masking

Our most recent studies into visual backward masking have taken advantage of the advances in fMRI technology to apply the masking paradigm to the fMRI scanner. We recently conducted a masking study during fMRI acquisition in a small sample of normal controls to demonstrate the feasibility of using our masking paradigm in a scanner and to determine the initial regions of interest to explore when comparing normal controls and schizophrenia patients (Green et al., 2005).

We examined the effects of SOA (SOAs of 34, 68, and 102 ms) in masking within several regions of interest (ROIs) in cortex in normal controls. We used two approaches to identify regions. In one approach, we selected regions a priori based on reference scans that used previously validated stimuli designed to activate

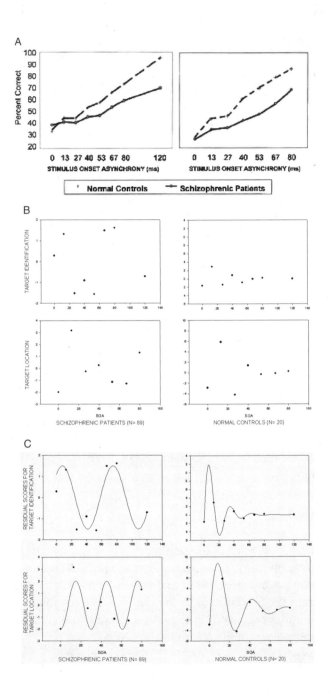

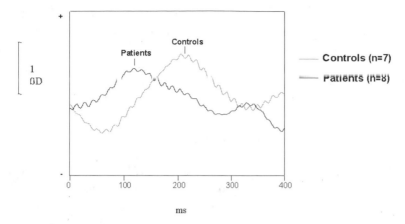

Figure 10.3
Event-related gamma activity (averaged across parietal and occipital sites) for masked trials for schizophrenia patients and normal control subjects. Data are in z-score units, with the size of one standard deviation noted by the bar on the left. (Reprinted from *Biological Psychiatry*, Vol. 53, Green, M. F., Mintz, J., Salveson, D., Nuechterlein, K. H., Breitmeyer, B. G., Light, G. A., & Braff, D. L., Visual masking as a probe for abnormal gama range activity in schizophrenia, pp. 1113–1119, Copyright 2003, with permission from Society of Biological Psychiatry)

specific visual areas—for example, V1 and V2, lateral occipital (LO) cortex, and human area MT (hMT+). In addition, we used a data-driven approach to identify ROIs in which we selected regions that were generally active during the backward masking task (all intervals of masking minus rest) and then determined which areas showed the predicted pattern of greater activation with longer SOA.

Results of the behavioral performance of subjects in the scanner showed a consistent SOA-dependent masking effect, reflecting that masking could indeed be successfully implemented during a functional imaging sequence. Among the regions identified with the ROI approach, ventral LO and, to a lesser degree, dorsal LO showed the largest hemodynamic response to the longest SOA and the smallest response to the shortest SOA.

Figure 10.2
Nonlinear modeling of masking performance data. (*A*) Performance data for patients and comparison subjects for two of the backward masking tasks (target identification, left; target location, right). In both tasks, patients showed poorer performance compared with control subjects. Stimulus onset asynchronies (SOAs) are indicated on the *x*-axis and performance on the *y*-axis. (*B*) Reisduals (after detrending) of the backward masking data for each group by masking task. (*C*) Results of the curve fitting of the residual scores for each masking task. The comparison group was fit with a damped (four-paramter) sine wave. The patients were fit with an undamped (three parameter) sine wave. (Reprinted from *Biological Psychiatry*, Vol. 53, Green, M. F., Mintz, J., Salveson, D., Nuechterlein, K. H., Breitmeyer, B. G., Light, G. A., & Braff, D. L., Visual masking as a probe for abnormal gama range activity in schizophrenia, pp. 1113–1119, Copyright 2003, with permission from Society of Biological Psychiatry)

Using the data-driven approach, ROIs were identified using a difference map in which all SOAs were contrasted with a resting state. Six regions were identified based on activity to masking stimuli regardless of sensitivity to SOA: inferior parietal, anterior cingulate, precentral, insula, thalamic, and occipital regions. A time-course analysis on each of these areas showed an increased hemodynamic response to weaker masking in the thalamus (primarily localized to the pulvinar), inferior parietal, and anterior cingulate.

The main goal of this study was to identify regions that are sensitive to the interval between the target and mask, thus reflecting the neural substrates of the visual backward masking effect. The results showed that the ventral LO region, and not earlier visual cortex, consistently exhibited SOA-dependent hemodynamic responses, making this a likely source of the neural masking effect. We hypothesize that LO is the first location in cortex that contains a sufficiently large number of neurons that respond differentially to our target versus mask stimuli and that integrate information over a minimum of 30–60 ms of our short SOAs.

The data-driven approach also identified several areas that show SOA-dependent activity, notably the inferior parietal region, the thalamus (pulvinar), and the anterior cingulate region. We hypothesize that these regions are more related to higher level attentional processes. Specifically, we hypothesize that these regions may be reflective of reentrant processing (the theory that higher level cortical processes influence low-level perceptual activity) that provides feedback to early visual processing centers (Enns & Di Lollo, 2000; chapter 9, this volume).

While this study had some limitations (small sample size, small range of SOAs, unequated unmasked targets), it allowed us to initially identify areas in the brain that show masking-related regional activation. As part of our larger program of research investigating early visual processing deficits in schizophrenia, this study will allow us to examine in better detail exactly where in the stream of visual processing schizophrenia patients show reduced brain activation.

10.6   Functional Significance of Masking Deficits in Schizophrenia

One of the main goals of our laboratory has been to explore the variables that contribute to functional outcome in schizophrenia. We have shown previously that specific domains of neurocognition—namely, secondary verbal memory, working verbal memory, and executive functioning measured with the Wisconsin Card Sorting Test—are consistently related to functional outcome (Green, 1996). We recently explored the relationship between visual backward masking and social cognition, which may be a mediator between neurocognition and social and functional outcome in schizophrenia (Green & Nuechterlein, 1999). *Social cognition* refers to the ability to perceive, interpret, and process information about oneself and others in social situations (Penn et al., 1997). It has been found that tests of early visual processing, such as the Span of Apprehension Test, are related to social perception (Corrigan et al., 1994). In an initial study in this area, we tested whether backward masking is related to social perception in schizophrenia (Sergi & Green, 2003). We found that patients with poorer social perception performed significantly worse (i.e., showed larger masking effects across SOAs) on tests of backward masking than those with better social perception. This study supports an association between social cognition and neurocognition in schizophrenia (e.g., Addington & Addington, 1998; Corrigan et al., 1994; Kee et al., 1998), which is an important step in understanding the neurocognitive deficits involved with poor social functioning in schizophrenia.

10.7   Future Directions

For the past 15 years, the focus of our research program has been to gain a better understanding of the nature of the early visual processing deficits exhibited by schizophrenia patients and first-degree relatives through the use of visual backward masking. We have learned a considerable amount about the nature of the deficit and have recently begun to explore new avenues to shed light on the visual processing abnormalities in schizophrenia. We are now shifting our focus to include studies of how early attentional processes might affect visual processing in schizophrenia. We mention two examples: common-onset four-dot masking and the attentional blink.

As mentioned in our discussion of fMRI findings on backward masking, we hypothesize that certain brain regions (i.e., thalamic, anterior cingulate, and inferior parietal regions) may show SOA-dependent activity that reflects allocation of attention to the mask. These processes may reflect reentrant processing of the target in the presence of the mask. Given the possibility that masking deficits in schizophrenia could be due, at least in part, to reentrant processes, we are currently assessing this possibility empirically using common-onset four-dot masking adapted from Enns and Di Lollo (1997, 2000). In addition, we intend to further assess the interactions between attentional processes and visual masking in schizophrenia through the use of the attentional blink paradigm (Chun & Potter, 1995; Raymond et al., 1992). These are both examples of taking well-validated paradigms from the experimental literature and using them to understand abnormalities in visual processes.

10.8   Conclusions

A defining goal of our research program has been to gain a better understanding of the nature of the early visual processing deficits exhibited by schizophrenia patients. We now have a better understanding of the neurophysiological deficits associated with masking deficits (i.e., poorer target detection across SOAs that persists longer than that of normal subjects) in schizophrenia through the examination of transient and sustained channels and their role in backward masking. Incorporating the latest theories of masking and neurophysiology, we have also found that schizophrenia patients are unable to exhibit neural synchronization in the gamma range, which may contribute to their masking deficits. Finally, we have made progress in understanding the neural structures associated with backward masking using functional neuroimaging in normal subjects. This area of research will allow us to examine which specific areas in the brain are linked to abnormal masking in schizophrenia.

Our program of research has been dependent on advances in studies of early visual processing in normal controls. It has been our goal to utilize the advances of basic behavioral researchers who study early visual processing in normal controls and apply those methods to gain a better understanding of the visual processing deficits seen in schizophrenia. The refinement of the basic science of early visual processing has allowed us to better direct our research program in schizophrenia. Given the presence of subtle visual processing abnormalities in siblings of patients, these advances may eventually lead to a greater understanding of the genetics of schizophrenia and provide clues for more effective pharmacotherapies. It is through the continued translation of basic behavioral to clinical science that we will be able to gain a better understanding of the nature of early visual processing deficits in schizophrenia.

Acknowledgments

The research and preparation of this chapter was supported by National Institute of Mental Health (NIMH) Grant MH-43292 to Michael F. Green and by the Department of Veterans Affairs, Veterans Integrated Services Network 22 Mental Illness Research, Education, and Clinical Center. Jonathan K. Wynn was supported during preparation of this chapter by NIMH National Research Service Award Training Grant MH-14584 (principal investigator: Keith Nuechterlein).

IV TEMPORAL ASPECTS OF ATTENTION

11 The Operation of Attention—Millisecond by Millisecond—Over the First Half Second

Steven J. Luck

11.1 Chapter Overview

This chapter reviews two decades of progress in mapping out the time course of visual attention over the first half second. In particular, the chapter will examine what kinds of attention-related processes operate at various times after the onset of a stimulus. Traditional behavioral methods do not typically directly reveal the precise time at which attention operates, and the chapter will therefore emphasize techniques that provide a continuous, millisecond-level measure of processing, especially the event-related potential (ERP) technique.

11.2 The ERP Technique

Because the ERP technique is not as well-known as some other techniques, it is worth spending a few words on the essential aspects of this technique, particularly with respect to its temporal properties. ERPs almost exclusively reflect postsynaptic potentials that occur when neurotransmitters bind with receptors, causing ion channels to open or close (see Allison et al., 1980; Nunez, 1981). This contrasts with single-unit and multi-unit recordings, which measure the action potentials that occur if the summed postsynaptic potentials across many synapses reach the neuron's threshold for firing. Thus, ERPs reflect the inputs to a neuron, whereas single-unit and multi-unit recordings reflect the outputs from a neuron.

Postsynaptic potentials in neurons are accompanied by changes in the local electrical field, and a nearby electrode can easily measure these *local field potentials*. The electrical potentials elicited by different neurons combine together by simple addition, and if postsynaptic potentials occur in many similarly oriented neurons at the same time, the sum of the local field potentials will be large enough to record at a distance. Local field potentials can therefore be recorded from within the cortex or from the cortical surface in patients undergoing exploratory neurosurgery. The brain is a highly conductive medium, and the electrical fields resulting from post-synaptic potentials at one location therefore spread throughout the entire brain, although they diminish in size as the recording electrode is moved away from the source. The skull has a higher resistance than the brain, and electricity follows the path of least resistance, so much of the electrical activity spreads laterally when it reaches the skull. However, some of the activity does pass through the skull to the scalp, where it can be recorded noninvasively.

The electrical potentials recorded on the scalp or the cortical surface are termed the *electroencephalogram* (EEG). The EEG reflects the summed activity of many different brain systems operating in parallel to perform various tasks, and when an experimenter presents a stimulus, only a small portion of the overall EEG reflects the processing of this stimulus. Consequently, if the scalp EEG following a single stimulus is examined, it is difficult to extract the response to the stimulus from the other, unrelated sources of electrical activity. The simplest way to extract the stimulus-related activity is to average together the EEG segments from a large number of stimulus presentations. Any consistent stimulus-evoked activity should be present on every trial, whereas any unrelated EEG activity will sometimes be positive and sometimes be negative. Consequently, the consistent stimulus-related activity will remain in the average, but unrelated EEG activity will cancel out and approach zero if enough trials are averaged together. In the experiments described in this chapter, at least 100 trials were averaged together for each condition in each subject. The resulting averaged waveforms are called *event-related potentials* because they are electrical *potentials* that are *related* to a specific *event*, such as the presentation of a stimulus.

Figure 11.1 shows an example of the ERP waveform elicited by a flashed visual stimulus. Note that time zero represents the onset of the stimulus and that, by convention, negative is plotted upward. A series of positive and negative peaks can be observed following the onset of the stimulus, reflecting the flow of information through the visual system and into higher cognitive and response systems. The peaks are also called *waves* or *components*, and they are typically labeled with a *P* or *N* to indicate whether the peak is a positive- or negative-going one, along with a number to indicate timing (e.g., *P1* for the first major positive peak, or *P115* to indicate its precise latency of 115 ms). For visual stimuli, an early component arising from area V1 is often observed, and this component is often called *C1* because it may be either positive or negative, depending on the spatial location of the evoking stimulus (the variations in C1 polarity are caused by the distinctive folding pattern of area V1 in the human brain). The C1 component is followed by P1 and N1 components that are modality specific. That is, the P1 and N1 waves elicited by a visual stimulus are completely unrelated to the P1 and N1 waves elicited by an auditory stimulus (they have the same names across modalities only because of their

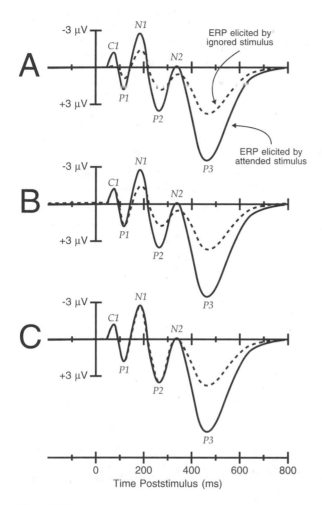

Figure 11.1
Examples of early (*A*), intermediate (*B*), and late (*C*) effects of attention on the visual event-related potential (ERP) waveform. Each waveform shows how voltage varies over time. By convention, negative is plotted upward. Time zero represents the moment of stimulus onset.

temporal order and polarity, not because of any functional relationship). By the time of the P2 and N2 waves, a combination of modality-specific and modality-independent activity is present, and the P3 wave is largely modality independent.

11.3 Spatial Resolution and Magnetic Recordings

Cognitive neuroscience techniques are often described along the dimensions of temporal resolution and spatial resolution. The ERP technique has relatively poor spatial resolution. One factor that contributes to this is the high resistance of the skull, which causes the electrical field to spread laterally. To avoid this, it is possible to record the magnetic field that accompanies the EEG, which is called the magnetoencephalogram. Electrical dipoles are always accompanied by magnetic fields, and changes in the magnitude of the electrical potential lead directly to changes in the strength of the magnetic field. Consequently, one can obtain essentially the same information by recording magnetic rather than electrical activity, and the same averaging approach can be used, yielding event-related magnetic fields (ERMFs) rather than ERPs. The advantage of ERMF recordings is that the skull is transparent to magnetism, eliminating the spatial blurring that is present in ERP recordings and providing improved spatial resolution. However, the magnetic fields are extremely small, especially in comparison to the Earth's magnetic field, and recording ERMFs requires extraordinarily sensitive and extremely expensive equipment. In addition, ERP/ERMF localization is much more indirect than, for example, localization of the blood oxygen level dependent (BOLD) signal in functional magnetic resonance imaging (fMRI) experiments. In particular, ERMFs and ERPs are localized by means of mathematical modeling techniques, and the models are evaluated by testing their ability to fit the observed pattern of data. The models typically have very large numbers of free parameters (tens, hundreds, or even thousands), and a given data set can potentially be fit by an infinite number of models. Consequently, ERP/ERMF localization models are not usually definitive. That is, they provide a useful suggestion about the likely generator source of a given signal, but it is not usually possible to provide a margin of error, a likelihood ratio, or some other quantification of confidence in the localization.

11.4 Temporal Resolution of ERPs

Although the ERP technique does not have high spatial resolution, it has very high temporal resolution. Electrical potentials pass through conductors essentially instantaneously, so fluctuations in voltage recorded at the scalp provide a precise index of fluctuations of neural activity within the brain. The bioelectric properties of the brain, skull, and scalp presumably lead to some temporal distortion of scalp-recorded ERPs, but the temporal resolution can be in the submillisecond range under optimal recording conditions. In most attention experiments, the effective resolution is probably on the order of 5–10 ms. This lower resolution is caused by several factors, including the use of filters to attenuate high-frequency electrical noise. However, this level of temporal resolution is entirely sufficient to answer most questions about attention, and higher temporal resolution is possible when necessary.

Although many writers have praised the temporal resolution of ERPs, raw temporal resolution is not really the main advantage of this technique. After all, it would be trivial to record button-press reaction times (RTs) with submillisecond resolution. The key advantage of ERPs over behavioral and neuroimaging measures is that ERPs provide a high-resolution and *continuous* measure of processing. That is, whereas an RT measure provides no information about processing between the time of the stimulus and the time of the response, ERPs provide a continuous measure of processing between the stimulus and the response (and even after the response). Neuroimaging methods can also provide a continuous measure of processing, potentially sampling at relatively high rates. However, current methods primarily measure the consequences of changes in blood flow, and these changes are very slow, so the effective temporal resolution of current neuroimaging methods is typically on the order of a few seconds (although resolution on the order of a few hundred milliseconds may be possible under certain conditions). Consequently, ERPs and ERMFs provide the only mainstream techniques for providing noninvasive, continuous measures of processing with high levels of temporal resolution.

11.5   Limitations of the ERP Technique

Although the ERP technique has many advantages over other techniques, it also has some significant limitations. First, as already mentioned, ERPs do not provide a direct means of determining the neuroanatomical sites of activation. Second, ERP waveforms are almost always based on averages of tens or hundreds of trials, and any trial-to-trial variations in the operation of attention may be lost in the averaged waveforms. In a visual search task, for example, attention might shift in a different spatial pattern on each trial, and this would be difficult to see in an averaged ERP waveform (note, however, that this problem is not entirely impossible to solve—see Woodman & Luck, 1999, 2003b). In addition, activity that is evoked by the stimulus but varies randomly in phase will average to zero in the averaged ERP waveforms (but this can be addressed by spectral analysis methods—see, e.g., Tallon-Baudry et al., 1996). Third, the observed ERP waveform consists of a set of internal components that sum together, and it can be very difficult to determine exactly which ERP component is influenced by an experimental manipulation. For example, attended auditory stimuli elicit a more negative response than ignored auditory stimuli in the time range of the N1 wave, but it has been difficult to determine whether this effect reflects an amplification of the sensory-evoked N1 wave or the addition of overlapping endogenous brain activity (Hansen & Hillyard, 1980; Naatanen, 1975; Woldorff et al., 1993). Finally, like the BOLD signal in fMRI experiments, the relationship between scalp-recorded ERPs and specific neural events is somewhat indirect, and it is therefore challenging (although not impossible) to draw precise conclusions about the information-processing transactions represented by a given ERP effect.

11.6   Measuring the Time Course of Attention

A straightforward way to study the timing of attentional processes is to examine the ERP waveform elicited by a given stimulus when it is attended and when it is ignored, determining the time point at which the waveform differs due to the allocation of attention (for classic examples, see Eason et al., 1969; Hillyard et al., 1973; Van Voorhis & Hillyard, 1977). As illustrated in figure 11.1A, attention might suppress the response to an ignored visual stimulus relative to an attended stimulus beginning in area V1, leading to a reduced C1 amplitude (and reductions in all of the subsequent ERP components). In contrast, attention may have no effect on the initial sensory response, influencing activity beginning at the time of the N1 wave (see figure 11.1B). Or, as proposed by late-selection theories of attention, attention may have no effect until the time of late, modality-independent ERP components, such as the P3 wave (see figure 11.1C). Given that visual information processing does not consist of a set of discrete, serially ordered stages, it is also possible that attention could influence some early components without influencing all of the later components.

In this manner, ERPs can be used to pinpoint the time at which attention begins to influence processing. Two caveats are necessary, however. First, the absence of an early effect does not by itself imply that attention only operates at late stages. Only a fraction of neural activity can be detected with ERP recordings, and it is always possible that an early effect is present but cannot be observed with ERPs (e.g., the individual local field potentials may be oriented in a manner that causes them to cancel out).

A second caveat is that raw timing is of limited use unless it can be linked to specific processes. Given what we know about the time course of information processing in visual cortex (see, e.g., Schmolesky et al., 1998), it is usually safe to conclude that any effects of attention arising from visual cortex within 100 ms of stimulus onset reflect a modulation of perceptual processing rather than modulations of higher level cognitive processing (although some prefrontal activity begins this early—see Foxe & Simpson, 2002). And given the use of brief stimuli, any effects of attention after 300 ms poststimulus can be assumed to reflect modulations of higher level processing and not perceptual modulations. However, this leaves a large ambiguous range (100–300 ms), and it makes more sense to treat the perceptual–cognitive distinction as continuous rather than categorical. Consequently, it is important to supplement raw timing information with other sources of evidence about the specific nature of the attention effects. The next sections will summarize what has been learned about the effects of attention in this type of experimental paradigm, in which attention is explicitly directed toward or away from a given stimulus source. We will begin with studies in which the stimulus source is defined by its location and then move on to other feature dimensions.

11.7 Visuospatial Attention: Timing and Neural Substrates

Many ERP experiments have examined visuospatial attention using variations on the sustained attention paradigm illustrated in figure 11.2A. In this paradigm, subjects fixate a central point, and fixation is monitored to ensure that covert rather than overt attention is manipulated. Stimuli are flashed in a rapid, random sequence to locations in the left and right visual fields, and subjects are instructed to monitor one of the two locations for target stimuli for a period of a few minutes. Most of the stimuli are nontarget stimuli, and the targets are defined by a subtle difference in some dimension, such as size. Subjects make a button-press response when they detect targets in the attended location, and they are told to ignore all stimuli in the other location. They attend to one location on some trial blocks and attend to the other location on other trial blocks, making it possible to compare the response to a given stimulus when it is attended versus when it is ignored. Because the task is identical for the attend-left and attend-right conditions and the order of stimuli is unpredictable, the subject's state of arousal is equated across conditions. Thus, any differences in the ERPs elicited by a given stimulus when it is attended compared to when it is ignored can be attributed to specific spatial attention effects.

This experimental paradigm is similar to the spatial cuing paradigm that is popular among behavioral attention researchers, but it differs in two key ways. First, after attention is directed to a specific location, only one stimulus is presented in the spatial cuing paradigm, whereas a long stream of stimuli is presented in the sustained attention paradigm (and attention must be sustained to the cued location through the entire stream). The use of a long stream of stimuli is helpful in ERP

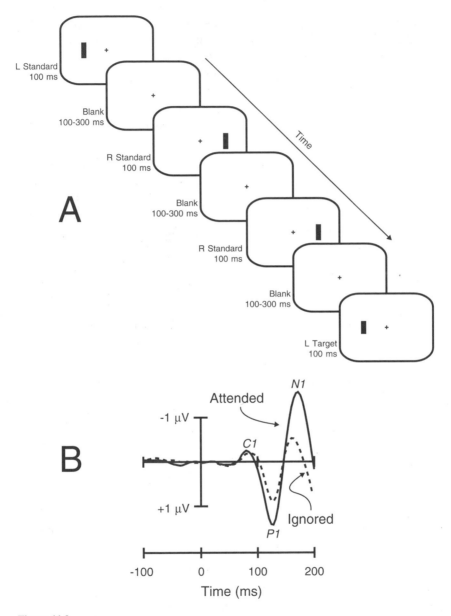

Figure 11.2
(*A*) Schematic version of sustained attention paradigm that is commonly used to assess the time course of attention in event-related potential experiments. Subjects are instructed to attend to the left or right visual field at the beginning of each trial block and press a button when slightly shorter target stimuli are presented at that location. Subjects are also required to maintain fixation on the central fixation point at all times, and accurate fixation performance is monitored. (*B*) Typical results from this type of experiment (from the study of Gomez Gonzales et al., 1994). The C1 component is not influenced by the direction of attention, but the P1 and N1 components elicited by a stimulus are larger when that stimulus appears on the attended side than when that stimulus appears on the unattended side.

research because it allows many more stimuli to be presented in a given amount of time (i.e., less time is "wasted" on presenting cues). This is important for achieving reasonably low-noise averaged ERP waveforms. The second difference is that subjects in the spatial cuing paradigm are instructed to respond to targets in the uncued locations as well as targets in the cued location, whereas subjects in the sustained attention paradigm are instructed to respond to targets only in the cued location. Responses to uncued targets are simply unnecessary when ERPs are recorded. These differences do not seem to have a substantial impact on attentional processes, because the same basic pattern of results has been obtained in both types of paradigms (see, e.g., Mangun & Hillyard, 1991).

In most studies using the sustained attention paradigm, the P1 and/or N1 components have been found to be larger for attended-location stimuli than for ignored-location stimuli, whether the stimuli are targets or nontargets. Some of these studies were also designed to evoke a C1 wave (from area V1), and these studies have demonstrated that the C1 wave is not influenced by attention. An example of this is shown in figure 11.2B (from the study of Gomez Gonzales et al., 1994). The P1 effect typically begins between 70 and 100 ms poststimulus, indicating that attention influences perceptual processing in this paradigm. The lack of a C1 effect suggests that attention does not influence processing in or prior to area V1, although it is possible that attention influences some sort of V1 response that does not contribute to scalp-recorded ERPs.

Heinze and his collaborators attempted to localize the P1 attention effect by combining ERP recordings with positron emission tomography (PET) imaging in a paradigm similar to that shown in figure 11.2A (Heinze et al., 1994). The PET data indicated an effect of attention in the fusiform gyrus, along the ventral surface of the occipital lobe. Mathematical modeling procedures demonstrated that this location was a plausible source of the P1 attention effect. Specifically, a pair of electrical dipoles located in the left- and right-hemisphere fusiform gyri could explain 96% of the scalp distribution of the P1 wave. More recent studies combining ERPs with fMRI have replicated this finding but have also shown that a portion of the P1 wave appears to arise from dorsal extrastriate areas (e.g., dorsal V3—see Martinez et al., 2001). Less work has focused on localizing the N1 attention effect (see Clark & Hillyard, 1996). This is due, in part, to the nature of mathematical modeling procedures: The N1 effect is overlapped by the P1 effect, and small errors in localizing the P1 effect could lead to larger errors in localizing the N1 effect.

Research using this paradigm has also been conducted with monkeys, using single-unit recordings (Luck et al., 1997a). Consistent with the human ERP studies, no effects of attention were observed in area V1. Attention effects were observed in areas V2 and V4. One key finding was that the effect of attention in V4 began at 60 ms poststimulus, which was the onset time of the sensory response in that area.

This is consistent with the proposal that visuospatial attention may serve as a sensory gain control, increasing or decreasing the feedforward transmission of information through extrastriate cortex (Hillyard et al., 1998). Another key finding is that a given neuron's activity was modulated by attention only when both the attended and ignored locations were inside that neuron's receptive field (typically separated by no more than 3° of visual angle). The human ERP studies have typically used very distant locations that would never fit within a V2 or V4 receptive field, suggesting that the P1 and N1 effects arise from a region such as inferotemporal cortex, where the receptive fields are very large.

Together, these studies indicate that visuospatial attention does not influence neural responses in area V1 but does change the gain of feedforward sensory transmission in extrastriate visual areas within the first 100 ms after stimulus onset. In contrast, several fMRI studies have found effects of attention in area V1 (e.g., Gandhi et al., 1999; Somers et al., 1999). There are two likely explanations for this discrepancy. First, it is possible that the fMRI studies used a task that was more appropriate for engaging attentional mechanisms in area V1. Second, it is possible that the fMRI effects reflect some kind of feedback signal rather than a modulation of feedforward sensory activity. Current evidence points to the second of these possibilities. First, a single-unit study using the curve-tracing paradigm has shown that attention effects are present in area V1 but that these effects begin more than 200 ms after stimulus onset (Roelfsema et al., 1998). Second, Martinez and her collaborators recorded both fMRI and ERP data from a group of subjects engaged in a spatial attention task similar to that shown in figure 11.2A, and they found an attention effect in area V1 in the fMRI recordings but no modulation of the C1 wave in the ERP recordings. Because the same task was used for both types of recordings, task differences cannot explain the discrepancy between the fMRI V1 results and the ERP C1 results. Third, additional studies using ERMFs or a combination of ERPs and fMRI have confirmed the finding of no effect on the initial sensory response in area V1 but have shown a V1 effect beginning around 150 ms (Di Russo et al., 2003; Martinez et al., 2001; Noesselt et al., 2002). Thus, the evidence so far indicates that any attention effects in area V1 reflect a feedback signal of some unknown origin rather than a modulation of feedforward sensory activity. We are just beginning to understand the role of feedback in area V1 (see, e.g., Lamme, 1995), so the functional role of this feedback effect is not yet known.

11.8   Visuospatial Attention: Enhancement Versus Suppression

Although these data suggest that attention operates like a gain control within extrastriate cortex, this is probably an oversimplification. For example, it is not the case that all of the ERP components from the P1 wave onward are decreased by a constant factor for ignored-location stimuli compared to attended-location stimuli. Indeed, it is possible to obtain a P1 modulation without an N1 modulation and vice versa. Some studies have therefore attempted to provide a more detailed characterization of the nature of the P1 and N1 attention effects. Several dissociations between the P1 and N1 effects have been described, and these differences led to the proposal that the P1 effect reflects a mechanism that suppresses activity at unattended locations to avoid interference, whereas the N1 effect reflects a limited-capacity discrimination mechanism that is applied to the attended location (see the review by Luck, 1995).

The proposal that the P1 effect reflects distractor suppression whereas the N1 effect reflects target enhancement was based, in part, on studies in which a neutral attention condition was included (Luck & Hillyard, 1995; Luck et al., 1994). In one study, for example, attention was directed to one of four locations on each trial by a central arrow cue, and neutral trials were included in which all four locations were cued. The P1 wave was found to be suppressed on *invalid* trials, in which one location was cued and the target appeared at a different location, compared to *neutral* trials, in which attention was distributed over all four locations. However, when compared to the neutral trials, no enhancement of the P1 was observed on *valid* trials, in which one location was cued and the target appeared at the cued location.

Another important difference is that P1 attention effects are observed primarily when the target discrimination might be impaired by distracting information, whereas N1 effects are observed when a discrimination is being made, regardless of whether distraction is likely. For example, the P1 effect was observed in a task that required subjects to combine two features of a target that were individually present in the distractors (Luck et al., 1993), but this effect was eliminated in a nearly identical task in which the target was defined by the presence of a single feature (Luck & Hillyard, 1995). This fits with the idea that attention is necessary to combine features but not to detect them (Treisman & Gelade, 1980). The N1 effect was present in both of these conditions, but it was eliminated when subjects made a simple detection response rather than a discriminative response (Mangun & Hillyard, 1991). Further studies have shown that the N1 wave is larger when subjects perform discrimination tasks than when they perform detection tasks, even if all of the stimuli are presented at a single, attended location (Ritter et al., 1979; Vogel & Luck, 2000) and that this effect arises from ventral–lateral regions of occipito-temporal cortex (Hopf et al., 2002).

11.9   Nonspatial Features

Spatial location plays a distinctive role in visual representation. Beginning with the lenses of the eyes and continuing through area V1, the visual system uses special mechanisms and considerable resources to coding space precisely and explicitly. Space has also been accorded a special status in several theories of attention (e.g., Logan, 1996; Nissen, 1985; Treisman & Gelade, 1980). ERP studies have supported a special status for space in visual attention, because spatial attention effects typically begin earlier than nonspatial attention effects.

Early studies of attention to nonspatial features used tasks that were analogous to the spatial attention paradigm shown in figure 11.2A, except that some other feature dimension replaced the dimension of spatial location (see, e.g., Anllo-Vento et al., 1998; Harter & Guido, 1980; Harter & Previc, 1978). In the study of Anllo-Vento et al. (1998), for example, subjects were instructed to monitor a stream of foveal stimuli, some of which were red and some of which were blue, attending to one color and ignoring the other color. The ERPs elicited by a given color when that color was attended were then compared to the ERPs elicited by that color when it was ignored. Feature-based attention effects have not been found to modulate the P1 wave; instead, the effects typically begin in the latency range of the P2 and N2 components. The most common pattern is a more negative-going waveform that begins around 150 ms poststimulus and lasts for 100–300 ms (this effect is often called a *selection negativity*).

Hillyard and Münte (1984) combined spatial and nonspatial attention within a single experiment to further define how they are related. Subjects attended to a particular color at a particular location, making it possible to examine the responses elicited by a stimulus that was attended along both dimensions, along only one dimension, or along neither dimension. Space was found to dominate color. Specifically, attended-location stimuli were found to elicit larger P1 waves than ignored-location stimuli, regardless of whether the color was attended or ignored. In contrast, a selection negativity was observed for attended-color stimuli compared to ignored-color stimuli, but only for attended-location stimuli. Unattended-location stimuli of the attended and ignored colors elicited nearly identical ERP waveforms. Thus, attention appeared to operate hierarchically, with location-based selection occurring first and color-based selection occurring only for attended-location stimuli. However, this pattern may obtain only if attention is strongly focused in advance of stimulus onset: As will be discussed later, feature-based attention may often be used to guide spatial attention to likely target objects.

11.10   The Visual Search Task

In sustained attention and trial-by-trial cuing paradigms, attention may be focused on a location prior to stimulus onset, making it possible for attention to modulate the initial feedforward wave of sensory activity evoked by the stimulus. In many real-world situations, however, attention shifts among items that are already present, guided by feature information. Imagine, for example, that you are eating a meal in a restaurant and that you would like to eat a green bean. To select a single bean as the target for your fork, you will shift first the spatial focus of attention to the pile of green beans to determine which bean to eat. In this situation, you will likely use both the color of the green beans and your knowledge of their general location on the plate to shift attention appropriately.

In the laboratory, visual search tasks are used to approximate this sort of real-world situation. Subjects are told to search for a target defined by a particular set of features (e.g., a long green line), and then an array of objects is presented that may or may not contain the target. In most cases, subjects press one of two buttons to indicate whether the target was present or absent. Feature information is typically used to guide attention to likely target objects (e.g., subjects might shift attention to each green item to determine whether it is the long, green target). Spatial information can also be used to guide attention (Chun & Jiang, 1998).

11.11 The N2pc Component

In ERP studies of visual search, the focusing of attention is associated with a component called *N2pc* (N2–posterior–contralateral), which occurs in the N2 latency range (200–300 ms) and has a posterior, contralateral scalp distribution. This component was first observed by Luck and Hillyard (1990), and it was also observed in two other studies published in the same year (Heinze et al., 1990; Luck et al., 1990). The evidence linking this component with the focusing of attention was provided by several subsequent studies (Luck et al., 1997b; Luck & Hillyard, 1994a, 1994b).

The typical paradigm for eliciting an N2pc component is shown in figure 11.3A. Subjects are instructed to attend to one color at the beginning of each trial block, and for each stimulus they must indicate whether the item drawn in that color is an upright *T* or an inverted *T*. Two distinctively colored items are present in each array, one in each hemifield, and subjects attend to one of these colors on each trial block. This makes it possible to examine the ERPs elicited by identical stimuli but with differing directions of attention. When left-hemisphere ERP waveforms are examined, the voltage from approximately 200–300 ms is found to be more negative for right-hemifield (contralateral) targets than for left-hemifield (ipsilateral) targets (see figure 11.3B). When right-hemisphere ERP waveforms are examined, the voltage is more negative for left-hemifield (contralateral) targets than for right-hemifield (ipsilateral) targets (see figure 11.3C).

The stimuli and tasks used in N2pc experiments are usually somewhat different from those used in behavioral experiments. There are two reasons for this. First, in

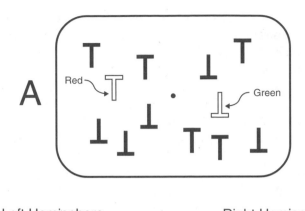

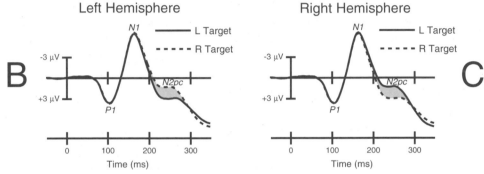

Figure 11.3
Experimental paradigm (*A*) and results (*B–C*) from a typical N2pc component. Subjects are told to attend either to red or to green at the beginning of each block of trials, pressing one of two buttons on each trial to indicate whether the item drawn in the attended color is an upright *T* or an inverted *T*. The positions of the items are randomized from trial to trial, so the subjects do not know which side will contain the attended color prior to stimulus onset. ERPs are recorded from electrodes over left and right posterior cortical areas. For left-hemisphere electrode sites (*B*), the response is more negative going (i.e., less positive) when the target is in the right hemisphere than when the target is in the left hemisphere. For right-hemisphere electrode sites (*C*), the response is more negative going when the target is in the left hemisphere than when the target is in the right hemisphere.

ERP experiments it is important to avoid low-level sensory confounds by comparing the responses to physically identical stimuli and vary only the instructions (e.g., attend red vs. attend green). Second, in many behavioral search tasks, the target is difficult to distinguish from the distractors, leading to a great deal of variability in the amount of time required to focus attention onto the target. This latency variability can be problematic for ERP recordings, because the ERPs are time locked to the stimulus rather than to the moment at which attention is focused on the target. Latency variability results in a temporal smearing of the N2pc component, making it look like a low-amplitude, long-duration deflection (even though it was presumably a large-amplitude, short-duration deflection on the individual trials).

Consequently, most ERP studies of visual search use stimuli similar to those shown in figure 11.3A, which allow subjects to rapidly and reliably shift attention to the target location. However, it is possible to observe an N2pc component with the types of stimuli used in typical behavioral experiments (see, e.g., Luck & Hillyard, 1990).

Several sources of converging evidence support the hypothesis that the N2pc component reflects the focusing of attention. First, a large N2pc is observed for non-targets that require careful scrutiny to be distinguished from the target, but little or no N2pc is observed for nontargets that can be rejected on the basis of salient feature information (Luck & Hillyard, 1994a, 1994b). Second, the N2pc component is larger for targets defined by conjunctions of multiple features than for targets defined by the presence of a single feature (Luck et al., 1997b), which corresponds to the greater attentional requirements of conjunction-defined targets (Treisman & Gelade, 1980). Third, even though an N2pc component is often observed for targets defined by a single feature, the process reflected by the N2pc component is not necessary for accurate feature detection but appears to be necessary for accurate conjunction discrimination. Specifically, when an attention-demanding central task is used to discourage subjects from focusing attention onto a concurrently presented visual search target, the N2pc component is no longer present for feature targets but is still present for conjunction targets (Luck & Ford, 1998). Fourth, the N2pc is larger when distractors are presented close to the target than when distractors are more distant (Luck et al., 1997b), which corresponds to behavioral observations of greater attentional demands when distractors are presented close to the target (Cohen & Ivry, 1991). Fifth, the N2pc component is larger in tasks that require target localization (Hyun & Luck, submitted; Luck et al., 1997b), which corresponds with the hypothesis that target localization requires focused attention (Treisman & Gelade, 1980).

In addition to the N2pc's being linked to attention in general, other evidence suggests a link to the more specific process of filtering out distractor stimuli so that they do not interfere with target identification. One piece of evidence for this more specific hypothesis is that the N2pc component is eliminated when no distractors are present (Luck & Hillyard, 1994b). Eimer (1996) demonstrated that an N2pc component is present if only one distractor is present, even when it is on the other side of the display from the target, and a similar result was obtained by Luck et al. (1997b). However, neurons at high levels of the visual system have very large receptive fields that would have encompassed both the target and the distractor in these experiments, so these results are not really evidence against the hypothesis that the N2pc component reflects a distractor-suppression process. Two additional findings provide support for this hypothesis by demonstrating that the N2pc component is eliminated if the distractors are not a real source of interference. First, if all the items in the search array are identical, the items do not conflict with each other and no N2pc is observed (Luck & Hillyard, 1994b, experiment 4). Second, if the target is defined as the one item that differs from the other items in the array, such that the distractors are actually necessary for determining that a target is present, no N2pc component is observed. Specifically, the target could be either a single vertical item among several horizontal distractors or a horizontal item among several vertical distractors. Consequently, identifying the orientation of the discrepant item was not useful, but determining that this item actually differed from the surrounding items was necessary, so filtering the surrounding items would have been counterproductive. No N2pc was observed under these conditions (Luck & Hillyard, 1994b, experiment 2).

The N2pc component may be an ERP manifestation of attention effects that have been observed in single-unit recordings from extrastriate and inferotemporal areas of monkey visual cortex (Chelazzi et al., 1998; Chelazzi et al., 2001). When monkeys perform visual search, neurons in the object recognition pathway initially respond solely on the basis of the stimulus properties of the visual search array, but the presence of a target begins to influence activity around 175 ms poststimulus (which is quite close to the typical onset time of the N2pc component). For example, a neuron that is selective for red stimuli will initially respond if the search array contains a red item inside the neuron's receptive field, whether or not the target is red. Beginning around 175 ms, however, the neuron's response will fade away if the target for that trial is not red, but it will be sustained if the target is the red item. This single-unit effect is larger for complex target–nontarget discriminations than for simple discriminations, just as the N2pc component is larger for conjunction targets than for feature targets. The single-unit effect and the N2pc component are also both increased when a distractor item is located near the target, and both are increased when subjects must make an eye movement to a target rather than making a manual response (for details, see Luck et al., 1997b). In addition, an ERMF study demonstrated that the magnetic field distribution corresponding to the N2pc component is consistent with a generator source in ventral occipitotemporal cortex (Hopf et al., 2000).

11.12   Using Features to Guide Spatial Attention

How are spatial and nonspatial forms of attention related? As discussed earlier, the first nonspatial attention effects typically occur around 150 ms poststimulus, whereas the first spatial attention effects typically occur between 70 and 100 ms poststimulus. However, the early spatial attention effects are observed only when subjects know which location is to be attended prior to stimulus onset. In most visual search tasks, subjects know in advance what features are to be attended (i.e., the features that define the target) but not the location of the target. It would therefore make sense that the feature-based effects that occur around 150 ms poststimulus reflect the processes that guide spatial attention to the target location around 200 ms poststimulus (as indexed by the N2pc component).

This possibility has been supported by single-unit and ERP/ERMF experiments. In a single-unit study, Motter (1994) found that color-selective neurons in extrastriate cortex responded differentially beginning at approximately 150 ms poststimulus, depending on whether the color of the stimulus inside the neuron's receptive field matched or mismatched the target color. Importantly, this effect occurred even when spatial attention was directed to a location outside the neuron's receptive field (see also Treue & Martinez Trujillo, 1999). A similar pattern of results has been observed in an ERP/ERMF study (Hopf et al., 2004). In this study, the presence of nontarget items containing target features led to a change in the neural response at approximately 140 ms poststimulus with an estimated neural origin in ventral occipitotemporal cortex, even when these features were at an ignored location. This was followed by an N2pc component at approximately 170 ms that was contralateral to the location of the actual target. Thus, feature-based attention precedes—and is presumably used to guide—spatial attention in visual search tasks.

11.13   Effects of Attention on Sensory Processing

Once attention is focused onto the target location, how is the processing of visual information changed at that location? To address this issue, Luck, Fan, and Hillyard (1993) flashed task-irrelevant *probe* stimuli at the location of the target or a distractor; the probe was presented 250 ms after the onset of the search array, during the period of the N2pc component. The ERP elicited by this probe stimulus was used to assess the status of processing at the target location relative to the distractor location at the time of the N2pc component. The probe-elicited P1 wave was found to be enhanced when the probe appeared at the location of the target compared to when it appeared at the location of the distractor, indicating that attending to the target causes a change in sensory responsiveness at the target location relative to the distractor location. Follow-up experiments (Luck & Hillyard, 1995) demonstrated that this effect was due to a suppression of responsiveness at the distractor location rather than an enhancement of responsiveness at the target location, consistent with the proposal that the N2pc component reflects a distractor-suppression process.

11.14   Serial Shifts of Attention

In the visual search experiments described so far, the target contained a distinctive feature and could therefore be localized very rapidly. In many behavioral visual search experiments—and in many real-world situations—the target is more difficult to localize and attention does not shift rapidly to the target. For decades, attention researchers have argued about the nature of the processing that occurs in these situations (for a review, see Chelazzi, 1999). One possibility is that attention shifts serially from one object to the next—identifying each attended object—until the target is found or the subject decides that no target is present. Another possibility is that all of the objects are attended and identified in parallel, but that this is a limited-capacity process that becomes slower as more objects must be processed. Behavioral experiments have provided evidence that parallel processing occurs under some conditions (Eckstein, 1998; McElree & Carrasco, 1999; Mordkoff et al., 1990), but this does not rule out the possibility that serial processing is used under other conditions.

It is extremely difficult to distinguish between serial processing and limited-capacity parallel processing on the basis of behavioral methods (Townsend, 1990). The problem is that behavioral measures cannot directly index the spatial focus of attention at each point in time following the presentation of a search array. In contrast, the contralateral distribution of the N2pc component makes it possible to use this component to assess which hemifield is attended, millisecond by millisecond, during visual search. That is, if attention shifts rapidly from an item in the left visual field to an item in the right visual field, then the N2pc component should shift rapidly from the right hemisphere to the left hemisphere. This is exactly what was found by Woodman and Luck (1999, 2003b).

To measure shifts of attention from one item to another using the N2pc component, it is necessary to know the order in which items are attended. Otherwise, trials with different patterns of attentional shifts will be averaged together and cancel out. To avoid this problem, Woodman and Luck (1999, 2003b) developed tasks that biased subjects to search the stimulus arrays in a known order. In one experiment, each display contained four distinctively colored items, one of which was the target on 75% of trials (called the C_{75} *color*) and another of which was the target on 25% of trials (called the C_{25} *color*). If search is serial, then subjects should attend to the C_{75} color first and then shift attention to the C_{25} color; consequently, the N2pc component should rapidly switch from the hemisphere contralateral to the C_{75} color to the hemisphere contralateral to the C_{25} color. However, if search is parallel, then subjects should simply devote more attention to the C_{75} color and less attention to the C_{25} color, with an overall larger N2pc contralateral to the C_{75} color and no change over time. When the C_{75} and C_{25} colors were in opposite hemifields, the N2pc component was found to appear over the hemisphere contralateral to the C_{75} color from 200–300 ms poststimulus and then to shift to the hemisphere contralateral to the C_{25} color from 300–400 ms, consistent with a serial search process with a dwell time of approximately 100 ms.

In another set of experiments in this study, two potential target items of the same color were present in each array, but one was close to fixation and the other was more peripheral (size was scaled according to the cortical magnification factor to equate discriminability). Previous studies have shown that subjects tend to search near items before searching far items (Carrasco et al., 1995; Wolfe et al., 1998); accordingly, the N2pc component was observed contralateral to the near item from 200–300 ms and then shifted to the hemisphere contralateral to the far item from 300–400 ms. These experiments provide direct evidence that attention shifts serially from object to object under some conditions.

11.15   The Time Course of Attention in Visual Search

Taken together, the results of these visual search experiments indicate that visual search unfolds over time in the following manner. When a visual search array is presented, the first feedforward wave of activity in the visual system simply reflects the physical properties of the stimulus array. If an item containing target features is present, neural activity is increased beginning 120—150 ms after stimulus onset. This activity is used to guide spatial attention to the location of the potential target item, which is reflected by the N2pc component (and changes in single-unit activity) beginning 175–200 ms poststimulus in occipitotemporal areas of visual cortex. This makes it possible to determine whether the attended item is actually the target, which will trigger a motor response. If the attended item is not a target, then attention may be shifted to another potential target item after a delay. The amount of time from the onset of attention to the first item and the onset of attention to the second item presumably depends on task difficulty and was found to be approximately 100 ms for a fairly difficult target–nontarget discrimination. Presumably, attention keeps on shifting from item to item until the target is found or the subject decides that no target is present.

11.16   Summary and Conclusions

This chapter has summarized the time course of attentional selection over the first half second. ERP studies—in combination with ERMF, neuroimaging, and single-unit studies—have revealed the following picture of the timing of attentional processing.

When attention is directed to a location before stimulus onset, spatial attention influences the feedforward transmission of sensory information through extrastriate cortex beginning 60–100 ms poststimulus. In contrast, attending to nonspatial features does not appear to influence feedforward sensory transmission in this manner; instead, feature-based attention begins to influence activity beginning approximately 150 ms poststimulus (for a potential counterexample, however, see Valdes-Sosa et al., 1998). But when the target location is not known in advance (as in many real-world situations), these feature-based attention mechanisms are used to guide spatial attention to objects that contain relevant features. When the target contains a salient feature, the salient feature is detected within 150 ms poststimulus and spatial attention is directed to its location 25–50 ms later. When the target does not contain a unique and distinctive feature, attention may be shifted to one or more nontargets before it shifts to the target. Under such conditions, attention sometimes operates serially, focusing on one object for approximately 100 ms before shifting to another object (although the dwell time may depend on stimulus discriminability).

12 Competition for Attention in Space and Time: The First 200 ms

Mary C. Potter

The goal of the research reported in this chapter is to understand how competing stimuli in a temporal stream attract and hold attention in the first 200 ms after onset. In normal circumstances, visual perception is continuous, a cycle of saccades and fixations. Yet, until recently, perception has been studied almost exclusively by presenting a single stimulus array, perhaps preceded by a fixation point and followed by a mask.

In an early study of more continuous perception, I tested memory for pictured scenes in a rapid serial visual presentation (RSVP). The goal was to study processing at durations in the range of normal fixations, presenting a different picture on each "fixation" so that we could subsequently measure recognition memory for that fixation. We found that memory for the pictures was excellent at a rate of 1/s, but that more than half the pictures were forgotten at a rate of 3/s, a rate typical of eye movements (Potter & Levy, 1969). Subsequent studies showed that detection of a named target picture (e.g., *small boats on beach*) within an RSVP stream was possible at a presentation rate of 3/s, showing that picture meaning can be extracted much faster than memory for pictures can be consolidated (Intraub, 1980, 1984; Potter, 1975, 1976). Similar experiments using words instead of pictures showed that meaning is extracted even more rapidly from a briefly presented word in an RSVP stream, permitting detection of a target word defined by a category such as *animal* (Lawrence, 1971) at rates of presentation too high for retention of even a short sequence of unrelated words (Potter, 1982, 1993).

These RSVP studies show that words or pictures in a continuous stream can be understood rapidly, but competition from subsequent items leads to forgetting of most of the items. If, however, the items in a stream are words in a meaningful sentence, the sentence (and thus all of the words) can be understood and reported at presentation rates of 12 words/s or even higher (Forster, 1970; Potter, 1984; Potter et al., 1980; Potter et al., 1986). Words in a sentence have meaningful connections to one another that can be computed on the fly, creating an integrated structure that supports reportable memory.

For words presented in a rapid temporal stream, meaningful connections can only be discovered if there is some form of memory for at least the several most recent words. I termed this mediating representation of individual items *conceptual short-term memory* (CSTM) and suggested that CSTM retains meaningful items briefly, permitting integrated structures to be formed (Potter, 1993, 1999). Such structure building requires not only identification of each word in a sentence but also the momentary retrieval of a large number of conceptual associations from which the relevant ones are selected. This process is largely unconscious, as illustrated by our normal lack of awareness that we have selected the context-appropriate meaning of an ambiguous word.

12.1   Competition for Attention Over Time: The Attentional Blink

A limitation on our capacity to process a rapid stream of stimuli leads to competition between items for attention. Although extensive research has been carried out on competition for attention over space, only recently have researchers begun to study competition for attention over time. In these studies investigators have presented RSVP sequences containing two or more items that have been designated as targets the viewer is to report—for example, two letters in a stream of digit distractors. By placing the second target at different serial positions in the sequence, the stimulus onset asynchrony (SOA) between the targets is varied. An early finding was that there is a brief temporal gap in reported perception shortly after attention has been directed to a particular target stimulus, and that if a second target appears during this interval, it is likely to be missed (Broadbent & Broadbent, 1987; Weichselgartner & Sperling, 1987). This transient negative effect on the second target was called an *attentional blink* by Raymond et al. (1992). Raymond et al. showed that the effect was maximal at an SOA between targets of about 200 ms and diminished as the SOA increased, disappearing by about 500 ms. Thus, the *attentional blink* is standardly defined as interference from an initial target (T1) with the processing of a second target (T2) that appears between 200 and 500 ms later. Figure 12.1 shows a typical attentional blink pattern, in an experiment in which viewers attempted to report the two letters in a sequence of digits presented at 10 items/s (Chun & Potter, 1995). Conventionally, performance on T2 is shown conditional on correct report of T1 and is plotted as a function of the lag, or SOA, between T1 and T2.[1]

Raymond et al. (1992; see also Chun & Potter, 1995, experiment 3) found that removing the distractor item immediately following T1 and replacing it with a blank frame reduced or eliminated the attentional blink on T2. This effect of unmasking T1 suggested that the attentional blink is the result of interference produced by an

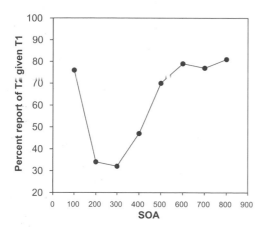

Figure 12.1
A characteristic attentional blink result, in which performance on target 2 (T2) is reported as a function of stimulus onset asynchrony, conditional on correct report of target 1 (T1). (From Chun & Potter, 1995, figure 2) T1 and T2 were letters, and the distractors were digits.

immediate visual event after T1, which slows processing of T1, thus interfering with processing of T2. Another effect noted by Raymond et al. (1992) was that when T2 appeared immediately after T1, T2 was often easier to report than when there was an intervening distractor (see figure 12.1). This effect, termed *lag 1 sparing* because T2 is spared when it lags one step behind T1, is found only when there is no major task shift between T1 and T2 (Potter et al., 1998; Visser et al., 1999).

12.1.1 The Two-Stage Model of the Attentional Blink

Chun and Potter (1995) developed a two-stage model of the attentional blink in which detection and identification of T1 take place in the first stage (lasting about 100 ms). Once identified, T1 is represented in CSTM while a second, serial, stage of consolidation into short-term memory begins (Potter, 1976; Jolicoeur & Dell'Acqua, 1998). This second stage, which is required for report of the item, may take 200–400 ms, so that if T2 appears during this time it will only be processed in stage 1 and will have to wait in CSTM for stage 2 to become available. CSTM is volatile and is subject to interference from subsequent stimuli. Thus, T2 may be momentarily detected and identified but may be forgotten before it can enter stage 2. A number of studies have provided evidence for the claim that an unreported T2 is nonetheless identified (e.g., Luck et al., 1996; Maki et al., 1997; Shapiro et al., 1997).

The Chun–Potter model explains lag 1 sparing as follows. Detection of a target opens an attentional gate, but closure of the gate is inexact or sluggish, and so the immediately following item is also attended (e.g., Weichselgartner & Sperling, 1987;

Raymond et al., 1992) and the two items enter stage 2 together. When the following stimulus is a distractor, it must be suppressed, but when it is also a target, the two targets are processed together in stage 2, with some resulting competition. Consistent with this account, performance on T1 was lower at lag 1 than at longer lags (suggesting competition), and the order of report of the two targets was frequently reversed (Chun & Potter, 1995). As will be seen, a different account of lag 1 sparing emerged from studies with shorter SOAs and shorter exposure durations, leading to a modification of the Chun–Potter (1995) model.

12.2   Short SOAs

Until recently, research on the attentional blink used presentation rates of about 10 items/s to ensure that T1 was likely to be perceived. The focus was on T2, and (as noted) performance on T2 was scored conditional on correct report of T1. To investigate performance at SOAs shorter than 100 ms, Potter et al. (2002) used a rate of about 19 items/s (53 ms per item). By approximately doubling the rate of presentation that had been used in most previous attentional blink studies, we were able to disentangle the effects of SOA and of lag. Whereas in earlier studies lag 1 was coincident with an SOA of about 100 ms, in Potter et al.'s studies lag 2 occurred at an SOA of 107 ms, and lag 1 at an SOA of 53 ms. The targets were four- and five-letter words (different on every trial), and the distractors were strings of keyboard symbols.

In our first experiment we presented a single stream of stimuli, and the SOAs between the two targets were 53, 107, or 213 ms. The results are shown in figure 12.2A, which shows performance separately for T1 (the black dots) and T2 (the white dots). Note first that the T2 results for SOAs of 107 and 213 ms were like those in earlier attentional blink studies: At an SOA of 107 ms there was sparing of T2, and at an SOA of 213 ms there was a sizable attentional blink. At an SOA of 53 ms (the actual lag 1 in this experiment) T2 was easily reported. In contrast, at an SOA of 53 ms T1 showed a substantial deficit: There was a marked crossover interaction

Figure 12.2
(*A*) Accuracy in report of each target (T) word (T1 and T2) among symbol strings presented in a single rapid serial visual presentation stream at stimulus onset asynchronies (SOAs) of 53, 107, or 213 ms. Error bars represent standard errors. (From Potter et al., 2002, figure 1) (*B*) Accuracy in report of each target word when targets were presented in separate streams, one above the other, at SOAs of 40, 107, or 213 ms. Error bars represent standard errors. (From Potter et al., 2002, figure 3) (*C*) Accuracy in report of a given word at SOAs of 53, 107, or 213 ms when there were two words on a trial (solid lines) and when there was only one word on a trial (dotted lines). On the one-word trials, T1 and T2 designate target words in the same serial positions as the corresponding words in the two-word trials. Error bars represent standard errors. (From Potter et al., 2002, figure 5)

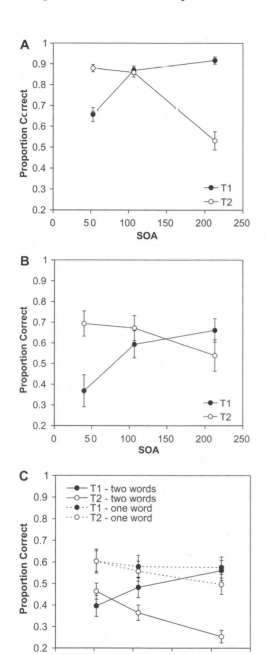

between target (T1 vs. T2) and SOA. That is, there was not only sparing of T2 at short SOAs but also marked interference with T1.

A possible reason for the poor performance on T1 at lag 1 was that T2 simply masked T1 more effectively than distractors did (a confound at lag 1 that was present in most previous attentional blink studies). In subsequent experiments, Potter et al. (2002) used two streams of stimuli, one directly above the other, with the two targets in separate streams. (The first target appeared randomly in the upper or lower stream.) This method not only avoided the differential masking problem (because the item immediately following each target in its stream was always a distractor) but also allowed for SOAs shorter than 53 ms, including simultaneous presentation. Figure 12.2B shows the results of one experiment with SOAs of 40, 107, and 213 ms. Overall performance was lower with dual streams, but the pattern was similar to that with a single stream. In particular, there was a marked crossover at the shortest SOA, with performance on T1 much lower than on T2. Evidently the masking confound noted in the one-stream experiment was not the sole reason for the crossover.

To show that the pattern resulted from mutual interference between the two targets, in a subsequent experiment with dual streams we omitted one of the two words on a random two thirds of the trials. The results are shown in figure 12.2C. The two lower curves show accuracy for each target when both were presented, with a crossover interaction. The dashed upper curves show the result for each target when only one of the two targets was presented and the other was replaced with a distractor. Overall accuracy in the two-target condition was 42%, compared with 57% in the one-target condition. This difference was significant for every condition except for T1 at an SOA of 213 ms: In that condition T1 performance was the same whether or not a T2 was presented. That is, performance on T1 was immune from interference from T2, presumably because after 213 ms T1 was already in stage 2. Moreover, in the one-target condition there was no evidence for the crossover pattern seen with two targets, showing clearly that the pattern was the result of mutual competition, not serial position or a prior allocation of attention to one of the two streams.

12.3   The Two-Stage Competition Model of Attention

Neither the Chun–Potter (1995) two-stage model nor other models of the attentional blink can account for the crossover between T1 and T2 (i.e., the advantage of T2 over T1) at very short SOAs. Chun and Potter had noted that in their experiments T1 and T2 showed evidence of competition at lag 1 (with an SOA of 100 ms). The two-stage competition model of Potter et al. (2002) was proposed as a modification and extension of the Chun–Potter two-stage model. The main new claim of the competition model is that competition arises in Stage 1 after detection of a potential target (e.g., a string of letters), but before identification of the word. As in the original Chun–Potter model, detection of T1 initiates an attentional response. Whereas the Chun–Potter model proposed that the attentional response ushered T1 into stage 2, in the two-stage competition model the attentional response simply mobilizes processing resources needed for identification of the detected target in stage 1. It takes 50–100 ms to identify T1, and if T2 appears during this time, it competes for these resources. Once one of the targets has been identified, it alone enters stage 2 for consolidation, and then the other target must wait.

Because the attentional response to T1 takes time to reach its maximum (e.g., Shih, 2000; Weichselgartner & Sperling, 1987), T2 may benefit more than T1 when the SOA is short. In effect, T2 steals the attention that T1 activated, creating the crossover pattern that Potter et al. (2002) observed. In this model, "lag 1 sparing" is the result of approximately equal competition between T1 and T2 at an SOA of about 100 ms; with shorter SOAs, T2 tends to dominate T1.

Stage 1, detection and identification, of the two-stage competition model can be summarized as follows:

• A potential target is detected on the basis of some relevant feature (e.g., being alphabetic, when the target is any word among keyboard symbols) and attracts attentional resources required to identify it.

• If a second target appears during this stage, it will compete for resources while both targets are in stage 1.

• At short SOAs, T2 benefits from the prior triggering of attention and may be identified before T1.

• The target that is first identified enters stage 2.

• When one target is occupying stage 2, another target that is left waiting in stage 1 or that enters stage 1 may be identified. If so, it will be represented briefly in CSTM, but it may be be forgotten before it can enter stage 2.

Stage 2, consolidation, of the two-stage competition model can be summarized as follows:

• This stage is serial, capable of processing only one target at a time.

• Consolidation into short-term memory (STM), which can take 200–500 ms, is required for an item to be reported.

12.4   Location Uncertainty

One surprise in Potter et al.'s (2002) results is that the crossover effect, benefiting T2, was obtained even though T1 and T2 appeared in different spatial locations. In other studies (e.g., those reviewed by Visser et al., 1999, and a study by Breitmeyer et al., 1999), a shift in location almost always eliminated lag 1 sparing: That is, T2 showed a large attentional blink deficit at lag 1. Potter et al. always presented the two targets in different streams, so that participants knew as soon as T1 appeared that T2 would be in the other stream; there was no location uncertainty. In most earlier studies using more than one location, the location of T2 remained uncertain.

To test the effect of location uncertainty, Potter and O'Connor (2000) carried out a further experiment in which T2 was equally likely to be in the same or the other stream; the results are shown in figure 12.3. When the targets were in the same stream (see figure 12.3A), the results were like those of Potter et al. (2002) with a single stream (see figure 12.2A) or with two streams when the targets were always in separate streams (see figure 12.2B): There was a crossover interaction between T1/T2 and SOA ($p < .001$). However, when the targets were in separate streams in the uncertain location experiment, the results were very different from the separate-stream results in Potter et al. (2002): T1 was always much better than T2 (see figure 12.3B). There was still a significant interaction with SOA: T1 got better with longer SOAs; T2 got worse ($p < .002$). Clearly, when T2 appeared in the same stream as T1 on half the trials, viewers adopted a conservative strategy of maintaining attention on the T1 stream. As a result, lag 1 sparing at short SOAs was minimal when T2 appeared in the other stream, just as in previous studies with a location shift between T1 and T2.

Thus, the pattern of resource competition is determined in part by expectation, such that there is a bias to maintain attention at the location of the first target at the expense of a target appearing in the other location. Only when the two targets are always presented in different locations is a viewer readily attracted to a second target in the other location, and then only at short SOAs.

12.5   Modifying the Crossover Pattern: Unmasking and Semantic Priming

To test and extend the two-stage competition model, my colleagues and I examined the effects of two other variables on performance at short SOAs, using the same basic procedure of search for two word targets in separate streams of nonalphabetic distractors. The variables we investigated were unmasking (substitution of a blank for the immediate masking stimulus following one or the other target) and seman-

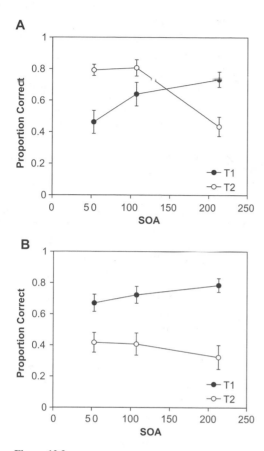

Figure 12.3
(*A*) Accuracy in report of each target (T) word in a two-stream presentation when the targets were in the same stream. Error bars represent standard errors. (*B*) Same, when the two targets were in different streams. SOA, stimulus onset asynchrony.

tic priming of one of the words. These manipulations were expected to boost performance on one of the two targets, allowing us to measure possible competitive effects on the other target.

12.6 Unmasking by Adding a Blank

Earlier work had shown that when a blank follows T1 (instead of a distractor), the attentional blink on T2 is reduced or eliminated (Raymond et al., 1992; Chun & Potter, 1995), presumably because processing of T1 is completed rapidly when there is no immediate visual mask. The presentation duration in those studies was about

100 ms/item, there was only one stream, stimuli were simple (typically, single letters), and performance on T1 was near ceiling even with no blank. In the present research items were presented for about 50 ms, the targets were words appearing in separate streams, and report of T1 was well below ceiling. In these conditions, we asked whether unmasking T1 or T2 would modify the crossover pattern. In particular, would unmasking bias the competition between T1 and T2 at short SOAs, favoring the unmasked target at the expense of the other target? And, at longer SOAs, would unmasking T1 reduce or even eliminate the attentional blink on T2?

12.6.1 Predictions of the Competition Model

We made the following predictions from the competition model:

1. Insofar as T1 and T2 compete in stage 1 at short SOAs (e.g., 53 ms), putting a blank after one or the other target will bias the competition in favor of the blanked target and will decrease the accuracy of reporting the nonblanked target. That is, there would be a benefit for the blanked target at the expense of the other target (a *competition pattern*).

2. At longer SOAs (e.g., 213 ms) unmasking T1 will not only increase report of T1 but will also diminish the attentional blink on T2 (as in earlier studies): That is, unmasking T1 will help both T1 and T2 at longer SOAs.

3. Unmasking T2 at longer SOAs (e.g., 213 ms or longer) will help T2 without a cost to T1.

12.6.2 Method and Results

The experiment (Potter et al., in preparation b) used the general method used by Potter et al. (2002). Presentation duration was 53 ms/item, and there were four SOAs: 53, 107, 213, and 427 ms.[2] Three conditions were intermixed randomly: a blank of 53 ms in the T1 stream immediately after T1, a blank in the T2 stream after T2, or no blank. The results for a blank after T1 and no blank are shown in figure 12.4A. In the no-blank condition we obtained the familiar crossover pattern. When T1 was followed by a blank, performance on T1 was markedly improved, more or less equally at all SOAs. Contrary to our first prediction, however, the competition pattern—a cost to T2—was absent at an SOA of 53 ms. (Similarly, when T2 was followed by a blank, there was no cost to T1—see figure 12.4B.)

Contrary to our second prediction, instead of a blank after T1's helping T2 at longer SOAs, the blank at SOAs of 107 and 213 ms interfered with T2 report, increasing the attentional blink. Thus, the results did not replicate previous studies (with slower presentation rates) in which a blank after T1 helped T2, reducing the attentional blink effect (Raymond et al., 1992; Chun & Potter, 1995). Rather, a blank after

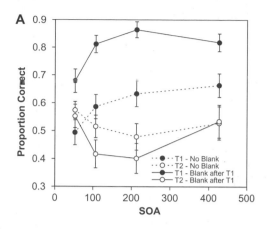

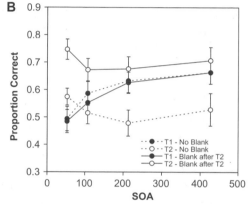

Figure 12.4
(*A*) Report of each target (T) word when T1 was immediately followed by a blank frame of 53 ms (solid lines) and when there were no blanks (dotted lines). Standard error bars are shown. (*B*) Report of each target word when T2 was immediately followed by a blank (solid lines) and when there were no blanks (dotted lines). Standard error bars are shown. SOA, stimulus onset asynchrony.

T1 hurt performance on T2 in the blink range, although not at an SOA of 53 ms nor at 427 ms. Only our third prediction was supported: A blank after T2 at longer SOAs helped T2 without affecting T1 (see figure 12.4B).

12.6.3   Discussion: Unmasking

What do the results say about the competition model? The claim of the model is that competition in stage 1 will only occur at a short SOA. If unmasking one of the targets biases the competition, that should be evident at an SOA of 53 ms, but no such competition pattern emerged. Instead, unmasking either T1 or T2 gave a consistent benefit to the unmasked target at all SOAs, with little effect on the other target except for an increase in the attentional blink on T2 at SOAs of 107 and 213 ms.

A possible explanation is that the unmasking blank came too late to affect competition in stage 1 (at an SOA of 53 ms). Consider the time course of events at an SOA of 53 ms. A blank after T2 began 100 ms after the onset of T1, probably too late to bias competition. However, a blank following T1 began at the onset of T2. If the two words were then processed in parallel, the blank after T1 should have helped it, relative to T2—but that is not what we found. There was no evidence of competition at an SOA of 53 ms, only a benefit for T1 without cost to T2.

12.6.4   A Winner-Take-All Competition in Stage 1?

In our initial competition model (Potter et al., 2002), stage 1 competition meant that resources were shared and that processing continued in parallel until one of the words was identified. A different assumption is that the onset of T2 has a certain probability of attracting all the resources initially accruing to T1. This probability decreases as SOA increases. In other words, the competition is all or nothing: Either attention shifts entirely to T2, or it stays with T1 until it is identified or fails to be identified. If this new hypothesis is correct, then it is not surprising that a T1 blank had no effect at SOAs of 53 ms or greater: At the time the blank began, T2 had appeared and the switch had happened (or not) without influence from the blank.

Why was there a cost to T2 when T1 was unmasked, at SOAs of 107 and 213 ms? In previous studies in which a blank after T1 helped T2, T1 was highly likely to be perceived even without a blank (and, indeed, performance on T2 was analyzed conditional on successful report of T1). Thus, any benefit to T1 would speed up its processing in stage 2 and therefore help T2. In the present experiments T1 was often missed, so a blank after T1 increased the probability that it would be identified and would enter stage 2, thus increasing the likelihood of an attentional blink on T2.

Further discussion of the time course of the unmasking effect is postponed until the results of experiments on semantic priming have been presented.

12.7   Semantic Priming

The second variable we investigated was semantic priming, to discover whether a priming word or phrase modulates the crossover pattern between T1/T2 and SOA. In the first of these studies (Potter et al., 2005, experiment 1, $N = 12$) the two target words were either associated in meaning (e.g., *zebra–horse*) or were unrelated. The targets were presented in separate streams as in Potter et al. (2002) and in the unmasking studies just described. Items were presented for 53 ms, and the SOAs between the two target words were 27, 53, 107, and 213 ms. Our predictions were as follows. We assumed that priming benefits flow from the prime to the target, over time, and so most of the priming benefit would be found in report of T2. However, at short SOAs the two targets are hypothesized to be in competition, with T2 at least as likely to be reported as T1. Thus, both T1 and T2 were predicted to show a benefit from priming at short SOAs. Figure 12.5 shows the results: Both predictions were supported.

For the unrelated pairs, although there was no crossover, there was a strong interaction between SOA and target (T1 or T2) as in the earlier studies. For the related pairs, T2 benefited greatly from its relation to T1 at all SOAs, but T1 benefited from T2 only at the shortest SOA, 27 ms. This is consistent with the evidence from the unrelated trials that T1 and T2 were equally likely to be reported at an SOA of 27 ms, but at longer SOAs T1 had an advantage over T2.

A clear implication of these results is that T1 is only semantically primed if T2 is identified first. Potter et al. (2005, experiment 2) also reported an independent experiment carried out in Italian, in which similar results were obtained.

Before considering the processing locus of this priming effect, I will describe two other priming studies in which two word targets were presented, as in the previous experiments. In one study (Davenport & Potter, 2005, experiment 1) a prime of one of the target words appeared just before each trial; the target word was an associate of the prime. We predicted that the related word would benefit from the prime in all conditions. The critical question, however, was whether there would be evidence of competition at a short SOA, such that the primed word would benefit at the expense of the unprimed word.

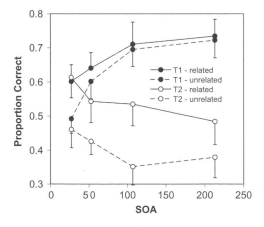

Figure 12.5
Report of each of two semantically related target (T) words (solid lines) or unrelated words (dashed lines). Standard error bars are shown. SOA, stimulus onset asynchrony. (From Potter et al., 2005, figure 2)

Figure 12.6A shows the familiar crossover pattern for the unprimed words, and (as predicted) a constant benefit to the primed word, regardless of SOA or T1/T2. Was there, however, a cost to the unprimed word when it accompanied a primed word? In one condition in the experiment the prime word was not related to either of the target words—neither word was primed. If priming one word biases the competition in stage 1, then the other word on that trial should suffer (at a short SOA), compared to the condition in which neither word is primed. As figure 12.6B shows, there was no significant difference between the two ways of not being primed— there was no evidence at any SOA that priming one of two words made report of

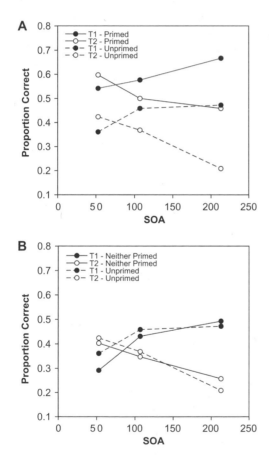

Figure 12.6
(*A*) Report of target (T) words preceded by a semantic prime (solid lines) and words unrelated to the prime (dashed lines) when one word in each pair was primed. SOA, stimulus onset asynchrony. (From Davenport & Potter, 2005, adapted from figure 2) (*B*) Report of target words preceded by a prime, when neither word was related to the prime (dotted lines) and when one word was unprimed (dashed lines) but the other word was primed. (From Davenport & Potter, 2005, adapted from figure 3)

the unprimed word less likely than in the neither-primed condition. (If anything, the result went in the opposite direction.)

We obtained a similar result in the third priming experiment, in which we used short, incomplete sentences as primes (Potter et al., in preparation a). One of the two target words was a good completion of the sentence, although not the most frequent completion that was generated by a norming group of subjects. The words of the sentence were presented at 107 ms/word in RSVP in a single stream, omitting the last word of the sentence (e.g., *She was late for the* . . .). The sentence fragment was followed immediately by two RSVP streams, as in the earlier experiments, with two target words (one of which was *party*, in this example). The SOA between the targets was 27, 53, 107, or 213 ms; the primed word was equally often the first or second word. The task was to report both words; the sentence fragment could be ignored.

Figure 12.7 shows the results, separately for T1 and T2, for the related and unrelated words. Once more, there was a crossover effect for unprimed words, and the priming effect was more or less constant over all conditions. In a replication of these results we included a condition in which neither word was related to the sentence; in that case, performance was almost identical to that of the unprimed word when the other word fit the sentence. That is, again there was no evidence that a priming benefit to one word was at the expense of the other word.

12.7.1   Discussion: Semantic Priming

To sum up the semantic priming results, priming from one target to the other was found only from T1 to T2, with the notable exception that at a very short SOA T2

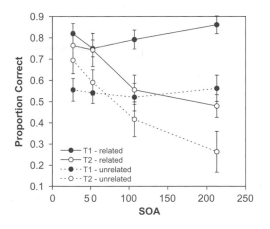

Figure 12.7
Report of target (T) words preceded by an incomplete sentence that was related to the word (solid lines) or unrelated (dotted lines). Standard error bars are shown. (From Potter et al., in preparation a)

was equally likely to prime T1 (Potter et al., 2005). When the prime came at the beginning of each trial, preceding both word targets, priming benefited the related target without cost to the unprimed word. For the primed word, the benefit was roughly constant across SOAs. The same pattern was found whether the prime was an associated word (Davenport & Potter, 2005) or a sentence fragment (Potter et al., in preparation a).

Semantic priming made it easier to see and report a difficult-to-see, masked word—a stimulus that seems to disappear completely when the mask arrives. Thus, there is reason to think that the semantic effect occurs very early in processing in this set of tasks, rather than reconstructively at the end of a trial. What does this tell us about the probable locus of the semantic priming effect? We can rule out an influence on the competition between T1 and T2 at short SOAs, in that if semantic priming biased this competition, the unprimed word should suffer, and it does not. However, if we assume (as we did earlier in discussing the unmasking results) that the competition consists of an all-or-nothing takeover of resources by T2 when T1 is in stage 1, then the competition stage would be over before either target has been identified. In that case, there would be no reason to expect semantic priming to affect the competition: Any effect would come later.

A likely time for a semantic prime to exert its influence is at the point of identification—that is, lexical access. It seems reasonable that an appropriate semantic context will increase the probability of successful word identification. Thus, even at a long SOA when T1 is likely to be identified first, priming T2 will increase its chances of also being reported.

Could the benefit come still later—for example, at the point of word retrieval at the end of the trial? We considered this possibility in the experiment in which the two target words were related on half the trials (Potter et al., 2005). Successful recall of one of the words could have increased recall of the other word because of their semantic relation. In that case, however, the priming benefit would be expected to be similar at all SOAs, whether T1 was recalled first and primed T2, or T2 was recalled first and primed T1. That was the case for the priming benefit to T2: It was found at all SOAs. However, strikingly, the benefit to T1 was only found at the shortest SOA, suggesting that priming effects occurred during presentation rather than at the point of retrieval.

12.8 General Discussion

A question on which I have focused is whether unmasking one of two targets, or semantically priming one target, would bias the competition between the two targets in stage 1, as predicted by the competition model of Potter et al. (2002). Both unmasking and priming had the expected positive effects on the target in question, but neither procedure resulted in a cost to the other target in the earliest stage of processing, contrary to our prediction.

A modification of the competition model's stage 1 is proposed to account for the failure to find a competitive cost for the other target. Instead of assuming that two targets presented very close in time compete in parallel for resources, my colleagues and I propose that the onset of the second target has a certain probability of shifting all the attentional resources to it, a probability that is greater the shorter the SOA. Thus, with an SOA of 27 or 53 ms, the second target is likely to cause a shift in attention on more than half the trials, whereas at longer SOAs a shift is less likely. In the unmasking condition, the positive effect of unmasking T1 cannot begin until the end of T1's presentation, but at that point T2 has just appeared (when the SOA is 53 ms) and the presumed switch occurs (or fails to occur) before any benefit from the blank following T1. That is, the blank comes too late to affect the probability of an attentional switch. In the case of a blank after T2, the effect begins even later (more than 100 ms after the onset of T1) and could have no effect on stage 1 competition.

For a different reason, the revised interpretation of stage 1 competition as an all-or-nothing switch of attention to T2 predicts that semantic priming (from an advance prime or sentence context) will not bias stage 1 competition. As the shift occurs before either target has been identified, semantic priming cannot bias this decision.

In both sets of experiments we obtained large benefits of unmasking and semantic priming. At what stage or stages of processing did these effects occur? In the case of semantic priming we proposed that the effects occur at the point of lexical access (word identification) at the end of stage 1. Is this also the point where the effects of unmasking occur? Unmasking makes a target easier to process, increasing the probability that it will be identified; this perceptual benefit could affect any stage of processing between the offset of the target and the point of identification. This effect can be expected to be approximately additive[3] with other factors such as SOA and whether the target is T1 or T2. Similarly, semantic priming facilitates lexical identification by increasing the accessibility of a related word, again somewhat independently of other factors. The result in both cases is that the increased accuracy for a primed or unmasked target is roughly additive with the effects of these other factors, as long as accuracy is below ceiling as it was in the present experiments.

12.9 The First 200 ms

The title of this chapter emphasizes the short time period over which competition between two briefly presented targets undergoes the changes shown in the experiments reported here. The competition in the first 100 ms (with an SOA of about

50 ms) favors the second target at the expense of the first; the two targets are more or less equal at an SOA of about 100 ms; and thereafter (at SOAs between 200 and 500 ms) the first target dominates, at the expense of the second target. (At still longer SOAs, not reported here, T2 performance may return to the level of T1 performance.) During the first 200 ms of processing, average accuracy in report of two targets is roughly constant; what changes is which target is more likely to be reported.

Unmasking one target or priming it with a semantically related context improves performance on the primed or unmasked target without otherwise affecting this pattern. Unmasking by inserting a blank frame makes it easier to see the unmasked target, but not in time to affect the competition between the two targets in stage 1 (before identification of either target). Competition once one of the targets has reached stage 2 takes a different form: The target undergoing consolidation monopolizes that stage of processing, forcing the other target to wait in CSTM, so that it is often forgotten before it gains access to stage 2. The fact that semantic priming facilitates target report is consistent with the idea that even under the present conditions, in which target words are very difficult to see, they are close to the point of lexical identification and access to meaning.

In accounting for this pattern of results, the earlier Chun–Potter (1995) two-stage model of the attentional blink was first modified and named the two-stage competition model (Potter et al., 2002) and here has been further modified by the proposal that the competition in stage 1 is not a matter of parallel sharing of limited resources but is instead an all-or-nothing, stochastic switch of attention from T1 to T2 that happens when T2 arrives while T1 is still in stage 1 (see also Davenport & Potter, 2005; Potter et al., 2005). We know that the probability of such a switch declines as the SOA between T1 and T2 increases. Further research will be required to discover whether other variables (such as contrast or hue) affect the likelihood of a switch in stage 1, producing the competition pattern that proved so elusive in the present studies.

Notes

1. Accuracy of report is measured, not response time, because report of the targets comes at the end of the trial, after both have been presented. Jolicoeur and his colleagues have shown that accuracy measures in an attentional blink paradigm are paralleled by reaction time measures in a modified psychological refractory period paradigm in which two stimuli in a trial are to be reported, but only the response to the second target is speeded (e.g., Jolicoeur & Dell'Acqua, 1998).

2. For 15 of the participants (out of 27), an SOA of 27 ms was included but is not reported.

3. Additivity in the sense of Sternberg's (1969) additive factors applies to measures of reaction time, not accuracy.

13 Effects of Masked Stimuli on Attention and Response Tendencies as Revealed by Event-Related EEG Potentials: Possible Application to Understanding Neglect

Rolf Verleger and Piotr Jaskowski

In the first part of this chapter, we will review our studies on attention-related effects of masked stimuli. In the second part, ideas derived from this research will be applied to research on neglect, which is a fascinating disorder of the mind caused by neurological damage. A common topic in both areas of research is that in both cases events do not enter awareness and nevertheless may have their effects on perception and action. A hypothesis will be put forward on how both phenomena might reflect the same underlying mechanism.

13.1   Effects of Masked Stimuli on Attention and Response Tendencies

13.1.1   Background

Our interest in visual masking derived from two sources: interest and experience in visual psychophysics, on the one hand (e.g., Jaśkowski, 1996), and interest in applying promising measures from electroencephalogram (EEG) potential research (see, e.g., critical reviews by Verleger, 1997, 1998), in this case the N2pc (Luck & Hillyard, 1994a,b), to new areas of research, on the other hand. We were attracted by the similarity between the stimulus configuration introduced to metacontrast research by Klotz and Neumann (1999) and stimulus configurations as used by us in research using the N2pc for investigating the relation between overt and covert shifts of attention (Wauschkuhn et al., 1998) or involuntary shifts of attention and motor preparation (Wascher et al., 2001), so we felt that applying these EEG potential methods to research on nonconscious perception might be a worthwhile enterprise.

13.1.2   Combining Metacontrast Masking With Choice Responses to Visible Stimuli

In the first study to be reported here, we used the task and stimuli developed by Klotz and Neumann (1999), drawing from the rich body of research in metacontrast

masking (see, e.g., Breitmeyer & Öğmen, 2000, for a review). These authors presented pairs of stimuli, with one stimulus left of fixation, and the other right. One
stimulus was a square; the other was a diamond (i.e., the square rotated by 45°).
Participants had to press the left or right key in response to the stimulus pair,
depending on which side the diamond was presented. (Actually, the diamond was
target for half of the participants only, and the square for the other half. For simplicity, the diamond will here be treated as target.) This main pair of stimuli was
preceded by a pair of smaller stimuli, each one of which fit within the inner contours of the main stimuli (see the layout of stimuli in figure 13.1), and therefore
could be masked by metacontrast; stimulus onset asynchrony (SOA) was 83 ms.
These preceding stimuli were either two squares (neutral) or one diamond and one
square, with the diamond either on the same side as in the main stimulus (congruent) or on the other side (incongruent). As Klotz and Neumann (1999) showed,
responses to the main diamond were speeded in congruent trials and delayed by
incongruent trials, although participants were unable to discriminate square and
diamond in the preceding stimuli when explicitly asked to do so. Therefore, the preceding stimuli acted as primes. Figure 13.1 shows this in our data (Jaśkowski et al.,
2002), replicating Klotz and Neumann's behavioral results for an SOA of 83 ms.
Indiscriminability of the targetlike shape in the primes was tested in the same experimental session by presenting the same stimuli and asking participants to decide
whether the target shape had occurred in the primes or not (i.e., a choice response
between congruent and incongruent primes, on the one hand, and neutral primes,
on the other hand). Discrimination accuracy did not differ from chance ($d' = 0.04$
on average, maximum = 0.27). We interspersed trials with longer SOAs between
primes and main stimuli (167 ms) as control stimuli to see what happens if the primes
are not indistinguishable any more, though still barely visible ($d' = 0.34$ on average).
Response effects became larger in these trials (see figure 13.1, upper middle panel,
"RT (ms)"), and more errors occurred when primes were incongruent, i.e., by perceiving the diamond in the prime on the other side, participants were led to press
the key on that side (see figure 13.1, upper right panel, "% correct"). Thus, in
summary, this paradigm combines the simple, elegant features of metacontrast
masking with choice response to visible stimuli. By repeating the same simple
stimuli throughout the task, the prerequisites are met for recording event-related
potentials (ERPs), which require replications over many trials because of their low
signal-to-noise ratio. Furthermore, by using stimuli and responses that are defined
by their left and right location, the methodology of contra-ipsilateral differences can
be used.

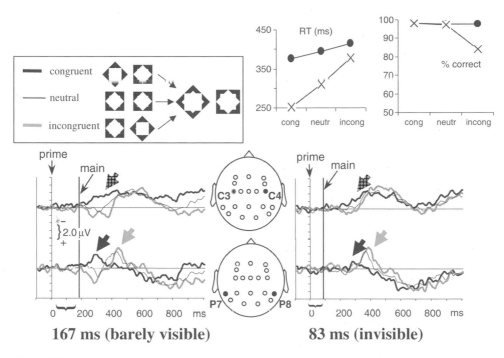

Figure 13.1
Priming effects of metacontrast-masked stimuli on response tendencies and attention. Sequences of primes and main stimuli with congruent (cong), neutral (neutr), and incongruent (incong) relationship are depicted in the upper left panel for main stimuli with the diamond left from fixation. Upper middle and upper right panels: Response times and percentage of correct responses for prime–main stimulus onset asynchronies of 83 ms (circles) and 167 ms (crosses). Means over the 12 participants are shown. Lower half: Grand means (12 participants) of contra-ipsilateral differences. Upper row: recordings from |C3-C4| overlying the motor cortices. Lower row: recordings from |P7-P8| overlying the visual system (roughly V4). The x-axis denotes milliseconds from prime onset (0 ms). Onset of the main stimulus is denoted by the solid vertical line, either at 167 ms (left part of the graph) or at 83 ms (right). The y-axis is in microvolts, with negative polarity contralateral to responding hand (i.e., to position of target stimulus in the main stimulus) plotted upward. Bold black lines are from congruent trials, thin lines from neutral, and gray lines from incongruent trials. Checked arrows denote priming of the lateralized readiness potential, black arrows N2pc evoked by the primes, and gray arrows N2pc evoked by the targets. (Data from Jaśkowski et al., 2002)

13.1.3 Using Contra-Ipsilateral Differences of EEG Potentials (Lateralized Readiness Potential and N2pc) to Study Effects of Masked Stimuli

All peaks of brain-potential waveshapes to be reported in the following occurred in the "first half second" indeed, thus underlining the appropriateness of the title of our symposium and of the resulting present book. Previous studies had already investigated effects of masked stimuli on motor activation, by recording the lateralized readiness potential (LRP). The LRP is the difference potential between the EEG recording sites overlying the motor cortex contralateral to the responding hand (therefore controlling the response) and the ipsilateral EEG sites, separately averaged across trials with right-hand and with left-hand responses. These difference potentials are then combined to remove everything not lateralized as well as any constant asymmetries (Coles, 1989). Any resulting difference must be related to the difference between activating one response to the disadvantage of the other response, because anything else is subtracted out. Thus, the LRP describes the specific state of response selection at any given moment—in our case between onset of the two stimuli in series (masked prime and main stimulus) and the eventual response. Investigations of the LRP in masked priming (Dehaene et al., 1998; Eimer & Schlaghecken, 1998; Leuthold & Kopp, 1998) had found that the LRP was affected by the masked prime. We replicated this (Jaśkowski et al., 2002) for the stimuli developed by Klotz and Neumann (1999), as can be seen in the |C3-C4| recordings in figure 13.1: About 200 ms after prime onset (see the checked arrows), the LRP starts to deviate from the LRP evoked by neutral primes, either (in the congruent case; black lines) in the "correct" direction, that is, the direction also needed for the response to the target, or (in the incongruent case; gray lines) in the "incorrect" direction. This divergence was significant 250–300 ms after prime onset not only with an SOA of 167 ms when primes were slightly discriminable but also with an SOA of 83 ms when primes could not be discriminated.

This finding, if considered in isolation, would fit the notion that nonconsciously processed stimuli exert their influence on behavior by activating the visuomotor system on the dorsal pathway (as reflected in the LRP effects) but do not activate the object-identification system on the ventral pathway.

However, recording from the motor cortices alone does not provide a full picture. We applied the same contra-ipsilateral difference calculation to recording sites overlying the visual cortex (|P7-P8| waveshapes in figure 13.1). A similar divergence of congruent and incongruent waveshapes is seen as in the LRP, with its peak at about 270 ms after prime onset (black arrows). However, at these posterior sites, this divergence is significant with distinguishable stimuli only (SOA = 167 ms). Having the same topographical focus and latency from stimulus onset as the above-mentioned N2pc, this peak was interpreted as an N2pc evoked by the relevant feature in the primes. If, being an N2pc, this peak reflects attention-controlled stimulus selection, following the interpretation given in many previous studies with nonmasked stimuli (e.g., Eimer, 1996; Wauschkuhn et al., 1998; Woodman & Luck, 1999), the diamond in the primes attracts attention, but only if it may be distinguished (SOA = 167 ms), not when completely masked (SOA = 83 ms). This findings fully conforms to the notion that masked stimuli exert their effects on motor processes only. However, a further peak occurs at 430 ms after prime onset with the 167-ms SOA and at 350 ms with the 83-ms SOA (gray arrows). Relative to target onset, this yields about 270 ms in both cases (430 – 160 and 350 – 80), so we interpret it as an N2pc again, this time evoked by the target; that is, this component reflects attention being attracted by the imperative diamond in the main stimulus. The effect is virtually identical with both SOAs: The component is present in neutral and incongruent trials and absent in congruent trials, both if primes were discriminable (SOA = 167 ms) and if not (SOA = 83 ms). The absence of an N2pc with congruent trials suggests that the relevant shape (the diamond) did not attract attention when preceded by a relevant shape at the same location, presumably because the attentional shift had already been primed by that preceding shape. Thus, these effects suggest that masked stimuli prime visual selective attention, in addition to their priming the motor system.

A control experiment (reported in Jaśkowski et al., 2002) confirmed that this effect on the N2pc over posterior scalp areas was not simply some volume-conducted effect from the more anterior motor-cortex scalp sites: When stimuli were above and below fixation rather than left and right of fixation, the motor effects seen in the LRP continued to occur (because responses still had to be performed by the left and right hand), but the N2pc effects were massively reduced. Thus, these findings converge with other recent data (Mattler, 2003; Scharlau & Ansorge, 2003; Schmidt, 2002) to support the assumption that masked stimuli have their effects both on motor and nonmotor processing.

13.1.4 How Can Masked Stimuli Be Prevented From Getting Control?

If indeed masked stimuli prime our actions and our attention, as illustrated by the LRP and N2pc effects, can such stimuli make us do things we do not want to? What will happen if we are influenced by many masked stimuli in sequence? Will their effects accumulate and become overwhelming?

We investigated this issue by presenting masked primes in series (Jaśkowski et al., 2003) using similar but simpler stimuli than in the preceding study. Stimuli were two squares, left and right of fixation; the target stimulus was the one square that had gaps (always in the middle of the left and right outlines). This imperative pair was preceded by a series of four pairs (see figure 13.2, top left). The first pair fit within the outlines of the second, the second in the third, and so on, such that every pair could be metacontrast-masked by the following pair. The SOA between each

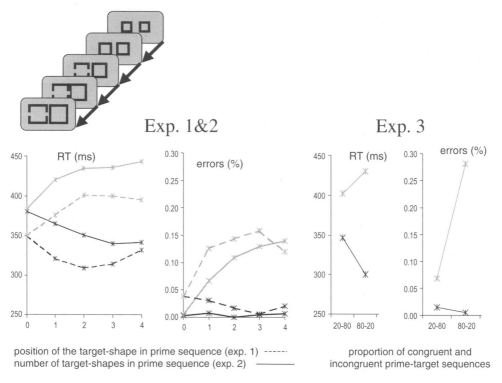

Figure 13.2
Cumulative priming effects of metacontrast-masked stimuli on behavior. The general layout of stimuli
is depicted on top: The main pair of stimuli was preceded by four metacontrast-masked primes. Primes
could include the targetlike shape (square with gaps), congruent or incongruent with the main stimulus.
Lower left panels: Results of experiments (Exp.) 1 and 2. Lower right panels: Results of experiment 3.
There were ten, nine, and nine participants in experiments 1, 2, 3, respectively. Note that y-scales are
equal across experiments for response times and errors, respectively. Black lines denote congruent trials;
gray lines incongruent trials. (Data from Jaśkowski et al., 2003)

pair was 35 ms. These preceding pairs were neutral (no gaps) or not (one member
of the pair had gaps). The square with gaps could be on the same side as the final
target square (congruent) or not (incongruent). In a first experiment, only one of
the four prime pairs contained a square with gaps (unlike in figure 13.2, top left),
so that we could be certain that responses to the target could be primed by targetlike shapes from each prime position. This was indeed the case, with a sufficiently
constant effect on response times of about 70 ms and a sufficiently constant error
rate in incongruent trials of about 15% (see figure 13.2, dashed lines). Therefore, in
the critical second experiment, the number of primes containing the target shape
was increased, varying from one to four between trials. We expected that the priming
effect would become overwhelming. Indeed, confirming this expectation, congru-

ence effects on error rates in incongruent trials and on response times became larger as the number of primes containing the target shape increased. However, even with four target-shape primes, these effects (see figure 13.2, solid lines) were not larger than in the previous experiment. Probably this was related to the overall speed of responses being slower in experiment 2 than in experiment 1. Therefore, we assumed that participants were more conservative in experiment 2, probably being aware that otherwise they would commit too many errors (although they did not perceive the reason for these errors). To test this hypothesis, we aimed at outwitting participants in experiment 3: The conservative strategy might be abandoned if the masked target shapes primed the correct response in most (80%) of the trials. Incongruent trials (20%) would then catch participants on their wrong foot. In comparison, if congruent trials were unlikely (20%), participants would be led to maintain a more conservative strategy. Thus, the proportion of congruent and incongruent trials was varied between blocks, being either 80/20 or 20/80. Indeed (see figure 13.2, lower right panels), when congruent trials were frequent, error rates in the few incongruent trials increased to 28% and prime effects on response times were large. In contrast, when incongruent trials were frequent, the error rate dropped to 7% and prime effects on response times were small. Note that the absolute number of errors remained approximately constant at 6% across blocks (28% of 20% incongruent trials is 5.6%, as is 7% of 80%), and this seems to be the subjectively relevant parameter for participants: If the number of errors becomes too high, for whatever reasons, subliminal or not, responses are selected in a more careful way. Thus, there is reason to hope that human subjects are not open to manipulation to an unlimited extent.

Prime discriminability was checked in these and the following experiments as follows. Two trials were presented, with primes containing gaps in one of the two trials only. Participants had to indicate which one of the two trials included the primes with gaps. To provide optimum conditions, we presented stimuli before this block in slow motion, and feedback was provided after each response. Participants whose d' score exceeded 0.25 were excluded.

Finally, we replicated experiment 3 and measured LRP and N2pc to see whether the "gate" that is opened and closed for the impact of masked stimuli can be localized in time and space. Have participants already rejected the effects of masked stimuli at a perceptual level, or is sensorimotor transmission reduced, or is the threshold elevated for the triggering of motor responses? As figure 13.3 shows, there were prime effects on the LRP (see the checked arrow), more extended in time than in figure 13.1, very probably because the four primes were also more extended in time than the one prime in figure 13.1. When "the gate is open" (the condition with 80% congruent trials; see the bold lines in figure 13.3) the prime effect on the LRP is significantly larger than when "the gate is closed" (the condition with 20%

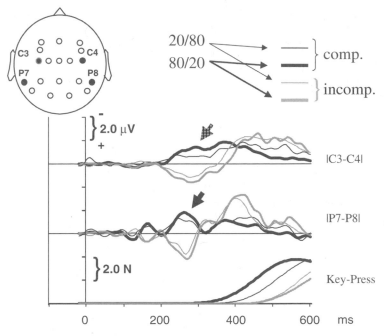

Figure 13.3
"Gate-opening" and "closing" for the effects of primes, as reflected in contra-ipsilateral event-related potential differences. Grand means over 11 participants. Upper row: recordings from |C3-C4| overlying the motor cortices. Middle row: recordings from |P7-P8| overlying the visual system (roughly V4). Lower row: recordings from the force-sensitive response keys, to display average times of response onset. The *x*-axis denotes milliseconds from onset of first prime (0 ms). Onset of the main stimulus, after four primes, was at 160 ms. There were three epochs of significant prime effects (differences between black and gray lines): 155–175, 205–325, and 355–475 ms after prime onset. These effects were moderated by proportion of congruent trials (differences between bold and thin lines) in the second and third epoch (with the second epoch of main interest). Checked arrows denote priming of the lateralized readiness potential in this epoch, black arrows of N2pc. (Data from Jaśkowski et al., 2003) comp., compatible; incomp., incompatible.

congruent trials; see the thin lines in figure 13.3). Of interest, this difference appeared to exist in figure 13.3 from the very beginning of the LRP effect, suggesting that not only did the gate become phasically active when some upper limit was exceeded by accumulated prime activation but prime effects on the motor system were generally attenuated.

When considering the recordings from visual areas (|P7-P8|), we notice an early prime effect at 170 ms, which did not occur in the previous experiment. This is probably an effect caused by the difference in simple visual features (i.e., the gap) between target-type and nontarget-type prime. This early prime effect was not affected by the gate. However, the following prime effect, peaking at about 270 ms (denoted by the black arrow in the figure) became smaller when the gate was closed (the condition with 20% congruent primes; see the thin lines). As in figure 13.1, we interpret this component as an N2pc evoked by the target-type prime, that is, as selection of the relevant feature in the prime. The gate effect on N2pc evoked by the primes suggests that the criterion for attentional selection was set more conservatively when primes were frequently incongruent with the final stimulus. (Note that this N2pc is not more extended in time than in figure 13.1, unlike the LRP, which fits well with the idea that attention cannot and need not be shifted any more when the shift has already been induced by the first prime. Only when the shape changes sides, as is the case with the main stimulus in incongruent trials, is a second N2pc generated in response to the main stimulus, at 400 ms, i.e., again about 270 ms after onset of the target, replicating the findings of Jaśkowski et al., 2002.)

We hope that readers will find these data as interesting as we do, but we would like to add some words of caution, to make clear that this field of ERP research is new, and so our interpretations of the waveshape peaks are hypotheses that may or may not be true. Comparing the |P7-P8| effects between figures 13.1 and 13.3 shows inconsistencies. We already mentioned the early effect at 170 ms, specific to the data in figure 13.3. Further, of some importance, masked primes did not evoke an N2pc in figure 13.1 but did so in the present experiment, even if the gate was closed (cf. also Woodman & Luck, 2003a). Again, a probable explanation is the layout of stimuli, which differed in shape in figure 13.1 (diamond vs. square) and in some simple feature in figure 13.3 (gap). To clarify matters, we are presently conducting control experiments, using both types of stimuli in the same tasks. A further interesting question is, Where is the "gatekeeper"? What we see in the ERP contra-ipsilateral differences probably is the functioning of the gate, but can we also see some area that surveys these processes? This gatekeeper need not be lateralized at all, so it may be suspected that some nonlateralized ERP components, such as N1, N2, and P3, are altered between 80/20 and 20/80 blocks. We did not find evidence for this (see figure 4 in Jaśkowski et al., 2003), but we recently started a functional magnetic resonance imaging experiment using this paradigm, hoping to localize more precisely the opening and closing gates and to find some evidence for the controlling action of a gatekeeper (Wolbers et al., in press).

13.2 Linking Research on Masking to Research on Hemineglect

The second part of this paper will describe research on the pathology of hemineglect. As will be detailed, masking and neglect have some things in common. First, in both cases events do not enter awareness but nevertheless may have priming effects on perception and action. Second, both phenomena share the common theme of visual attention. Evidence that this is true for effects of masked primes has been presented in the first part of this chapter. Some evidence for this hypothesis with respect to neglect will be discussed below.

13.3 Pathological Hemineglect

13.3.1 Introduction

Hemineglect is defined as a decreased tendency to respond to stimulation on one side (generally the left side) of space, of objects, or of one own's body (for recent reviews, see Driver & Vuilleumier, 2001; Kerkhoff, 2001; Husain & Rorden, 2003). This is a fascinating disorder because the affected patients no longer seem to share our common, agreed-upon model of the external world. In this respect, this pathology resembles psychiatric conditions, though evidently being due to neurological, somatic disease.

The most frequent cause of hemineglect is stroke, affecting posterior branches of the widely distributed middle cerebral artery (MCA). This artery supplies large regions of the cerebral cortex. The best known consequence of MCA infarction is paresis of one arm. This condition is due to infarction of anterior (or of small subcortical) branches of this artery. In contrast, if posterior MCA branches in the right hemisphere are affected, then a most likely consequence (at least in right-handers) will be neglect of the left side. The critical brain area to be affected is the junction of the right temporal and parietal lobes. It is controversial whether the focus is on the parietal side of the junction (Mort et al., 2003) or on the temporal side (Karnath et al., 2004). Patients with neglect might display bizarre behavior, sometimes misinterpreted in elderly patients as signs of dementia. Famous and illustrative are cases of florid neglect, where patients eat half the meal only, leaving the left half of their plate untouched, and complain about their portion being too small. Bisiach and coworkers (see Bisiach, 1993, for a review) beautifully demonstrated that *neglect* also refers to purely mental representations. For example, when asked to describe the buildings on the Piazza Duomo in Milan, patients enumerated buildings on the right side of their suggested viewpoint only, with the mentioned and not-mentioned buildings varying according to the suggested viewpoint.

As this evidence suggests, hemineglect can be clearly distinguished from hemianopia, which is defined as restriction of the visual field in the hemifield contralateral to the lesion. The most common cause of hemianopia is infarction of the posterior cerebral artery, leading to a lesion of the primary visual cortex situated in the occipital lobe. Hemianopia differs from hemineglect because (1) in hemineglect the visual field is intact, ideally; (2) hemineglect affects not only vision but also touch or even audition or smell; and (3) hemineglect patients do not seem to be aware of or to try to compensate for their deficit. In clinical practice, though, hemianopia may co-occur with hemineglect when areas supplied by the posterior cerebral artery and by posterior branches of the MCA do not neatly fit the standard brain (or, less frequently, when both arteries are affected).

A concept related to neglect is *extinction*, defined as a reduced tendency to respond to stimulation on one side *in the presence of stimulation on the healthy side*. It is often hard to tease apart what is neglect and what is extinction. For example, if the left half of food on the plate is not eaten, is this due to pure neglect, or are there some crumbs on the right side of the plate that lead to the left half's being extinguished? In fact, tests for extinction are the typical bedside tests for neglect, and, although neglect and extinction can be separately quantified in Posner's task (see below; Posner et al., 1984; Schürmann et al., 2003), extinction can be demonstrated without other signs of neglect in chronic patients (Friedrich et al., 1998) and thus might be conceived of as a residual, chronic symptom of former, more severe neglect. Therefore, although there have been suggestions to the contrary (e.g., Milner & Goodale, 1995, proposed that neglect is a disorder of the ventral pathway of visual processing, extinction of the dorsal pathway), extinction will here be treated as one (residual) symptom of the neglect syndrome.

13.3.2 Research Questions

Research on hemineglect has increased at a rapid rate in the past decade. Multiple connections to other areas of research have been developed, linking this research to experimental psychology as well as to cognitive neuroscience, in an attempt to account for hemineglect as a case of failure of mechanisms investigated in normal human subjects. While this approach has undoubtedly been fruitful, the precise mechanisms involved in producing neglect do not yet appear to be clear. For example, the extant literature does not provide a clear answer to the basic question of why neglect patients do not take a second look at those objects that they failed to focus their attention upon. The preferred answer still appears to be the one that was provided 20 years ago by Posner et al. (1984), who stated that these patients cannot withdraw their attention from the other, healthy side. Given that this is true, why do patients not realize that they have this problem?

13.3.3 Priming by Neglected Stimuli

A particularly fascinating aspect of the neglect disorder, suggesting its being related to perception of masked stimuli in healthy people, is that, although not consciously discriminated, neglected stimuli may have priming effects on subsequent behavior. Three examples will be given from recent literature. Schweinberger and Stief (2001) presented words left or right of fixation. In the "direct" task (our term, used here for convenience to match other literature), these words were followed by two words above and below fixation, one of which repeated the preceding lateral word. Patients showed severe hemineglect: They could indicate with only chance accuracy (50%) whether the upper or lower word repeated the preceding word when that word had been presented on the left side, in contrast to almost 100% accuracy when that word had been presented on the right side. In the "indirect" task, the lateral word was followed by a centrally presented word or nonword, and this central stimulus repeated the preceding lateral stimulus or did not. Patients were faster in making word–nonword decisions about the central word when it repeated the previous lateral word, by at least the same amount as healthy controls. Moreover, the positions of the preceding left and right words had no effect in the neglect patients (in contrast to hemianopic control patients). Thus, neglected left-side words did prime responses to following words.

Vuilleumier et al. (2002b) showed fragmented pictures of objects that either had been presented in a previous task or were novel. In that previous task, the objects had been briefly presented in the right, left, or both visual fields, and patients had not been able to respond to most left stimuli on bilateral presentation. Indeed, when asked in the fragmented-picture test whether such an object had been seen in the previous task (direct test), patients responded affirmatively as infrequently as to truly novel stimuli. Nevertheless, these pictures were better identified (i.e., when still on a more fragmented level) than novel stimuli (indirect test). Thus, extinguished left-side pictures did prime recognition of following pictures.

Manly et al. (2002) had patients perform the star cancellation task, which is part of a test battery for neglect. Patients have to detect stars printed on a sheet of paper amid several other stimuli and mark these stars with a pencil. Typical neglect patients mark only stars printed on the right side of the paper. Moreover, many patients seem to perseverate by putting several marks on those right-side stars. Manly et al. reasoned that this perseveration might in fact be a consequence of nonconsciously perceiving the unmarked stars on the left side. Therefore, these authors changed the test sheets, replacing stars on the left side by other, irrelevant stimuli. Indeed, the more stars, even though neglected, were replaced by other stimuli, the less those multiple markings of detected stimuli occurred. Thus, the direct measure indicated neglect of stars on the left side: They were not marked by patients. Yet an indirect measure indicated effects of the neglected stars on behavior: The more neglected stars were present, the more multiple marks of non-neglected stars occurred.

Thus, to summarize, although the priming effects found in these three tasks operate on very different time scales (more than 30 min from priming to the prime effect in Vuilleumier et al., 2002b; a few seconds in Schweinberger and Stief, 2001; simultaneous presence of the neglected stars in Manly et al., 2002), all the examples suggest that neglected stimuli, though not accessible to awareness, may affect behavior. This strikingly parallels the effects of masked stimuli in healthy people. Therefore, it might be assumed that neglect, rather than (or in addition to) being a failure of the mechanisms effective in healthy subjects, is an exaggeration, a caricature, as it were, of a neglect mechanism present in healthy subjects: Is pathological hemineglect not similar to normal behavior with masked stimuli?

13.3.4 Neglect Occurs Early in Perception and Depends on Focusing of Attention

In support of drawing this parallel between neglect and masked priming, we briefly review our own study with Posner et al.'s (1984) task in neglect patients, measuring ERPs and saccades (Verleger et al., 1996, 2002; for first data of a follow-up study, see Schürmann et al., 2003). In this task, two boxes are presented, left and right of fixation. Brightening of the outline of one box is the cue, followed 150 ms later by a cross in one of the boxes as the target. Participants have to make a simple keypress response to the target, irrespective of its side. All combinations of left and right cue with left and right target are equally probable. The important result in patients with right-parietal damage is the "extinction-type" deficit (Posner et al., 1984; see Schürmann et al., 2003, for linear separation of contributing factors), with misses and prolonged response times to left targets that are preceded by right cues. Figure 13.4 shows the ERPs evoked by targets from a group of 10 patients and 10 age-matched healthy subjects. The important feature, highlighted by arrows, is that patients display reduced early responses: Their N1 (peaking about 200 ms after target onset) is reduced to all stimuli but is virtually absent to the critical combination of right cue and left target. Thus, obviously, neglect occurs early in perception and is not due to some conservative response strategy on the part of the patients. (A thoughtful review on further ERP results in neglect patients was provided by Deouell et al., 2000b; cf. Deouell et al., 2000a).

Since we noticed in our electrooculographic recordings (originally recorded as a necessary control of ocular artifacts for EEG recording) that participants made systematic eye movements toward cue and targets in about 50% of all trials, we reanalyzed the response-time data, asking how patients' delay to right cue and left target is affected by the presence or absence of saccades. As figure 13.5 shows, the response-time delay to these targets (and other invalidly cued targets as well) is massively boosted by the presence of saccades. (Other details of these data cannot be discussed here, for brevity's sake; cf. Verleger et al., 2002.) It seems as if subjects used two different means of processing stimuli, one associated with saccades, the other not. One plausible dichotomy is between a distributed, diffuse mode of attention and a spatially selective, focused mode. In the distributed mode, subjects would perceive the stimuli on either side equally well. In the focused mode, attention would be positioned at a delimited location. This might either be the correct

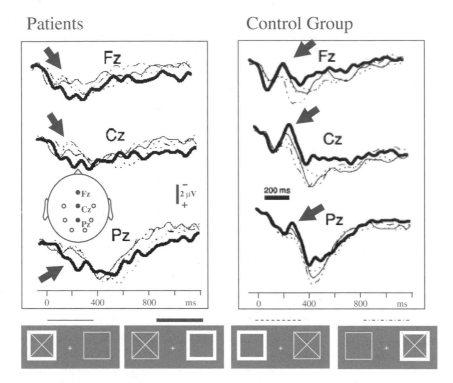

Figure 13.4
Event-related potentials evoked by targets in Posner et al.'s (1984) cuing task. Grand means over 10 patients with right-parietal lesions and 10 age-matched healthy participants. The x-axis is in milliseconds from target onset (onset of the cross in the left or right box). The cue (brightening of one box) occurred 150 ms earlier. The y-axis is in microvolts, with negative polarity (relative to linked earlobes) plotted upward. As symbolized by the schematic inserts of the boxes, the critical combination of right cue and left target is plotted in bold. Note the generally smaller N1 in patients and, in particular, the missing N1 to the critical combination. (Data are from Verleger et al., 1996)

position, in which case no shift of attention is necessary, or this might be an incorrect position, either with respect to the cue or to the target, in which case attention would have to be redirected to the presented stimulus. This redirecting would often be accomplished by a saccade. The point is that in this relatively undemanding task, the diffuse mode of attention would be entirely sufficient for performance. As soon as participants become more involved, focusing their attention on stimuli, performance deteriorates.

This hypothesis fits nicely the data published by Vuilleumier and Rafal (2000). By elegantly varying task demands with the same stimulus material, these authors found drastically differing rates of neglect, depending (in our interpretation of their data) on whether patients were led to use a diffuse distribution of attention ("How

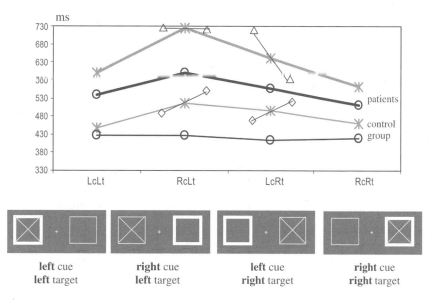

left cue | right cue | left cue | right cue
left target | left target | right target | right target

Figure 13.5
Response times in Posner et al.'s (1984) cuing task, depending on whether spontaneous saccades (eye movements) were made. Data from the same 10 patients with right-parietal lesions and 10 age-matched healthy participants as in figure 13.4. The *x*-axis denotes the four combinations of cue and target (LcLt, left cue and left target; RcLt, right cue and left target; LcRt, left cue and right target; RcRt, right cue and right target), as explained by the schematic inserts of the boxes; the *y*-axis denotes simple response times from target onset (cross in left or right box). Bold lines (slower responses): patients. Thin lines (faster responses): control group. Black lines with circles: trials in which no saccades were made. Gray lines with stars: trials in which saccades were made. The small left and right lines at the RcLt and LcRt combinations break the saccade trials further down into trials in which the first saccade went to the left or right. Note the generally drastic effect of whether a saccade was made or not. (See Verleger et al., 2002, for more details.)

many stimuli are there?") or a focused mode ("How many stars are there?"). Therefore, we, and others, have concluded that the important characteristic of neglect is a failure in the focusing of attention. The important link to be drawn here to research on masking is that the mechanism involved in this pathological failure of attention might be the same mechanism as is involved in lack of awareness normal people have for masked stimuli. Therefore, we will next address the question of whether neglect may be described in terms of a concept discussed as relevant in research on masking: *reentrant processing* (e.g., Di Lollo et al., 2000).

13.3.5 Is Reentrant Processing Deficient in Neglect?

As described in more detail elsewhere in this book, the empirical basis for reentrant processing is recordings from monkeys' visual cortex V1, showing that both masked and unmasked stimuli cause early activation in V1, peaking around 80 ms, and that

masked and unmasked stimuli differ in the amount of V1 activity from about
280 ms onward: This activity is reduced with masked stimuli (Bridgeman, 1980;
Lamme et al., 2002). Since rich feedback connections from "higher" visual areas
back to V1 have been described (Bullier, 2001), this later activity may be interpreted
as the result of recurrent processing: Higher areas "play back" some information to
V1, causing a second and a third pass of information through the visual system, refining the visual signal, which, by this very process, might reach conscious awareness
(Lamme, 2000; Di Lollo et al., 2000). Such second and third passes would not be
possible if stimuli are masked.

To prove the existence of reentrant processing in humans, it has to be shown that
the same location in visual cortex is passed at least two times with relevant stimuli.
Indeed, some evidence has been provided in support of this notion. Taking advantage of the opportunity to record directly from visual cortex in patients with med-
ically intractable epilepsy who were being evaluated for possible resection surgery,
Olson et al. (2001) found enhanced late activity (following unchanged early activity) in V1, V2, and other areas from 200 ms onward when the target in a visual search
display appeared at precued locations. Recording ERPs from the scalp in a demanding spatial-attention task and fitting the topographical distribution of their effects
to position emission tomography (PET) measurements from the same task,
Woldorff et al. (2002) replicated earlier findings of enhanced early activity (90–
160 ms) to spatially attended stimuli and added the new finding that later activity
to spatially attended stimuli (240–280 ms) had exactly the same topographical distribution, localized by PET to V2 and V3.

Differences between both findings do obviously exist and may be due to the different tasks, stimuli, and measurement methods. Further, we would have preferred
it if Woldorff et al. (2002) had found a more ventral topography for their reentrant
process at 270 ms, which would have made it easier to draw a parallel to research
on N2pc, as reported in the first part of this chapter, because N2pc probably originates from V4 and/or temporal occipital cortex (TEO) (Luck et al., 1997b; Hopf et
al., 2000; Oostenveld et al., 2001; cf. De Weerd et al., 2003). Nevertheless, in spite of
these problems, the results of Olson et al. (2001) and Woldorff et al. (2002) can be
interpreted (and were, in fact, interpreted by the authors of both papers) as evidence for the existence of reentrant processing in the human visual system.

The function played by reentrant processing has been interpreted as rechecking
the product of the first pass through the visual system with the original data stored
in V1. This might indeed be an adequate description of perceptual processing in
most of our experimental studies, where stimuli are only briefly flashed. In everyday life, however, objects tend to be more constant, so the data store does not need
to be in V1 but can reside in the outside world, and visual awareness can be
described as something we *do* with objects in the outside world (O'Regan & Noë,

2001). In this vein, the function played by reentrant processing may be interpreted as rechecking the product of the first pass through the visual system with the next perceptual input entering V1 from the same object. To get a second input from the same object, attention must be redirected to that object, as a product of the first pass through the system, and this implies (perhaps as a result of the following pass through the system) that the eyes become fixated on relevant parts of the object and (perhaps on subsequent passes) that the object is grasped.

The present proposal to explain neglect in these terms is that the right-side temporo-parietal junction plays an important part in controlling reentrant processing, possibly, in line with the above-mentioned remarks, by controlling the directing of attention. To the extent that this controlling center is damaged, only results from the first pass through the system will be available for further processing, as is probably the case with masked stimuli in healthy people, and this is possibly the reason for patients' behavior in studies exemplified above by the research of Schweinberger and Stief (2001), Vuilleumier et al. (2002b) and Manly et al. (2002). This would provide an answer to the question asked above: Why do neglect patients not take a second look at those objects that they failed to focus their attention upon? Because this is precisely the ability that is damaged in these patients.

Acknowledgments

Research reported in this chapter was supported by grants from the Deutsche Forschungsgemeinschaft, in particular Ve110/7-2 and -4.

V TEMPORAL CHARACTERISTICS OF FEATURE AND OBJECT PERCEPTION

14 Perceptual Consequences of Timing Differences Within Parallel Feature-Processing Systems in Human Vision

Harold E. Bedell, Saumil S. Patel, Susana T. L. Chung, and Haluk Öğmen

The transmission of information in sensory systems and within the brain occurs primarily via neural action potentials, which take time to generate and transmit. For example, the conduction velocities of mammalian unmyelinated retinal axons range approximately between 1 and 5 m/s, depending on the axon diameter. The conduction velocities of myelinated optic nerve axons also vary systematically with fiber diameter, ranging approximately between 5 and 30 m/s (Tolhurst & Lewis, 1992). As a result of the delays that are introduced by the elaboration and transmission of neural signals, information processing within the brain must always lag to a greater or lesser extent behind the real-world events that this brain information represents.

In this chapter, we will focus on the temporal aspects of information processing within the primate and human visual systems. The earliest stages of visual information processing in the retina depend to some extent on the characteristics of the visual stimulus. For example, the earliest responses that are recorded in the optic nerve vary inversely with the luminance of the visual stimulus (Lennie, 1981; Lee et al., 1990). These stimulus-dependent differences in neural response time carry forward to produce the initial responses to visual events in the lateral geniculate nucleus and visual cortex (e.g., Maunsell & Gibson, 1992; Maunsell et al., 1999).

Two additional properties of the primate visual system generate additional difficulties for the timing of visual events. First, evidence exists that visual information is encoded and transmitted from the retina to the visual cortex in two (or three; see Dacey & Lee, 1994; Hendry & Reid, 2000) parallel pathways, with overlapping but different temporal characteristics (Maunsell & Gibson, 1992; Schmolesky et al., 1998; Maunsell et al., 1999). And, second, visual information processing in the brain appears to be largely modular. That is, information about many aspects of the visual stimulus (e.g., color, motion, depth, etc.) is processed in specialized brain centers (e.g., Zeki & Shipp, 1988; Livingstone & Hubel, 1988; van Essen et al., 1992; Tootell et al., 1996; however, for a different view see Lennie, 1998), each of which may require a different amount of time to complete its analysis. Although the various brain areas are richly interconnected (van Essen et al., 1992; Tootell et al., 1996), it is unclear to what extent the vision-related events that result from modular processing within different areas in the brain are synchronized.

Uniform neural conduction and processing delays should cause sensory events to be registered or perceived at some fixed time after they actually occur. Clearly, such delays are detrimental for accurate interaction with the physical world, much of which must occur "online" in real time. One general strategy to alleviate this problem is motor prediction (Kerzel & Gegenfurtner, 2003), that is, the generation of motor programs and responses to stimuli based on the recent previous record of sensory information. The accuracy of this approach can be monitored by the sensory feedback that results from motor events (cf. von Holst & Mittelstädt, 1950), such as the retinal position and velocity signals that occur during ocular tracking of visual targets or during manual reaching responses to moving stimuli (Goodale et al., 1986; Barnes & Asselman, 1991; Saunders & Knill, 2003).

Even more problematic are the *differential* timing errors that would be expected to result from the unequal conduction and processing delays within specialized neural streams and within brain areas that preferentially encode and process different characteristics of a stimulus. These differential processing delays raise the possibility that different stimulus attributes could reach perception at different times, which would be expected to lead to interesting, annoying, and sometimes dangerous errors in perception. One well-known illusion of this type is the *Pulfrich stereo-phenomenon*, wherein a longer conduction latency from one eye (as the result of unequal target luminance in the two eyes or of unilateral optic nerve pathology, e.g., Lit, 1960; Julesz & White, 1969; Rushton, 1975) produces substantial distortions of perceived stereoscopic depth during object or observer motion.

The goal of this chapter is to consider two visual illusions—the flash-lag phenomenon and color–motion perceptual asynchrony—that have been attributed by some authors to differences in relative neural timing. We will refer to this explanation based on a difference in neural timing as the *differential-latency hypothesis*. First, we will provide a brief description of the phenomenology associated with each illusion. Next, we will examine the influence of stimulus parameters and of the observer's task on each illusion. Finally, we will present a qualitative model to account for both illusions, which represents essentially an elaborated version of the differential-latency hypothesis.

14.1   The Flash-Lag Effect

The flash-lag effect (FLE) is the perception that a briefly flashed target is at an erroneous location with respect to a continuously moving target. In particular, the flashed target typically appears to lag spatially behind the moving target when both are presented simultaneously at the same spatial location (for reviews, see Krekelberg & Lappe, 2001; Nijhawan, 2002; Öğmen et al., 2004b). Most investigators agree that the FLE requires the image of the moving target to traverse across the retina (Brenner et al., 2001; Nijhawan, 2001; but also see Cai et al., 2000), although it appears to be immaterial whether motion of the retinal image results from object or eye motion (Mateeff & Hohnsbein, 1988; Nijhawan, 2001; van Beers et al., 2001). The spatial magnitude of the FLE increases linearly with the velocity of the moving target (Nijhawan, 1994; Krekelberg & Lappe, 2000), which implies that the FLE corresponds to a constant temporal delay of the flashed stimulus with respect to the moving target. This interpretation is consistent with the earliest explanations of the FLE in terms of a difference in the "sensation time" or "perception time" between the flashed and moving targets (e.g., Metzger, 1932). Our version of this differential-latency hypothesis assumes that the relative delay in determining the position of a moving compared to a flashed target is associated primarily with the characteristics of different neural streams that are hypothesized to process moving versus nonmoving (in this instance, flashed) stimuli. However, we do not assume that the delay in each processing stream is fixed but rather, as discussed below, that it varies systematically with characteristics of the target and the observer's task. As summarized, for example, in Krekelberg and Lappe (2001), Nijhawan (2002), and Öğmen et al. (2004b), a number of competing explanations have been proposed previously for the FLE.

The FLE still occurs when the flashed target occurs concurrently with the onset of motion (Khurana & Nijhawan, 1995; Eagleman & Sejnowski, 2000a; Patel et al., 2000). Initially, this result may be surprising, as a moving and a flashed target are physically indistinguishable right at the onset of motion. However, a moving target has been reported to become visible only after it traverses the earliest portion of its trajectory, presumably because of spatiotemporal interactions that are inherent in the early phases of motion processing. This phenomenon, known as the *Fröhlich effect*, could conceivably account for the presence of a flash lag when the flash is presented concurrently with the beginning of target motion (Eagleman & Sejnowski, 2000a). However, this possibility is not supported by findings that the Fröhlich effect can be substantially smaller than the FLE that occurs at the onset of motion (Whitney & Cavanagh, 2000; Müsseler et al., 2002; Kreegipuu & Allik, 2003).

The magnitude of the FLE depends on the retinal eccentricity of the targets (Baldo et al., 2002), and possibly also on whether the spatial position and timing of the flashed target are predictable (Khurana et al., 2000; Brenner & Smeets, 2000; Eagleman & Sejnowski, 2000b; Baldo et al., 2002; Namba & Baldo, 2004). For parafoveal flashed and moving targets that are approximately the same luminance, a typical magnitude of the FLE is 40–80 ms (e.g., Whitney et al., 2000; Krekelberg & Lappe, 2001).

Altering the detectability of the flashed and moving stimuli results in systematic changes in the temporal magnitude of the measured FLE. For example, making the flashed target dimmer increases the FLE, and making the flashed target brighter reduces the FLE (Purushothaman et al., 1998; Lappe & Krekelberg, 1998; Öğmen et al., 2004b). If the flash is very bright and the moving stimulus is dim, the flash lag can reverse to a flash lead (see figure 14.1; see also Purushothaman et al., 1998; Patel et al., 2000). The existence of a flash lead casts substantial doubt on several proposed explanations for the FLE—for example, those that require the position of the moving target to be sampled only *after* the flash is perceived (cf. Öğmen et al., 2004b).

The changes in the FLE with target luminance can be accounted for on the basis of latency changes in the visual system that occur with variations in the stimulus intensity. As noted above, physiological recordings indicate that the latency of visual responses increases systematically as the luminance of the stimulus is reduced (Lennie, 1981; Lee et al., 1990; Maunsell & Gibson, 1992; Maunsell et al., 1999). In addition to the Pulfrich stereo-phenomenon, another piece of psychophysical

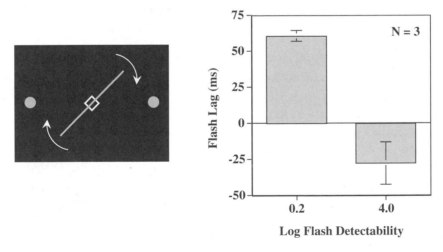

Figure 14.1
The flash-lag effect (FLE) can be determined as the temporal offset, with respect to the instant of *physical* alignment between a pair of briefly flashed dots and a rotating line, that yields the perception that the dots and line are in spatial alignment (left). The measured FLE changes from approximately a 60-ms lag (flashes presented *before* physical alignment with the moving line) to approximately a 25-ms lead (flashes presented *after* physical alignment with the moving line) when the luminance of the flashes increases from 0.2 to 4.0 log units above their detection threshold (right). The luminance of the rotating line was 0.5 log units above its detection threshold. (Data are the average of three observers ±1 *SE*, replotted from Öğmen et al., 2004b)

evidence for the dependence of visual processing latency on stimulus luminance is the *Hess effect*, wherein the dimmer of two moving stimuli is perceived to lag behind the brighter one, even though both stimuli are physically aligned. According to Williams and Lit (1983), the Hess effect corresponds to a delay of approximately 50 ms when the luminance of two relatively dim photopic moving stimuli differs by 2 log units.

14.2 Perceived Color–Motion Asynchrony

More recently, experiments using stimuli that change periodically in color and direction of motion have led to the inference that a temporal asynchrony exists between the processing of color and motion information in the brain (Moutoussis & Zeki, 1997a, 1997b; Zeki & Moutoussis, 1997). Consider the stimulus pictured in figure 14.2A, which is modeled after the stimulus used in the initial report of this phenomenon (Moutoussis & Zeki, 1997a). In order for the squares to be perceived as uniformly red when moving upward and uniformly green when moving downward, the change from upward to downward motion has to precede the change in color by between 80 and 140 ms (Moutoussis & Zeki, 1997a, 1997b; Zeki & Moutoussis, 1997; Arnold & Clifford, 2002; Nishida & Johnston, 2002; Bedell et al., 2003). Moutoussis and Zeki (1997a, 1997b) interpreted this result to mean that the neural processing of motion information lags behind the processing of color by this amount of time. Using a similar paradigm, the processing of stimulus orientation also was inferred to lag behind the processing of color (Moutoussis & Zeki, 1997b).

Altering the characteristics of the stimuli can substantially change the outcome of these temporal asynchrony experiments. For example, if the direction of motion change is less than 180°, then a much smaller temporal advance of the motion stimulus is required for stimulus color and motion to be perceived in correspondence. In particular, when the change in direction of motion is 45°, both Arnold and Clifford (2002) and Bedell et al. (2003) have reported that the apparent temporal asynchrony decreased from approximately 140 to 80 ms.

Changing the observers' task can cause the apparent temporal asynchrony between color and motion to vanish almost completely. Nishida and Johnston (2002) presented their observers with a stimulus on one side of fixation that changed in color from green to red and a second stimulus on the opposite side of fixation that changed in direction of motion from upward to downward. Both stimuli changed just once during each trial. Observers performed a temporal order judgment, by reporting whether the change in color or the change in direction of motion occurred first. The results indicate virtually no perceptual asynchrony when the color and direction of stimulus motion changed physically at the same time.[1]

A

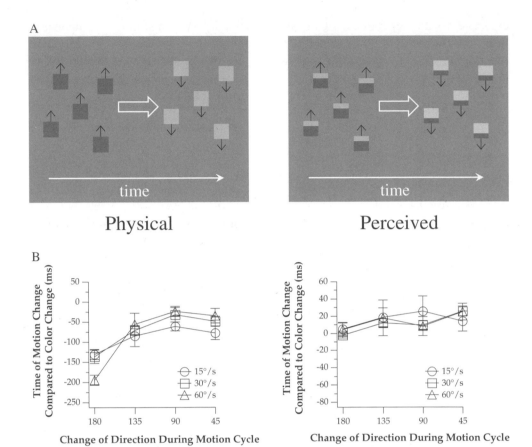

Figure 14.2

(*A*) A field of moving dots that synchronously changes color from red to green and direction of motion from up to down is perceived to change in color during both upward and downward motion. This stimulus, in which each dot undergoes both a color and direction-of-motion change, is referred to as the *conjunctive* stimulus in the text. Red and green colors are indicated by relatively darker and lighter shades of gray in the figure, but in our experiments both stimulus colors were adjusted to be equally above the detection threshold. (*B*) The temporal asynchrony between the change in color and the change in direction of motion that is required for perceptual synchrony between color and motion depends on the observers' task. Depending on the magnitude of the direction change, the direction of dot motion has to change between 50 and 150 ms before dot color in order for observers to perceive the motion and color of the dots to correspond temporally (left panel). Regardless of the magnitude of the direction change, the direction of dot motion and dot color have to change at approximately the same time for observers to perceive both changes to occur simultaneously (right panel). Data are the averages of four (left) or three (right) observers, for three velocities of dot motion (Bedell et al., 2003). The temporal period of each cycle of color and motion change was 706 ms.

We replicated this finding, using a single, composite stimulus like that used by Moutoussis and Zeki (1997a) for a range of motion-direction changes between 45 and 180 deg (see figure 14.2B). In one condition, the color and direction of motion of the stimulus changed just once during each trial. In another condition, the color and direction of motion changed repetitively, but the observers waited until the final half cycle of color and motion change, signaled by an auditory cue, to make the temporal order judgment. In neither of these conditions did the perceived temporal asynchrony between the change in color and direction of motion differ significantly from zero, regardless of the magnitude of the direction change. In contrast, the same observers judged the color and direction of motion of the repetitively changing stimulus to correspond when the change in direction of motion occurred 30 to 140 ms earlier (depending on the magnitude of the direction change) than the change in stimulus color. Clifford et al. (2003) reported a similar task-dependent outcome for stimuli that changed in color and orientation.

On the basis of the influence of target luminance on the FLE, we expected that changing the detectability of a stimulus that alternated in color and direction of motion should systematically influence the magnitude of the apparent temporal asynchronies in the color correspondence and temporal order tasks. To test this hypothesis, we modified our stimulus, so that the luminance of the color and motion components could be manipulated separately. The stimulus that we adopted was similar to the one described above for the temporal order experiment of Nishida and Johnston (2002) and, previously, by Moutoussis and Zeki (1997b). As depicted in figure 14.3A, a field of stationary 1.1 deg squares on the right side of fixation changed periodically (1.42 Hz) from red to green, and a field of yellow squares on the left side of fixation changed periodically between upward and downward motion at 30 deg/s. At the observers' viewing distance of 21 cm, each stimulus field subtended 11.3 × 11.3 deg, and the edge-to-edge separation between the right and left fields was 1.4 deg. In agreement with the results of Moutoussis and Zeki (1997b), the motion in the left field had to reverse in direction substantially earlier than the change in color in the right half field, in order for the observers to judge the color and motion of the stimuli to be in correspondence (see figure 14.3B). For other magnitudes of motion-direction change, this "disjunctive" stimulus yielded results that were similar, although not identical, to those obtained on the color–motion correspondence task using the original "conjunctive" color–motion stimulus (see figure 14.3B). As with our original, conjunctive stimulus, temporal order judgments made with the disjunctive stimulus showed no significant color–motion asynchrony.

In the experiment described above, each of the stimuli in the color–motion display were approximately 4.4 log units above the observers' detection threshold. Decreasing the luminance of the targets on either the right or the left side of the display produced the expected changes in timing in both the color–motion correspondence

A

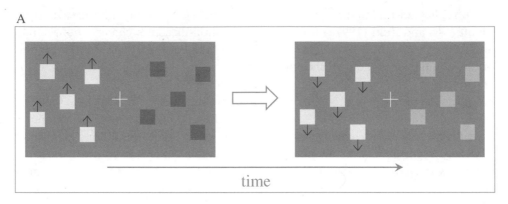

Physical

B

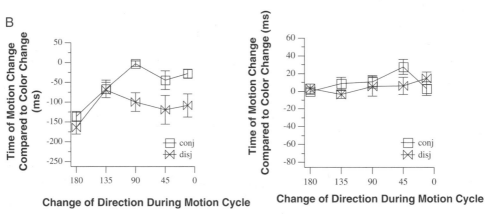

Change of Direction During Motion Cycle

C

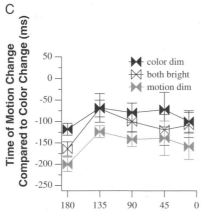

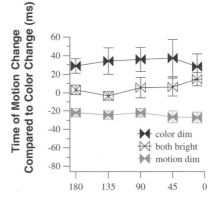

Change of Direction During Motion Cycle   **Change of Direction During Motion Cycle**

task and the temporal order task (see figure 14.3C). Specifically, when the luminance of the right-hand (changing-color) side of the display was reduced by 2 log units, the apparent temporal asynchrony in the color–motion correspondence task decreased by approximately 25 ms, for all tested directions of motion change. When the lumi-nance of the left-hand (changing-direction-of-motion) side of the display was reduced by 2 log units, the apparent temporal asynchrony between color and motion increased by approximately 40 ms. Across all directions of motion change, the absolute magnitude of the luminance-induced changes in apparent asynchrony does not depend on which side of the display was made dimmer, $(t(4) = 0.93, p = 0.40)$. Very similar changes, of approximately ±30 ms, were obtained for the temporal order judgments when the luminance of the color or the motion stimulus was decreased by 2 log units.

14.3   A Qualitative Model for Perceived Temporal Asynchronies

Figure 14.4 shows a qualitative model to account for the findings of experiments on the flash-lag and color–motion asynchrony, which are summarized in the sections above. Consistent with previous physiological and psychophysical data, we envision that the cortical processing of visual information is modular, with separate special-ized brain areas devoted to the processing of visual motion, color, static position, and so forth (Livingstone & Hubel, 1988; van Essen et al., 1992; Tootell et al., 1996). The model in figure 14.4 incorporates separate delays between the retina and each brain module, in order to represent the possibility that each of these retinocortical delays may not be the same. Rather, the delay for retinal information to reach each cortical module is likely to depend on the processing stream that is involved, the amount of preprocessing that is required before the information reaches each module (e.g., in early stages of V1), and on the characteristics of the stimulus (see below).

Figure 14.3
(*A*) The *disjunctive* stimulus consists of two fields of dots that straddle a central fixation target. The right-hand field of dots changes color and the left-hand field of dots changes direction of motion, both with a period of 706 ms. (*B*) Temporal asynchronies between the change in color and the change in direction of motion to achieve perceived temporal correspondence between color and motion vary similarly with the direction of motion change for the conjunctive (conj) and disjunctive (disj) stimulus (left panel). However, the direction of dot motion and dot color have to change at approximately the same time for observers to perceive both changes simultaneously, for both the conjunctive (conj) and disjunctive (disj) stimulus (right panel). Plotted data are the average of two observers, for a speed of dot motion of 30 deg/s. (*C*) A 2 log-unit decrease in the luminance of the dots that change in color or direction of motion produces a systematic shift in the temporal asynchrony that is required to achieve perceived temporal correspondence (left panel) or perceived simultaneity (right panel) between color and motion. Note that the *y*-axes are scaled differently in the left and right panels. The plotted data are the averages of the same two observers shown figure 14.3B, using the "disjunctive" stimulus and dot motion of 30 deg/s.

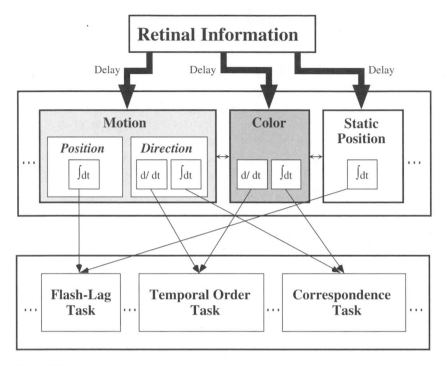

Figure 14.4
A qualitative model to account for the perceived temporal asynchronies between various stimulus attributes, for different perceptual tasks. The components of the model and their temporal properties are described in the text.

The color processing module in the center of the figure is subdivided functionally according to the temporal characteristics of the information processing that occurs. This module can provide sustained information about stimulus color, based on a relatively slow process that includes an obligatory stage of temporal integration. In addition, we propose that a different subdivision of the same color module can provide more rapid information about *changes* in color, based on operations that respond selectively to transients or variation in the chromatic content of the stimulus.[2] In our scheme, the rapid information about color change is not necessarily informative about the actual color that is present, which becomes available only after integration of the stimulus-related input in the slower, sustained subdivision of this module.

The motion processing module at the left of the figure is shown to include more than one functional component. One of these provides integrated, sustained information about the direction of motion, as well as more rapid information that specifies the occurrence of a change in the direction of motion. A second, presumably parallel component uses motion information to determine the position of a moving target. A separate module shown at the right of the figure provides sustained output about the position of nonmoving targets.[3]

Like the color module and the direction component of the motion module, other modules not shown in the figure (such as modules for processing orientation and depth) are envisioned to have a similar architecture, with the ability to provide separate information about sustained and transient features of various visual stimuli. Although the general characteristics of sustained and transient signal processing are presumed to be similar within each module, we do not believe that each module's temporal properties are identical (cf. the discussion of the FLE, below).

The final layer that is shown in the model represents a highly flexible level of processing that compares the information from relevant modules or module subdivisions, in order to meet the requirements of the observer's specific task. Based on the topics that we discussed in this chapter, the figure shows the proposed comparisons between visual information for just three types of tasks: (1) the perceived positions of a moving and a nonmoving target that give rise to the FLE, (2) target color and the direction of stimulus motion as in the color–motion correspondence task described originally by Moutoussis and Zeki (1997a, 1997b), and (3) *changes* in the color and the direction of motion of one or more stimuli as in the temporal order judgments reported by Nishida and Johnston (2002) and others. In the remainder of the chapter we will consider how the model in figure 14.4 accounts for the principal results that are reported for these three tasks. However, the model permits a much larger number of stimulus comparisons to be made, especially if one considers additional visual (and nonvisual) processing modules and divisions that are not currently represented explicitly in the figure.[4]

The main findings that the model can account for are:

1. The flash-lag paradigm requires observers to compare the temporally integrated position signals from the motion and static-position modules. We assume that this comparison occurs at the instant the flash becomes visible, as specified by a transient signal of target brightness or contrast that is not depicted explicitly in this representation of the model (see Öğmen et al., 2004b). Presumably, the FLE occurs because retinal information is delayed less in reaching the motion module compared to the static-position module and/or because, for a continuously moving stimulus, the processing of motion into a signal of target position occurs more quickly than the generation of a static-position signal. Systematic variations in the magnitude and direction of the FLE for targets of different luminance are attributable primarily to luminance-dependent changes in the delays that retinal information undergoes before it reaches the cortical modules that analyze motion and static position. In contrast, the reported modulation of the FLE according to the predictability of the flashed target (Khurana et al., 2000; Brenner & Smeets, 2000; Eagleman & Sejnowski, 2000b; Baldo et al., 2002; Namba & Baldo, 2004) could reflect an unequal

facilitation of position processing by attentional mechanisms within the motion and static-position modules.

2. In the model, judgments of color–motion correspondence require a comparison between the temporally integrated information from the color–processing module and the subdivision of the motion-processing module that determines the direction of target motion (Bedell et al., 2003). As indicated above, the apparent temporal asynchrony between color and motion is appreciably longer when the motion stimulus reverses its direction, compared to when the change in the direction of motion is smaller than 180 deg (Arnold & Clifford, 2002; Bedell et al., 2003). To interpret this result, we note a moving stimulus that reverses in direction will sequentially stimulate a pair of opponent motion channels, whereas a stimulus that changes direction by an appreciably smaller angle (e.g., 135 deg or less) will not. When opponent motion channels are activated one after the other, the response to the first direction of motion may have to be terminated before a response to the opposite direction of motion can begin. Consequently, the generation of an integrated signal to indicate the direction of motion would be expected to include a longer delay within the motion-processing module when a pair of opponent motion channels are activated than when opponent channels are not involved (i.e., for direction changes that are less than 180 deg). A similar added delay could accrue when opponent *color* channels are stimulated in succession, but the results of color–motion correspondence experiments suggest that this delay must be relatively small. Possibly, motion information is integrated over a longer period of time than color, in order to generate a reliable steady-state signal for the direction of motion. Clifford et al. (2003) offered a similar interpretation of their data on the apparent perceptual asynchronies between color and orientation changes, namely, that differences in the integration properties for different dimensions of the stimulus would be expected to produce an effective phase shift in perceived temporal correspondence.

3. In contrast to judgments of color–motion correspondence, temporal order judgments do *not* require integrated information about either the current stimulus color or its direction of motion. Consequently, these judgments can be based on the detection of transients that occur in association with a change in stimulus color or direction of motion. In the model, information about changes in the color and direction of motion of the stimulus are available from the transient subdivisions of each processing module. Because the transient signals for color and direction change do not require temporal integration (and, specifically, do not involve the relatively slow integration of information within opponent motion channels), each module can provide these signals quickly and with very little *relative* delay.

Nishida and Johnston (2002) reported that the apparent temporal asynchrony between color and motion varies systematically with the temporal frequency of the color and motion changes. Specifically, when the color and the direction of motion of their stimuli alternated at 2 Hz, observers judged these changes to occur in phase if the direction of motion changed physically about 100 ms earlier than the change in color. In contrast, when the color and direction of motion of their stimuli changed at 0.25 Hz, the observers' judgments about relative phase were close to veridical. Our interpretation of these data is that their observers used information from the transient subdivisions of the color and motion modules to make temporal order judgments when the temporal frequency of color and direction changes was low. When the temporal frequency of color and direction changes increased, it may have been difficult for the observers to compare the resulting transients accurately for the same half cycle. If so, then the observers would have been forced to rely on the temporally integrated information about color and direction of motion to make a comparison, thereby switching to a color–motion correspondence judgment.

4. Reducing the luminance of either the color or the motion component of the stimulus introduces comparable changes in timing, both for judgments of color–motion correspondence and of temporal order. Analogous to our discussion of the influence of target luminance on the FLE, above, the most parsimonious interpretation of these results is that a decrease in the luminance of one component of the stimulus increases the neural delay before information about that component reaches the cortical module that analyzes color or motion.[5] This analogy between the effects of target luminance in the color–motion asynchrony and the FLE paradigms can also be examined quantitatively. As shown in figure 14.3, a decrease in the luminance of the color or the motion target from approximately 4.4 to 2.4 log units above its luminance detection threshold produced approximately a 30-ms change in timing. In agreement with this result, we reported recently that the FLE also increases by approximately 30 ms when the luminance of the flashed target decreases from 4 to 2 log units above its detection threshold (Öğmen et al., 2004b). The correspondence between these values is striking, as the luminance-dependent changes in delay that occur in these different experiments involve different cortical modules as illustrated in the model in figure 14.4.

14.4   Summary and Conclusions

The principal points in this chapter may be summarized as follows:

1. The relative timing of perceived visual events is influenced by the characteristics of the neural channels and mechanisms that respond to specific stimulus characteristics. For example, the FLE suggests that the processing of position for a moving stimulus occurs more quickly than the processing of position for a flashed stimulus.

2. The relative timing of perceived visual events varies also with stimulus parameters that influence the delay involved in low-level visual processing, such as luminance and retinal eccentricity.

3. The observers' task also influences the relative timing of perceived events, based on the type of information and information processing (e.g., temporally averaged vs. transient) that is required to perform the task.

Acknowledgments

Preparation of this chapter and the studies that are reported in it were supported by Research Grants R01 EY05068 (to Harold E. Bedell), R01 MH49892 (to Haluk Öğmen), and R01 EY12810 (to Susana T. L. Chung) from the National Institutes of Health. We thank our collaborators, Gopathy Purushothaman and Kaan Camuz, who were instrumental in collecting some of the data that we describe.

Notes

1. Viviani and Aymoz (2001) reported a nonzero temporal asynchrony between a change in color and a change in motion using a temporal order task. However, in their experiment the changes in color and motion occurred at different retinal eccentricities, which may have introduced an additional timing difference (see Bedell et al., 2003).

2. However, even the transient subdivision includes a finite period of integration, which places an upper limit on the temporal frequency of visual changes to which it can respond.

3. Although not represented in the figure, the static position module and the position component of the motion module could include transient as well as sustained functional subdivisions.

4. Our representation of the model is *not* meant to suggest that separate sites are required for each possible comparison between stimuli. Although it remains unclear how and where such comparisons occur, the model stipulates only that the comparison site(s) must be able to observe simultaneously the outputs of the relevant processing modules.

5. The smallest change in the direction of motion that we presented in our experiments was 11.3 deg (the right-most data points in each panel of figure 14.3B and 14.3C). This value is only about four times the threshold for discriminating a change in the direction of motion for this stimulus. Based on the difficulty of discriminating such a small change in the direction of motion, one might expect that the apparent temporal lag between motion and color would increase, compared to conditions in which the change in the direction of motion is larger. This expectation is supported by findings that reaction times are prolonged substantially when observers are asked to respond to small compared to larger changes in the direction of stimulus motion (Mateeff et al., 1999; Genova et al., 2000). Nevertheless, our results indicate that the apparent temporal lag in the color–motion correspondence task is similar for changes in the direction of motion from 11.3 deg to 135 deg, and that the perceived temporal order between color and motion is similar for changes in the direction of motion from 11.3 deg to 180 deg. Our explanation for these results, which may be applied also to other reported dissociations between judgments of temporal order and reaction times (e.g., Williams & Lit, 1983), is that an additional delay can be introduced for stimuli of low discriminability *after* the stimuli are processed by the cortical color and motion modules, at the level where the module outputs are compared. Clearly, this additional delay is task specific and therefore presumably represents an operation, such as thresholding (e.g., Sternberg & Knoll, 1973), that is implemented differently in the reaction time and temporal order tasks.

15 The Relationship of Visual Masking and Basic Object Recognition in Healthy Observers and Patients with Schizophrenia

Michael H. Herzog

Despite more than 100 years of research, the mechanisms underlying visual masking are still largely unknown. Most explanations of masking rely on either low-level energy or high-level object recognition based models. Using the recently discovered feature inheritance and shine-through effects, I review psychophysical evidence that visual masking can also be related to the basics of object recognition such as grouping, figure–ground segmentation, and feature binding. Computer simulations suggest that masking effects can occur when redundant stimulus elements are eliminated from further processing when grouping elements to objects and segmenting these objects from the background. Surprisingly, even if targets are masked completely, some of their features can still be visible, being "inherited" to elements of the mask. This inheritance effect is attributed to the binding of features to objects. In schizophrenic patients, compared to healthy observers, visual masking can exert much stronger effects. Our results (Herzog et al., 2004b) indicate that grouping and figure–ground segmentation processing are intact even under masked conditions. Our studies suggest that visual information processing in schizophrenics may be attributable to influences we are just beginning to explore.

15.1 Introduction

The deteriorating effects of a mask on a target are, classically, explained in terms of integration and interruption masking (e.g., Breitmeyer, 1984; Bachmann, 1994; Breitmeyer & Öğmen, 2000). *Integration masking* can be described by a temporal low-pass filtering caused by the limited temporal resolution of the visual system, that is, target and mask are processed as *one* stimulus. Deteriorated performance occurs since the target contrast is reduced or the target is camouflaged by the mask. In integration masking, usually, mask and target spatially overlap as occurs for pattern, noise, and light masks. The later the presentation of the mask, the weaker is the masking effect.

Interruption masking means that the mask interferes with the *processing* of the target. Whereas integration masking is described by a rather unspecific lumping of mask and target, recent approaches to interruption masking employ sophisticated interactions of target and mask processing. For example, transient channels interact with sustained channels (Öğmen & Breitmeyer, this volume), unspecific thalamic facilitation interacts with specific cortical processing (Bachmann, this volume), or the high-level representation of the target is substituted by the mask representation (Enns et al., this volume). Interruption masking is also often explained by an interference of contour processing of the mask with the target as it occurs with spatially nonoverlapping metacontrast masks (e.g., Werner, 1935; Alpern, 1953).

Here, I will introduce two masking paradigms, feature inheritance and shine through, that cannot be explained by the common integration and interruption masking mechanism. I will argue that these two effects are related to the fundamental processes of object recognition such as object grouping, figure–ground segmentation, and feature binding. These object recognition processes are often assumed to involve complex, high-level processing characteristics. However, modeling results show that lateral interactions of simple low-level mechanisms can explain the basic masking effects in shine through. Moreover, the shine-through paradigm can be used as a versatile tool in schizophrenia research, showing that basic object recognition processes, such as object grouping, are fast and intact.

15.2 Review of Major Findings

15.2.1 Feature Binding and Feature Inheritance

In the feature inheritance effect, features of a single preceding element, such as vernier offset, orientation, or apparent motion, are bound to a following masking grating (see figure 15.1[1]). The grating appears to be offset, oriented, or "moved" in the direction of the preceding element (see figure 15.1). Since a single, "parental" element "bequeaths" its features to a number of elements in a subsequent "filial" generation, we called this effect the *feature inheritance effect*. In the inheritance effect, the preceding element remains largely invisible.[2]

How can these inheritance effects be explained? For the following scenario, let us focus on the case of motion inheritance (see figure 15.1C). Visual information processing is highly parallel—that is, the different attributes of an object, such as its shape, color, and motion, are analyzed in different parts of the brain. How these elements are bound together is known as the *binding problem* (for a review, see Roskies, 1999). Because of this parallel processing, the "apparent" motion of the

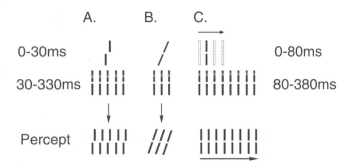

Figure 15.1
Examples of feature inheritance. (*A*) A vernier stimulus—that is, two lines of the same orientation that are slightly separated from each other—is followed by a grating comprising five verniers without offset. The grating appears to be offset in the direction of the vernier. (*B*) A clockwise tilted vernier followed by a grating, comprising three straight elements, results in the percept of a clockwise tilted grating. (*C*) A vernier is presented at four consecutive locations for a duration of 20 ms each, that is, 80 ms altogether (see the time scale on the right). Afterward, a grating comprising eight lines follows. Even though all grating elements are displayed simultaneously, observers perceive a grating in which the elements are drawn one after the other in the direction of the apparent motion of the preceding vernier. Verniers were 1260 arc sec long. The distance between grating elements was 200 arc sec. (Adapted from Herzog & Koch, 2001)

preceding vernier may elicit responses in the "motion area" MT, whereas the line structure of the vernier may be analyzed in the primary visual cortex V1. The following grating provokes no responses in MT since the grating is static. However, the grating may elicit neuronal signals in V1 or V2 (in V2, neurons were found that are dedicated to second-order structures such as gratings; e.g., von der Heydt, Peterhans, & Dursteler, 1992). We suggest that the representation of the *individual* elements of the grating is *suppressed* in favor of a representation of the grating as a *whole*. This may be achieved by lateral or recurrent (Ma et al., this volume; Hamker, 2004) connections in or between areas V1 and V2. During the suppression process of the single grating elements the preceding vernier is also inhibited, since it is a single element. Hence, the preceding vernier is invisible. Only the existence of the grating is signaled. However, the motion of the preceding vernier is not masked by the grating and, hence, may be attributed to the grating by virtue of the binding power of the human brain. The very same binding processing would occur if the grating was in motion and there is no preceding vernier: The grating's motion would be analyzed in MT, whereas its second-order structure would be processed in V1 or V2. Both would be linked by the binding mechanisms of the human brain.

Motion inheritance is much more easily performed than is vernier offset inheritance. This suggests that the motion is processed in area MT quite distinct from the spatial processing of V1 and V2 where vernier offset analysis may also be carried out. Since the vernier has to be masked for successful feature inheritance, the vernier offset may also be partly masked.

The feature inheritance effect shows that features, such as motion, orientation, or vernier offset, can be freed from their carriers and can be bound to different objects. Feature inheritance–like effects are often observed with metacontrast masks (e.g., Werner, 1935; Enns, 2002; Breitmeyer, personal communication). Wilson and Johnson (1985) showed that a gap in a line can be bequeathed to a following non-interrupted line. Stewart and Purcell (1970) found an analogous result for a broken ring and a following annulus.

15.2.2   Grouping and Shine Through

In the feature inheritance effect, only one entity, the grating, is perceived, to which the features of the preceding vernier are bequeathed. Surprisingly, adding more elements to the grating renders the preceding vernier visible as a shine-through element that appears to be superimposed on the grating (figure 15.2A; Herzog & Koch, 2001; Herzog et al., 2001a). The shine-through element inherits the vernier offset. Hence, two independent entities are perceived, the grating and the shine-through element. Just by adding more elements to the grating, the state of feature binding has changed. Improved performance for extended versus small masks occurs also for classical light, noise, and metacontrast masks (Herzog et al., 2003b) and has been shown for simultaneously presented pattern masks, too (Wehrhahn, Li, & Westheimer, 1996; Li et al., 2000).

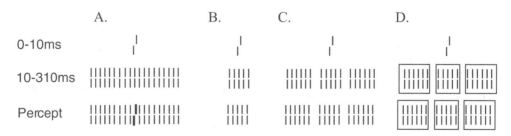

Figure 15.2
(*A*) The shine-through effect. A vernier is presented for a short duration and followed by a grating comprising more than seven elements. The preceding vernier appears to be superimposed on the grating and to look wider, brighter, and, for some observers, even longer than it is in reality. Presentation time can be as short as 10 ms for trained observers. (*B*) For a grating with five elements and a duration of 10 ms, no shine through occurs. Also, almost no inheritance occurs, since presentation time of the vernier is too short. (*C*) No shine through occurs for an extended grating with gaps. (*D*) We suggest that the gaps initiate grouping of the elements to three gratings: two peripheral gratings and a central one with five elements. Because of grouping, the vernier precedes a small five-element grating that does not yield shine through. Hence, no shine through occurs for the extended "gap grating." The rectangles indicate grouping of the single grating elements into coherent entities. In the quantitative experiments, observers had to indicate the offset direction of the vernier. We determined thresholds by an adaptive method. (For details, see Herzog et al., 2001a)

If a grating with 25 elements contains two gaps, singling out a center grating with 5 elements, performance is comparable to a 5-element grating, that is, dramatically worse than with a 25-element grating without gaps (see figure 15.2C). Why is performance so different if a 25-element grating contains gaps? Very likely the gaps initiate *grouping* of the center 5 elements as one small grating and the remaining elements as two peripheral gratings. Since the center grating, following the vernier, is small, no shine-through effect occurs. Hence, it seems that the spatial layout of the grating, related to grouping elements to objects, determines the shine-through effect. To show that, indeed, grouping and segmentation are the relevant factors for the shine-through effect, simpler mechanisms have to be ruled out as explanations.

Figure 15.3 shows various masks that follow the vernier. The masks shown under (A) yield significant better results than the masks shown under (B). First, low-level orientational aspects are unlikely to explain the effects in shine through per se. For example, single vertical contextual lines, as well as interrupted horizontal lines, yield a strong deterioration of performance compared to the standard condition (see figure 15.3, masks A1, B2, B3). However, when the collinear, vertical and the interrupted, horizontal lines are embedded in vertical contextual gratings or uninterrupted, horizontal lines, performance is comparable to the standard condition without contextual lines—even the single lines are part of the extended gratings or lines (see figure 15.3, masks A1, A2, A3; see also Herzog & Fahle, 2002; Herzog et al., 2004a).

Second, low-pass filtering of the grating is an unlikely mechanism to explain shine through. Assume that small spatial differences are blurred, for example, the spatial difference between the vertical contextual lines in the contextual gratings. A horizontally elongated object would occur (see figure 15.3, masks A2, A3; see also Herzog & Fahle, 2002). However, such blurring should also blur the breaks in the horizontal "broken" lines and yield performance comparable to the uninterrupted horizontal line (see figure 15.3, masks A3, B3). However, this is not the case. Shine through is also strongly diminished if the spacing of the standard grating is irregular—also arguing against the idea that low-pass filtering plays an important role in shine through (Herzog et al., 2003b). Moreover, the grating elements are subjectively clearly visible. For example, their individual orientation can be clearly determined (see also Intrilligator & Cavanagh, 2001). Finally, if low-pass filtering of the 25-element grating would result in an extended light-mask-like structure, the same would happen to the 5-element grating. However, deterioration of performance for small versus extended light masks is much weaker than for small versus extended grating masks (Herzog et al., 2003b).

Third, edge and line ending processing per se cannot explain the shine-through effect, that is, edges and line endings per se do not deteriorate performance. Small contextual gratings yield performance comparable to the standard condition if there

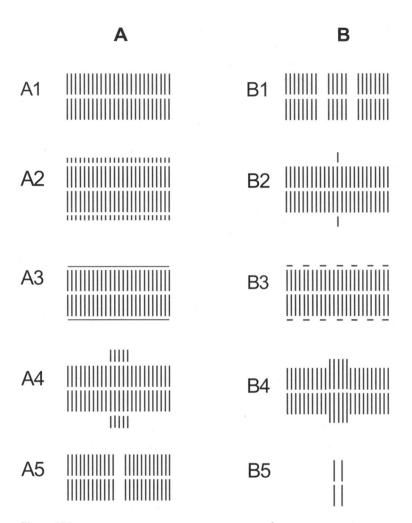

Figure 15.3
A vernier (not shown) precedes masks of various types. Masks labeled *A* yield better results than the corresponding masks labeled *B*. (*A*) Masks that yield performance comparable to the standard shine-through effect (A1): standard grating with 2×25 contextual lines (A2), standard grating with two long horizontal contextual lines (A3), standard grating with small contextual gratings (A4). A metacontrast grating with 24 elements (A5) yields performance significantly worse than in the standard shine-through effect (A1) but significantly better than in the metacontrast condition with two elements (B5). (*B*) Masks that yield performance significantly worse than the corresponding masks shown in (*A*): a grating with gaps (B1), standard grating with two collinear contextual lines (B2), standard grating with horizontal lines with breaks (B3), standard grating with small contextual gratings that are attached to the standard grating (B4), and a two-element metacontrast grating (B5).

is a vertical gap between the standard and the contextual gratings (see figure 15.3, mask A4). Removing this gap, that is, attaching the contextual gratings to the standard grating, exerts strong suppression compared to the nonattached conditions (see figure 15.3, masks A4, B4; see also Herzog & Fahle, 2002). Hence, removing line endings deteriorates performance in this condition, whereas removing line endings improves performance in other conditions, for example, the horizontal lines with breaks versus no breaks (see figures 15.3, masks A3, B3). Since low-pass filtering seems not to explain the effects, the edges of the 5-element, 25-element, and gap grating are second-order edges, that is, these edges indicate the beginning or ending of an array of homogeneous lines rather than a change of luminance of a contiguous object. However, no claim is made that edge detection plays no role in the shine-through effect. Quite to the contrary, with the detection of the second-order edges of the grating, the proposed grouping and figure–ground segmentation processes are initiated by highlighting edges as a transition from figure to ground. The paramount role of edges has been revealed in psychophysical experiments and physiological recording studies (MacKay, 1973; McCarter & Roehrs, 1976; Sagi & Hochstein, 1985; Macknik et al., 2000). It seems that not only grouping of the standard grating elements but also the spatial layout of the context, that is, contextual modulation, is important for the shine-through effect.

Fourth, the simple proximity of the vernier target to the mask contours, often proposed as a mechanism in interruption and metacontrast masking, cannot explain the effects of mask extension. Figure 15.3, masks A5, B5 shows two extreme cases: a 24- and a 2-element metacontrast grating. For both gratings, the distance from the vernier target to the central contours of the masks is identical, since the 2-element grating is part of the 24 element grating. However, performance differs strongly (Herzog et al., 2003b; see also Breitmeyer, 1978).

Fifth, (B-type) masking is often attributed to interactions between a fast transient and a slower sustained system related to the magnocellular and the parvocellular visual systems (Öğmen & Breitmeyer, this volume). It is assumed that the transient response of the mask catches up with and suppresses the sustained response of the target, thus deteriorating performance. Since we are not changing the timing of the stimuli, we would expect identical effects of the standard and the gap grating, especially if we take into account that the transient system is assumed to be inert vis-à-vis spatial changes such as inserting gaps. However, this is not the case, indicating an involvement of parvocellular system and integration rather than interruption masking.

Sixth, in the retouch account of masking, unspecific subcortical facilitation elicited by the target improves performance of the mask rather than the target since the unspecific facilitation is delayed compared to *specific* cortical processing (Bachmann, this volume). As argued before, we would not expect a difference in performance between the standard and the gap grating, since the unspecific system should treat both masks equally "unspecific ally."

Seventh, an analogous argument applies to substitution masking in which the masks substitutes for the target on a higher object recognition level. Why should an inhomogeneous grating substitute for the vernier but not a homogeneous one? (Note that the center of both gratings is identical.) Moreover, object substitution occurs mainly outside the focus of attention, whereas in the shine-through paradigm no attentional uncertainty is involved. Finally, we applied transcranial magnetic stimulation (TMS) over the occipital lobe (Kammer et al., 2003). A strong deterioration of performance occurs in the range of 120–160 ms after vernier onset, indicating the involvement of early areas in the shine-through effect (see also Ro, this volume).

Eighth, local contrast and camouflage effects cannot play an effective role for shine-through since the center of the masks is constant in most conditions.

Dynamics of the Shine-Through Effect

Performance improves strongly when a 25- compared to a 5-element grating follows the vernier. We related this effect to the role of edges and subsequent grouping of grating elements. As shown by combining both gratings, edge and grouping processing can be induced with very short presentation times (Herzog et al., 2001b). After the vernier, we presented a grating with 5 elements for a variable duration that was followed by a grating composed of 25 elements for 300 ms. As figure 15.4 shows, performance already strongly deteriorates for a duration of the 5-element grating of only 10 ms. Therefore, the human brain seems to process the contours of the 5-element grating with a 10-ms duration only (please note that we do not claim that processing is achieved in 10 ms).

Modeling

Since our TMS study suggests that occipital areas are involved in shine-through processing, we used one of the most simple models, namely, a Wilson–Cowan type model that is often used for modeling early visual processes. We focus on a one-dimensional version of the model. Since in a one-dimensional model the vernier *offset* cannot be defined, we focus on the visibility of the preceding vernier that corresponds to a dot in this one-dimensional simulation.

The model comprises only two layers, an excitatory one and an inhibitory one. Neurons in each layer and between the two layers are interconnected. The closer the neurons are to each other, the stronger are their mutual excitatory and inhibitory interactions. The dynamics of the network are determined by a set of differential equations (for the mathematical details, see Herzog et al., 2003a).

We tested four conditions: a vernier followed by a 5-element, 25-element, or gap grating, and the temporal condition in which a 5-element grating follows the vernier

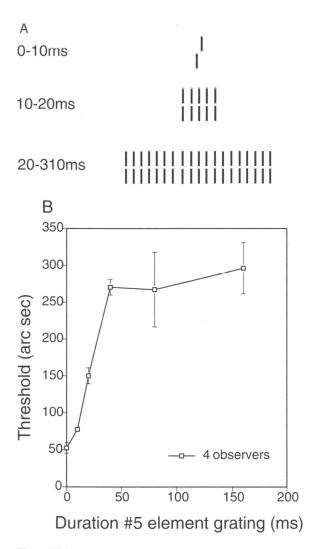

Figure 15.4
The vernier was followed by a 5-element (#5) grating for a variable duration (*x*-axis) followed by the 25-element grating presented for 300 ms minus the duration of the 5-element grating (a 10 ms duration of the 5-element grating is shown as an example on the left). A duration of 0 ms indicates that only the 25-element grating was displayed. Surprisingly, a 10-ms duration of the 5-element grating significantly already deteriorates performance. Observers had to discriminate the offset direction of the shine-through element. We determined thresholds of 75% correct responses via an adaptive method. (Adapted from Herzog et al., 2001b)

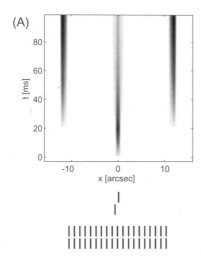

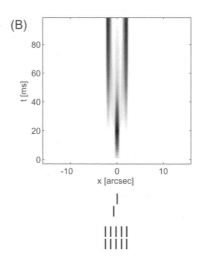

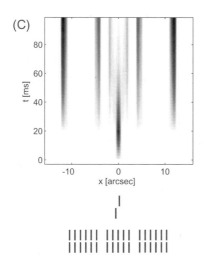

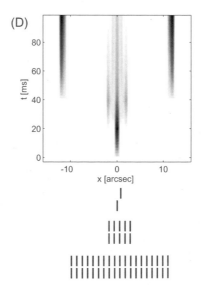

for 20 ms preceding a 25-element grating (see figure 15.4). We found a good correspondence between the model and the empirical data (figure 15.5). Analogous results have been obtained with a two-dimensional model (Zhaoping, 2003). We suggest that shine though occurs because the inner grating elements exert strong mutual inhibition on each other. Elements at the edges are strongly enhanced since they have only one neighboring element instead of two (one on each side) for inner grating elements. If edges are close to the vernier, as with the 5-element or the gap grating, this enhanced activity suppresses vernier activity. For a 25-element grating, edges are remote and, thus, vernier activity is less strongly suppressed. We interpret this inner-grating-element inhibition as a removal of redundant elements. Hence, a grating may be represented just by its second-order edges.

15.2.3   Schizophrenia Research

Visual backward masking studies have revealed strong deficits in the schizophrenic patient, likely related to early visual processing deficiencies (e.g., Braff & Saccuzzo, 1981; Cadenhead et al., 1996; Cadenhead et al., 1998; Green et al., 1999; Green et al., 1994a, 1994b). These results are interesting, since low-level processing deficits may cause, by virtue of error propagation, deficits at higher processing levels such as those governing cognitive functions. It is, therefore, interesting to analyze at which processing stages deficits occur first. In this section, we show that object grouping, that is, one of the very basic aspects of object recognition, is fast and intact in schizophrenic patients, whereas strong backward masking effect are still found.

A vernier was followed by a 25- or a 5-element grating as in the experiments described above. To avoid confusion between masking effects and a deteriorated vernier discrimination in patients, we first determined a vernier duration without mask for each observer to yield results comparable across all observers. Second, to determine the effect of masking, an interstimulus interval was inserted between the

Figure 15.5
We used a neural network of the Wilson–Cowan type to show that the basic aspects of the shine-through effect can be explained by simple mechanisms. The model is one-dimensional, neglecting the vertical extension of the stimulus. Results of computer simulations with this network are shown. On the x-coordinate, the activity of neurons corresponding to the horizontal extension of the stimulus is shown (0 indicates the position of the vernier; -10 and 10 indicate the position of the tenth element either to the left or right, respectively). On the y-axis, the time course of activation is shown. The stronger the activity of neurons, the stronger the gray values are. (A) A vernier is followed by a 25-element grating. Activity at the position where the vernier was presented rises strongly after stimulus onset and decays slowly afterward, lasting until the end of the presentation. Analogously, a strong enhancement of activity occurs at the edges of the grating, whereas for inner grating elements activity stays on a constant, vanishing level of activation. (B) For a 5-element grating, vernier activity is strongly diminished after the strong onset activation and does not last until the end of presentation. (C) Analogous results occur for a grating with gaps. Here, a strong activation occurs for the outer edges of the grating and the edges making up the gaps. (D) A 5-element grating following the vernier for 20 ms followed by the 25-element grating also yields a strong suppression of shine through related to a fast increase of activity corresponding to the edges of the briefly displayed 5-element grating. In this condition, vernier related activity lasts longer than in the preceding two conditions but is still deteriorated compared with (A).

vernier and the grating (see figure 15.6; for details, see Herzog et al., 2004b). As in the previous experiments, observers had to indicate the offset direction of the vernier that had a constant offset of 75″ for all observers. We determined the stimulus onset asynchrony (SOA) for which 75% correct responses occurred adaptively. Hence, we determined masking effects in one block. The following grating could contain either 25 or 5 elements and lasted for 300 ms. Patients show for both gratings immense, prolonged SOAs compared to healthy controls (see figure 15.6).

Whereas processing of the vernier target is strongly prolonged, grouping or figure–ground segmentation seems to be fast and intact (figure 15.7). Even though patients need very long SOAs between vernier and grating, they are very sensitive to the presentation of the display of the disturbing 5-element grating presented only for 20 ms. If detection of the 5-element grating were slow, the 5-element grating would be integrated with the 25-element grating—not suppressing shine through. Paradoxically, in this case performance would have improved (see also Place & Gilmore, 1980). Indeed, slightly better performance in the patients might indicate such a partially deteriorated performance; still the strongly deteriorated performance compared to the 25-element condition shows good object grouping in the patient—possibly related to the detection of the edges of the grating (see Herzog

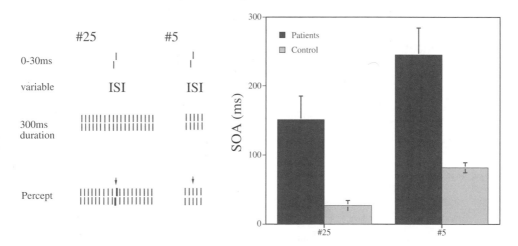

Figure 15.6
First, we determined a vernier duration to reach vernier discrimination with offsets lower than 40″ for each observer individually (no mask presented). Second, the vernier was followed by a blank screen (interstimulus interval; ISI) and a 25-element grating (#25) presented for 300 ms. We determined the stimulus onset asynchrony (SOA)—that is, ISI plus vernier duration—necessary to reach a performance level of 75% correct responses for a fixed vernier offset size of 75″. Third, the SOA for a 5-element grating (#5) was determined analogously. Clearly, performance is strongly deteriorated for schizophrenic patients compared to healthy observers for both gratings. Gratings of 25 elements yield better performance than 5-element gratings for patients and controls. (From Herzog et al., 2004b)

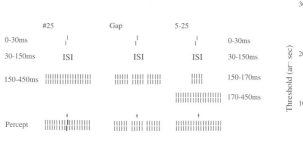

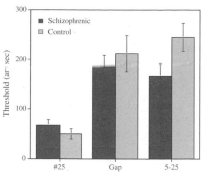

Figure 15.7
Three types of gratings were used: a 25-element grating (#25), a gap, or a 5–25 grating. In the 5–25 grating condition, a 5-element grating was presented for 20 ms after the vernier and the interstimulus interval (ISI). Afterward, the 25-element grating was displayed for 280 ms. In the last experiment, each observer reached an individual stimulus onset asynchrony (SOA) for an individual vernier duration (see figure 15.6). This SOA and the vernier duration were used in this experiment for each observer individually (an SOA of 150 ms is shown as an example). We determined the vernier offset size adaptively. Since vernier duration and ISI were individually adjusted, performance should be comparable across all observers when a 25-element grating follows the vernier and the individual ISI. This was, indeed, the case, indicating that our normalization procedure of vernier duration and ISI was successful. When a gap or a 5–25 element grating follows, performance significantly deteriorates for both patients and controls. This indicates that schizophrenic patients and healthy observers are both sensitive to the spatial as well as the temporal inhomogeneities of the grating. It is important to note that the 5-element grating in the 5–25 element grating condition was presented only for 20 ms for all observers, that is, presentation was very short. Usually, its existence does not even reach the conscious level. Still, this 5-element grating exerts a strong performance-deterioration effect. This implies that the grating is detected by the visual system as a small grating. Since small gratings do not yield shine through, performance deteriorates. Hence, grouping and figure–ground segmentation seem to be fast and intact. (From Herzog et al., 2004b)

et al., 2001a). It seems that one of the most fundamental processes of object recognition, object grouping, is fast and intact.

Whereas we find intact grouping in schizophrenic patients, in other paradigms deteriorated performance occurs (e.g., Silverstein et al., 1996; Place & Gilmore, 1980). It may be that grouping in our paradigm is more related to early visual processing than was the case in these other studies.

Deficient processing is often attributed to an overactive transient system (e.g., Wynn & Green, this volume; Breitmeyer, 1984; Cadenhead et al., 1998; Green et al., 1994a, 1994b; Slaghuis & Curran, 1999; however, see Keri et al., 2000; Saccuzzo et al., 1996; Slaghuis & Bakker, 1995). Our results partly favor and partly challenge this hypothesis. Patients are very sensitive to the edges of the 5-element grating preceding the 25-element grating even though it is presented for only 20 ms (see figure 15.7). This short duration of presentation may be evidence for the involvement of the overactive transient visual system. On the other hand, the "frequency" of the masking gratings corresponds to 18 cyc/deg being assumed to be related to sustained rather than transient system processing (Slaghuis & Curran, 1999; Schechter et al., 2002).

Our results with schizophrenic patients may have also implications for masking research in general. Enns et al. (this volume) showed that *all* masks exert identical masking for SOAs longer than about 150 ms. However, schizophrenic patients reveal mask-specific effects even for SOAs of more than 150 ms (see figure 15.6).

15.3 Discussion

Classical interpretations in terms of integration and interruption masking cannot explain the results in the shine-through and feature inheritance effects. Integration masking related to a change of contrast or camouflage cannot play an important role, since the center of the masking gratings stays constant in most conditions (see figures 15.2 and 15.3). Moreover, extended gratings with a higher "overall" luminance and a possibly higher potential of camouflage yield better performance than smaller gratings.

Moreover, it seems that interruption masking accounts cannot explain the shine-through phenomenon. Interruption masking by neighboring contours is an unlikely approach, since performance can change significantly even if neighboring contours are kept constant (see figure 15.3, masks A5, B5). In contrast to the results for object substitution (Enns et al., this volume), our masking elements do not have to be outside of the focus of attention to exert their strong suppressive effects (for more details, see Herzog et al., 2003d). Moreover, the striking differences in performance between the standard and the gap grating condition are difficult to explain. The same argument applies to the transient and sustained system (Breit-meyer, 1984; Öğmen et al., this volume) and the retouch (Bachmann, this volume) approach.

It is important to note that we do not claim that integration and interruption are unimportant for masking research. Quite to the contrary, both integration and interruption are two fundamental aspects of masking. We simply state that other aspects related to the basics of object recognition can play an important role in masking as well.

Object recognition comprises at least three stages: object grouping, object segmentation, and feature binding. In object grouping and segmentation, an object is grouped from single elements and segmented from its background and other objects. In the next stage, features are bound to this object. Processing in these stages is achieved in a dynamic way and not instantaneously. Accordingly the masking effects of shine through and feature inheritance can be best explained in relation to these basic object recognition processes.

Shine through occurs for extended homogeneous gratings but not for small or extended, inhomogeneous gratings. As argued above, the human brain tries to eliminate redundant information, such as the inside of textures, by inhibiting neural activity—for example, that related to inner grating elements. Only edges and inhomogeneities are highlighted, since these may indicate the transition from figure to ground or from one to another figure (see figure 15.5). These results extend to the classical masks, such as pattern, noise, light, and metacontrast masks, used for more than a century (Herzog et al., 2003b).

The question of what constitutes a strong mask has to be reconsidered in the shine-through paradigm, since the global layout of the mask is more important than energy aspects per se (see also Francis and Cho, this volume). However, the global layout of an object is not easy to define. Thus, it is difficult to say what a strong mask is. A weak mask may be easier to define: A weak mask is a mask in which masking elements strongly inhibit each other and so interfere less with the target. The shine-through mask is a particularly weak mask since all inner grating elements are inhibiting each other (see figure 15.5).

Changes of the spatial layout can change not only the strength of masking but also the state of feature binding. In this sense, our terminology refers to the binding states rather than the masking effects per se. We use the term *feature inheritance* since features are bequeathed from the preceding, parental, to the subsequent, filial elements. We use the term *shine-through effect* since features are not misbound and the shine-through element does not result from fusion of the vernier with the central grating element that otherwise occurs when only the central grating element follows the vernier (Herzog et al., 2003c). It seems that the mask–target relationship and the corresponding grouping and segmentation processes determine the type of feature binding—and masking. In this sense, masking can occur naturally by the suppression of elements during these object recognition processes, for example, by the elimination of redundant elements or the highlighting of edges. Depending on the processing, it can be the case that the existence of elements is strongly masked, whereas their features survive the masking.

The shine-through effect not only seems to be a versatile tool in basic vision science research but can also successfully be applied in schizophrenia research. We were able to show that patients have a subtle sensitivity to temporal changes in the stimulus and are, therefore, not simply slower. It seems that their spatial processing abilities, such as grouping, are spared. These results may allow researchers to study the "first" occurrences of abnormal processing in the schizophrenic patient.

15.3.1 Summary

Our results show that backward masking can dramatically change when the spatial layout of the following grating changes. These findings suggest a strong role of basic object recognition processes in masking such as grouping of elements to objects, segmenting these objects from backgrounds, and binding features to the objects. It seems that learning from object recognition may help us to understand masking and vice versa. Integration and interruption masking can hardly explain these results, since the center is always constant. Moreover, no attentional uncertainty is involved, since the vernier is always presented at the same central position. It seems that the shine-through paradigm is a new masking paradigm.

Acknowledgments

I would like to thank Marc Repnow for excellent technical support and Haluk Öğmen for helpful discussions.

Notes

1. For an animation of the stimuli, see: http://neuro.physik.uni-bremen.de/~vernier/vernier_english/vindex.html
2. However, we do not claim $d' = 0$ in a detection task with the preceding vernier being present or absent.

16 Neural Mechanisms Underlying Temporal Aspects of Conscious Visual Perception

Wei Ji Ma, Fred Hamker, and Christof Koch

In this chapter, we will examine dynamical aspects of conscious visual perception related to briefly presented stimuli, and their possible neural underpinnings. The time course of the contents of conscious perception usually reflects the time course of events in the world, but this correspondence is not absolute. As is illustrated in many examples in this book, it can break down in various ways: Physical events can get wiped out, stretched out in time, temporally blended, or modified. The last of these occurs in feature inheritance (Herzog & Koch, 2001), which we will study in some detail here. That these distortions do not seem omnipresent in daily life is because most of them occur at very short time scales of tens and hundreds of milliseconds. Their effects can often only be made apparent by presenting very specific, tightly controlled stimulus sequences. For a neuroscientist, these are exactly the interesting time scales. Because of the short duration of the stimuli involved, the stimuli can interfere with ongoing neural processing and hopefully reveal mechanisms used by the brain in more generality.

In studying temporal effects in perception, several quantities are of relevance. It is worthwhile to distinguish them clearly.

Perceived duration. How long do observers perceive an event of a given physical duration to be? While this question is hardly experimentally tractable, there is extensive literature on its active version, that is, how well humans estimate the passage of time (temporal cognition, interval timing). In the realm of millisecond stimuli, there is evidence for the existence of a minimal perceptual moment (Efron, 1970; Koch, 2004). For durations of seconds to minutes, our judgment of the subjective duration of a stimulus and its actual, physical duration can differ widely. Many studies show that the distribution of subjective durations (timed intervals) is invariant under scaling of the physical duration, a property that has implications for associative learning (Gibbon et al., 1997; Matell & Meck, 2000).

Temporal positioning of a percept. How long does it take before we see something, and do we think the event happens at the moment when we become aware of it, or earlier? Recent years have witnessed widespread interest in the temporal positioning of a percept. This has been fueled by research on the flash-lag effect, in which a flashed stimulus, when presented spatially aligned with a moving object, is perceived as lagging spatially behind the object (MacKay, 1958; Nijhawan, 1994). It has been postulated (Eagleman & Sejnowski, 2000a) that the percept that the brain associates with the flash depends on events following it, but this view has been challenged (Patel et al., 2000; Nijhawan, 2002). A similar proposal has been made in the context of filling in the perceptual gap during saccadic suppression (Yarrow et al., 2001).

Content of conscious perception.   What do we see? In this chapter, we will mostly be concerned with this topic. We will focus on two broad classes of perceptual distortions occurring in sequences of short stimuli. The first is *temporal integration*; the second is *backward masking*.

16.1   Perceptual Illusions for Short Stimuli

When a small green disk is presented on a screen for 10 ms, immediately followed by a red disk at the same location for 10 ms, observers perceive a yellow disk with a slight red hue (Efron, 1967, 1973). When either stimulus is presented by itself, it is perceived properly, that is, as either green or red. This shows that for very brief stimuli, the brain integrates stimuli over time to create a percept. This can be modeled by a convolution with a temporal filter. When the green–red sequence is presented for a sufficiently long period of time (for instance, both components for 500 ms), green is seen, followed by red. It is nontrivial to note that the sequence 10 ms green + 10 ms red, which by itself would be perceived as yellow, is now part of the stimulus sequence but nonetheless does *not* give rise to the *percept of yellow* in between the green and the red. This shows that the contents of perception are not always determined by a simple convolution; any linear filter would predict the intermediate percept of yellow. Related to this experiment is the everyday observation that a movie, recorded at 24 frames per second (i.e., each frame is 42 ms), is effortlessly perceived as a continuum.

A similar effect occurs for the rapid presentation of dot patterns (DiLollo, 1980). When a matrix of 5×5 dots is presented with one dot left out, it is easy to detect the gap. Now the same 24-dot display is split into two complementary 12-dot displays that follow each other in time, with a 10-ms blank interstimulus interval separating them. The first set of 12 dots is chosen randomly. The task of detecting which location was empty in both displays can become much harder, depending on the temporal parameters. If both halves are shown for 10 ms, they become perceptually blended and the observer will make few errors in detecting the missing dot. When the duration of the first display is increased, the percentage of errors increases, most steeply between 80 and 160 ms. Again, we conclude that integration occurs for very brief stimuli and also that in order to explain conscious perception, an additional mechanism is needed. The reason is that we know that the integration period can bridge the 10-ms interstimulus interval. Thus, in all conditions, right after the onset of the second display, both the first and the second display would contribute to the integration, and their superposition would be visible. The idea has been invoked of a threshold value that the integrated activity due to one stimulus has to exceed for a certain amount of time in order for this stimulus to be perceived (Herzog et al., 2003c; Koch, 2004; Dehaene et al., 2003). In this view, a long duration for the first display would cause it to be perceived; after that, some form of reset would occur, and the first and the second display would not become superimposed.

That linear temporal integration cannot be the whole story is also clear from the phenomenon of backward masking. In backward masking, the visibility of a stimulus is destroyed or reduced by another stimulus following it; thus, there must be some mechanism at work besides that of mere temporal integration. Masking studies support the concept of the formation of an "object" as central to visual perception, as reported by Enns in this volume and in earlier work with DiLollo and Rensink (DiLollo et al., 2000). The key idea of their *object substitution theory* is that sensory input is processed in two stages. First, a feedforward sweep originating in the retina subsequently causes activation in the lateral geniculate nucleus (LGN), primary visual cortex, after which it moves toward higher and higher areas in the visual hierarchy. In the areas sequentially activated in this propagation, the receptive fields of cells are larger, and more and more complex visual features are encoded. Then, a feedback sweep acts to compare the generalized pattern activation generated at a high level, a "hypothesis," with the ongoing, high-resolution activity at a (nonspecified) lower level (see also Lee et al., 1998; Ullman, 2000; Lee & Mumford, 2003). This would serve the purpose of resolving ambiguities within a pattern hypothesis and of binding patterns to specific locations. Only after confirmation of the perceptual hypothesis are its contents, an "object," perceived. In this framework, a mask can interfere with the feedback sweep and reset the entire process, after which only the mask is perceived.

16.2 Feedforward or Feedback?

From the perspective of neuroscience, backward masking and temporal integration raise questions about the processes determining whether a stimulus is consciously perceived. An important and long-standing issue in this context is whether feedback interactions are necessary for conscious awareness. Neuroanatomically, feedback connections are a dominant feature in visual cortex (Felleman & Van Essen, 1991), reaching all the way back into the LGN. Yet, their functions remain veiled. Some apparently complicated tasks, such as distinguishing animal pictures from nonanimal ones, can be performed by the brain very fast, suggesting—although most certainly not proving—that feedback is not necessary for those (Thorpe et al., 1996; VanRullen & Koch, 2003a). While classical models of backward masking (Breitmeyer, 1984; Breitmeyer & Öğmen, 2000; Öğmen, 1993) are based on local, lateral connections, object substitution theory posits feedback interactions as an essential ingredient. Several physiological studies in the macaque monkey show that in figure–ground segregation tasks, the awareness of the figure is correlated with a late component of V1 activity (Scholte et al., this volume; Lamme et al., 2000; Lamme et al., 2002; Lamme & Roelfsema, 2000). This has been taken to indicate that feedback into V1 is essential for visual awareness. However, on the basis of a computational study (Li, 2000) it has been argued that local V1 mechanisms can account for these figure–ground effects. In a study using transcranial magnetic stimulation, it was shown that the percept of a moving phosphene evoked in V1 can be masked by applying stimulation to V1 at a time that would interfere with feedback from MT (Pascual-Leone & Walsh, 2001). However, the biophysical effects of such stimulation are still poorly understood, and it should in addition be noted that rather than demonstrating the necessity of feedback, this result shows the necessary involvement of V1 at a later stage in conscious visual processing. As was pointed out in Öğmen et al. (2003), it is possible to have a graph-theoretically feedforward architecture with an anatomically descending connection, that is, from a higher to a lower area in the visual hierarchy (for instance, IT to V1). We will use such an architecture in our model ("Template" to "Object" in figure 16.1). In many studies, the distinction between anatomical and functional feedback is not properly drawn.

As a starting point to modeling the time course of visual perception, we take the above idea of *perceptual hypothesis testing*: Before an object can be consciously perceived, the brain first confirms its identity by comparing it with the sensory input at a later time. Especially when input is rapidly changing or when significant amounts of extrinsic or intrinsic noise are present, it is ecologically meaningful to ascertain whether the initial input reflects the current state of the world before engaging in a behavioral response. Models of consciousness often posit the necessity of a "coalition" of cortical areas, connected with each other through loops of feedforward and feedback connections (Koch, 2004; Baars, 2002; Baars et al., 2003; Grossberg, 1999; Dehaene et al., 2003). In these models, the main goal of a feedback circuit is presented primarily as a form of working memory rather than as a means of testing perceptual hypotheses; these two viewpoints may coincide.

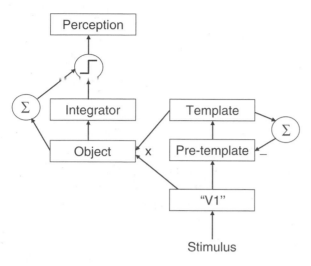

Figure 16.1
Schematic of the model. Images pass through orientation-selective filters in V1. The pretemplate–template subsystem creates an inert hypothesis about the stimulus. The hypothesis is tested against the later input into the object area. Finally, integration and thresholding determine the contents of perception.

   Perceptual hypothesis testing can be mathematically modeled in terms of neural populations. One starts by describing a visual stimulus as a bundle of perceptual features, such as position, orientation, color, and shape, which are together—and not necessarily independently—encoded in neural populations. This encoding is noisy, so a sharply defined input will give rise to a broad population response. Let us concentrate on a single feature dimension, say, orientation, at one particular point in the visual field. The task of the brain is to decode the value of this quantity from the noisy population response, possibly making use of prior knowledge. Each possible orientation can be regarded as a hypothesis. Because of the numerosity of the hypotheses, the problem is one of parameter estimation, and hypothesis testing will consist of comparing neural population responses.

16.3   Parameter Estimation

Parameter estimation based on population codes is an example of Bayesian inference, with population activity patterns representing uncertainty about stimuli in the form of probability distributions. Bayesian inference has been postulated to be a general operating principle of the brain (Pouget et al., 2003; Rao et al., 2002; Yuille & Bülthoff, 1996). The idea here is that the brain tries to infer the identity of a source Z of an event in the world by optimally making use of the noisy (probabilistic) information contained in the sensory input S. It does this using Bayes's rule:

$$P(Z|S) = P(S|Z)\frac{P(Z)}{P(S)}. \tag{16.1}$$

$P(S|Z)$ is called the *likelihood function*, and $P(Z)$ is called the *prior distribution*. The priors can contain many factors, including genetically specified biases, previous experiences, and response biases.

Psychophysical evidence that the brain performs Bayesian inference partly comes from studies of how the brain combines noisy cues from two sensory modalities, or two cues from the same sensory modality, into a single percept (for instance, see Knill & Richards, 1996; Ernst & Banks, 2002). In these combinations, the best estimate is obtained by multiplying the probability distributions obtained from the two different cues and of the priors, if any, and locating the peak of the product distribution. If we denote the two cues by S_1 and S_2, this is captured by

$$P(Z|S_1, S_2) = P(S_1|Z)P(S_2|Z)\frac{P(Z)}{P(S_1, S_2)}. \tag{16.2}$$

Our problem concerns two cues appearing at different times, and Z is the orientation to be inferred. We assume that the likelihood function corresponding to the cues is encoded in the population activity pattern, where each neuron signals the probability of the stimulus given the neuron's preferred orientation.[1] In the absence of priors—that is, if $P(Z)$ is a flat distribution—the best estimate based on the two cues is then obtained by multiplication of the activities at each cell in the population.

In our model, one can also regard multiplication of population activities as an implementation of Bayes's rule of equation 16.1, where the one population encodes the likelihood function and the other one contains the priors. This is valid if the bottom-up input is compared with an expectation that has been generated not from directly preceding stimuli but from previous experience.

There are several examples of neural circuits performing multiplication, varying from spatial receptive fields in the barn owl (Pena & Konishi, 2001), to gain fields in the monkey's posterior parietal cortex (Andersen et al., 1997), to motion-sensitive neurons in the blowfly (Egelhaaf et al., 1989). There is evidence for single-cell mechanisms able to execute multiplicative computations (Gabbiani et al., 2002). Salinas and Abbott (1996) showed that multiplicative responses can also arise in a network model through population effects.

Our model is based on the idea of optimal cue combination, but it is, strictly speaking, not Bayesian. The reason is that we use the magnitude of the product response across the population as information about the similarity of the two population activities that are multiplied: The higher the product activity, the more similar the two activity patterns were. The key idea is then to use the product activity in some higher visual area as representing an object. If earlier and later activity patterns match, the multiplication will produce a high outcome and the stimulus will be perceived. If the match is not good, because the first stimulus has been replaced by a dissimilar one, either masking or pure temporal integration occurs. The latter gives rise to a percept in which stimuli physically present at different times are perceived simultaneously, in a sort of superposition. It can also happen that the match is not perfect and the first stimulus is not perceived but still modulates the perception of the second stimulus. We claim that this is what happens in feature inheritance.

16.4 Feature Inheritance

In the orientation paradigm of feature inheritance (Herzog & Koch, 2001), detailed in chapter 15 (Herzog, this volume), a bar slightly tilted with respect to the vertical is presented for 30 ms (the target), immediately followed by a grating of 3–5 vertical bars, presented for 300 ms (the "mask"). The percept is a slightly tilted grating. The perceived tilt is much smaller than the actual tilt of the first stimulus, but always in the same direction as the (perceptually invisible) target. This illusion is surprising in several respects: first, the invisibility of the target; second, the spread of the tilt over the entire grating[2]; and finally, the long duration of 300 ms over which the effect extends.

We now consider what happens to feature inheritance when the temporal parameters are varied. When the duration of target presentation is increased to several hundred milliseconds, the target and the mask are perceived veridically, that is, as a sequence of two stimuli. When the target is flashed by itself, it is clearly perceived. When the mask is of very long duration (e.g., 1,000 ms), one first observes the illusory, feature inheritance percept, which subsequently changes into the veridical percept of the original mask. When the target and the mask are very different in orientation, both the mask and the target are visible (so-called shine through, although this term was originally coined to describe the case in which the masking grating has many lines). We would like to simulate each of these cases.

Some of the spatial characteristics of the shine-through effect that can give rise to the spread of the feature over the grating have been explained with a feedforward, two-layer neural network model (Herzog et al., 2003a) and with a system of interconnected excitatory–inhibitory neuron pairs (Li, 2003). The issue of feature inheritance, that is, of how the orientation is decoded and assigned to the mask, and how the target becomes invisible, has not yet been addressed. A crucial issue is the invisibility of the target, on the one hand, if and only if a mask follows, and the perception of a tilted mask, on the other hand. A feedforward system with lateral interactions would have difficulties in explaining how it is that the target is not perceived at all if a mask follows. This suggests that the earlier presented target influences the neural processing of the later presented mask in some kind of top-down fashion.

In our model, we focus on the temporal characteristics of visual perception. For simplicity, our only dimension is orientation space at the central location. We will see that with the mechanism sketched above, the temporal aspects of the inheritance process can be understood without any spatial interactions.

16.5   Model

The architecture of our model is shown in figure 16.1. It consists of early visual processing, a pretemplate and a template area, an object area, an integration area, and a perception area. We describe each area in terms of an analogue population activity. This is much cruder than a biophysical model, but we believe that this level of analysis will suffice for our purposes.

16.5.1   Early Visual Processing

Early visual processing, conveniently denoted as *V1*, although it is not necessarily limited to primary visual cortex, is modeled by convolving the black-and-white image of the oriented bar with a family $G_\theta(x,y)$ of two-dimensional Gabor filters, one for every integer number of degrees of angle θ. This describes the spatial receptive fields of cells with different orientation selectivities. We need a fine resolution in orientation space, because the effect we eventually want to show is rather subtle. The response in V1 to an image $S(t)$ is a 180-unit population activity pattern $(S(t) * G_\theta)(x,y)$ at each spatial location. Now we restrict ourselves to the central point ($x = y = 0$), where both the target and one bar of the masking grating are presented; this gives a population activity pattern $I(\theta,t)$. The half width at half height of this pattern is 13°. The pattern depends on time in a manner determined only by the stimulus sequence.

The temporal dynamics of V1 responses to visual stimuli is known to be affected by synaptic depression (Chance et al., 1998). This causes cells to initially respond very strongly (the *transient response*), followed by a decrease in sensitivity and a leveling off of firing rate (the *sustained response*). For our purposes, it can be modeled simply by a multiplicative factor in the input (Chance et al., 1998). The differential equation for the V1 response $A_{V1}(\theta,t)$ at angle θ and time t reads

$$\tau_{V1} \frac{\partial A_{V1}}{\partial t} = -A_{V1}(\theta,t) + \{1 - \alpha_d S(t)\} \cdot I(\theta,t), \qquad (16.3a)$$

where the synaptic depression $S(t)$ is governed by

$$\tau_S \frac{dS}{dt} = 1 - S. \tag{16.3b}$$

16.5.2 Pretemplate and Template

The template is a higher level area that receives and stores the input for comparison with the later input. This area has a biophysically very long time constant (200 ms), which can be obtained, for instance, by a local positive feedback loop or self-excitation. In order to encode a hypothesis, activity in this area should not be readily overwritten by new input. This is the purpose of the pretemplate area, a gateway that receives bottom-up input from V1 and global inhibition from the template area. A new input has to compete with the existing hypothesis before it can form a new hypothesis. The activity in the pretemplate area A_{PT} is determined by

$$\tau_{PT} \frac{\partial A_{PT}}{\partial t} = -A_{PT}(\theta, t) + [\alpha_{PT} A_{V1}(\theta, t) - A_{PT}^I(t)]_+, \tag{16.4}$$

where $[..]_+$ denotes rectification (i.e., the function value is zero when the argument is negative, and it is equal to the argument otherwise) and the inhibitory activity A_{PT}^I is determined by

$$\tau_{PT}^I \frac{\partial A_{PT}^I}{\partial t} = -A_{PT}^I(t) + \alpha_{PT}^I \sum_\theta A_T(\theta - \varepsilon). \tag{16.5}$$

Here, ε is a delay without which the inhibition would only amount to a subtractive normalization. The template is solely driven by pretemplate input,

$$\tau_T \frac{\partial A_T}{\partial t} = -A_T(\theta, t) + \alpha_T A_{PT}(\theta, t). \tag{16.6}$$

16.5.3 Object Representation

This area is where the comparison between template and low-level activity takes place. It receives bottom-up input from V1, which is multiplied by the activity in the template area. The activity A_O is described by

$$\tau_O \frac{\partial A_O}{\partial t} = -A_O(\theta, t) + \alpha_O A_{V1}(\theta, t) \cdot A_T(\theta, t). \tag{16.7}$$

16.5.4 Integrator

The governing equation of the integration area reads

$$\tau_I \frac{\partial A_I}{\partial t} = -A_I(\theta,t) + \alpha_I A_O(\theta,t). \tag{16.8}$$

This area implements the fact that evidence has to build up over time before neural activity is sufficient for perception. Neurons in this area may be comparable to neurons in parietal and prefrontal cortex integrating sensory evidence until a decision criterion is reached (Gold & Shadlen, 2001; Freedman et al., 2002). Although this integration is in dynamics similar to the one in the template area, it serves a different goal. Here it is a mechanism for evidence accumulation, while there it guarantees the sustaining of a hypothesis.

16.5.5 Perception

The population activity pattern in the perception area determines the contents of the percept: in our case, which orientation or orientations are seen. The activity in the integration area is thresholded as follows:

$$\tau_P \frac{\partial A_P}{\partial t} = -A_P(\theta,t) + \frac{[\alpha_P A_I(\theta,t) - T]_+}{1 + \sum_\theta A_P(\theta,t)}. \tag{16.9}$$

The denominator serves as a normalization. The threshold T is given by

$$T = \max\left\{ T_0, \alpha_{thr} \sum_\theta A_O(\theta,t) \right\}. \tag{16.10}$$

There is a baseline threshold T_0 and a threshold dependent on the total activity in the object area. In feature inheritance, no percept should be created before the multiplicative interaction in the object area has finished, although the stimulus is 300 ms long. On the other hand, any single 10-ms stimulus is perceived. This means that the perceptual threshold should be dependent on activity in a lower area. In this simple model, we take this activity to be the total activity in the object area. Such a dynamic threshold is equivalent to feedforward inhibition from the object area into the integration area.

The activity in the perception area is read out by registering sufficiently high local maxima, where "sufficiently high" at a certain point in time is taken to be at least 50% of the highest overall activity in the perception area until that moment. The duration of sufficiently high activity in the perception area is interpreted as the duration of the percept. Whether this is realistic is an open question. It has been noted that distinguishing the simultaneous presence of multiple distinct stimuli from the population noise intrinsic to the encoding of a single stimulus can be a problem (Sahani & Dayan, 2003), but we do not address that issue here.

16.6 Results

We presented this network with an oriented bar at an angle of 80° with respect
to the horizontal for 30 ms, followed by a vertical bar for 300 ms. We tuned
the parameters in the model such that it produces the desired phenomenology.
Figure 16.2 shows the activity in each of the areas in the model when the target is
oriented at 80°. The model produces a single peak at an orientation of 87°, corresponding to the percept in feature inheritance. The target is rendered invisible.
Figure 16.3 shows the multiplication of V1 with template activity in the object area
at $t = 200$ ms.

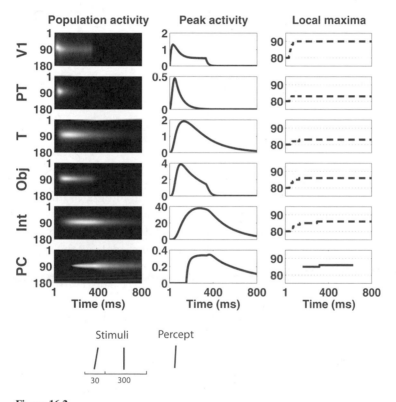

Figure 16.2
Feature inheritance. In all figures, the left column shows plots of the activity in each area as a function
of time (*x*-axis) and orientation (*y*-axis). The second column shows the maximum activity in each area
as a function of time. The third column shows the location of the local maxima in orientation space. Only
for the perception area (PC), the third column shows all sufficiently high local maxima. Activity units
are arbitrary but are consistent throughout the simulations. The diagram at the bottom shows the time
course of stimulation (in milliseconds) and the resulting percept. Int, integrator; Obj, object; T, template;
PT, pretemplate.

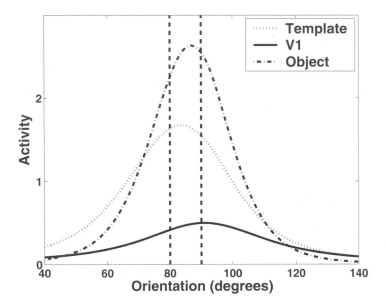

Figure 16.3
The multiplicative interaction occurring in the object area, taken at time $t = 200$ from figure 16.2. The dotted vertical lines represent the target and mask orientations.

A single short stimulus (10 ms) is perceived even though the activity it produces in the integration area is much lower (figure 16.4). Because of the integrator, the perceived duration is much longer than the stimulus duration. Figure 16.4b shows the effect of varying physical duration on perceived duration. The graph has a plateau at a value of about 250 ms. Because of the many parameters in our model and the ad hoc readout rule, we cannot reliably use this as a quantitative test, but it is qualitatively in accordance with the concept of a "minimal perceptual moment" (Efron, 1970).

A sequence of long-duration stimuli gets perceived veridically because the match between template and bottom-up activity is good (figure 16.5a). We compared a target at 80° (figure 16.5a) with one at 40° (figure 16.5b). The first one produces a smooth transition between the percept of target and mask, because the orientations are close enough together that the template activity representing the target can interact with the mask activity. This can be interpreted as apparent rotation. (In the real experiment [Herzog, this volume], observers were presented with an entire grating rather than with a single bar; the grating could serve as a perceptual cue against apparent rotation.) In the second case, we find a sudden transition. We do not know of any psychophysical studies of the strength of apparent motion as a function of spatial and temporal distance for rotations, although there have been such studies of linear motion (Korte's laws, and Burt & Sperling, 1981).

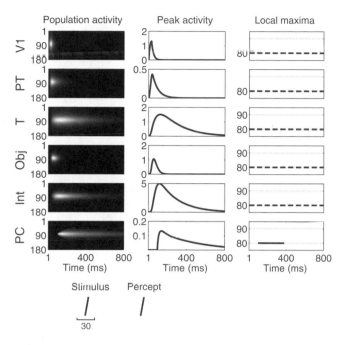

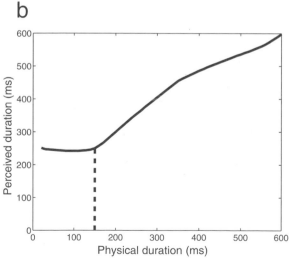

Figure 16.4
(*a*) A single 30-ms stimulus is perceived. PC, perception area; Int, integrator; Obj, object; T, template; PT, pretemplate. (*b*) The model qualitatively reproduces the "minimal perceptual moment": up to a certain physical duration, perceived duration has a constant value. This value is higher than the physical duration and is between 200 and 300 ms.

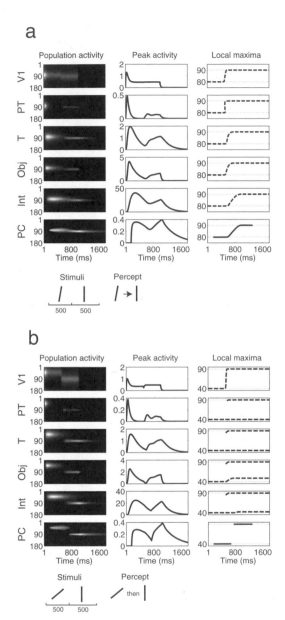

Figure 16.5
(*a*) Target and mask are presented sequentially, each for 500 ms, with a small orientation difference. They are perceived sequentially, with apparent rotation. (*b*) If two orientations with a large orientation difference (target, 40°; mask, 90°) are presented for the same durations (500 and 500 ms), they are observed sequentially, without any apparent motion. PC, perception area; Int, integrator; Obj, object; T, template; PT, pretemplate.

For two brief stimuli (both 20 ms), the percept also depends on the orientation difference. The model shows that when the difference is small, a single line with the average orientation is perceived (figure 16.6a). This is different from feature inheritance in that it does not involve any hypothesis testing; the line is also predicted to be at a slightly different orientation. When the difference is large, two lines superimposed on each other will be perceived (temporal integration; see figure 16.6b). This percept is essentially different from the one in figure 16.5b, while, physically speaking, the 20 + 20-ms stimulus sequence is contained within the 500 + 500-ms sequence. A condition that the model can also deal with is that of a target at 40° for 30 ms, followed by a masking grating for 300 ms, that is, the temporal parameters at which feature inheritance would occur were the target at 80°. In this case, a sort of superposition is observed (see figure 16.7). In the cases of figures 16.6 and 16.7, we can again not interpret the onsets and durations as quantitative predictions. In the superposition percepts, different perceptual durations for the components do not necessarily mean that an observer will see them superimposed only part of the time.

Table 16.1 shows the impact of leaving out certain aspects of the model on the reproduction of the phenomenology in three conditions, on the existence of a minimal perceptual moment, and on consistency with object substitution theory.

16.7 Discussion

Modeling the contents of perception based on neuronal population activity usually requires many simplifications. With our approach, we merely hope to outline a mechanism that can simultaneously explain the temporal characteristics of feature inheritance, backward masking, and temporal integration. The key properties of our network, which—so we claim—give rise to a visual percept, are as follows:

- a Bayes-motivated comparison interaction between a dynamic template and bottom-up input, leading to the formation of an "object"
- linear temporal integration, followed by a threshold
- feedforward inhibition proportional to the strength of an "object"

Speculations about the existence of both a threshold and an integration period for perception are supported by neurosurgical experiments (Libet, 1966, 1973, 1993; for an overview, see Koch, 2004).

If we examine the architecture of the model, we see that there is no loop between the model areas V1, template, and object; thus, there is no feedback in a graph-theoretical sense. However, it is possible that the template area is higher in the cortical hierarchy than the object area. Thus, a physiologist may characterize this interaction as a feedback interaction, although there is no recursion involved (cf.

a

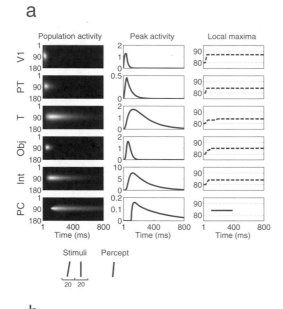

b

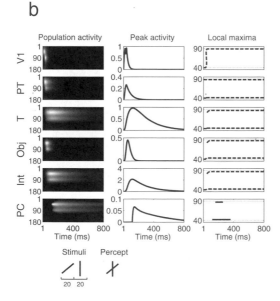

Figure 16.6
Perception of two 20-ms stimuli immediately following each other is determined by temporal integration. (*a*) When the orientation difference is small, a single line at the average orientation is perceived. This is an effect different from feature inheritance. (*b*) When the orientation difference is large, the two lines are perceived simultaneously and separately. PC, perception area; Int, integrator; Obj, object; T, template; PT, pretemplate.

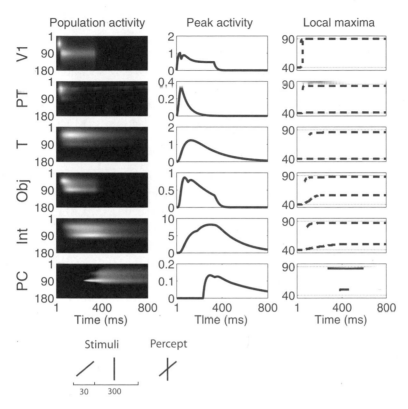

Figure 16.7
With a large orientation difference and the same timing as in feature inheritance, a superposition is observed. PC, perception area; Int, integrator; Obj, object; T, template; PT, pretemplate.

Table 16.1
Impact of leaving out selected aspects of the model on the reproduction of phenomenology

	30/300 orientations close, figure 16.2	30/300 orientations far apart, figure 16.7	20/20 orientations far apart, figure 16.6b	Minimal perceptual moment? figure 16.4b	Consistent with object substitution theory?
Full model	X	X	X	X	X
Template constant (linear feedforward)			X	X	
Short τ_T				X	X
No pretemplate			X	X	X
No integrator	X				X
Fixed threshold		X	X		X

Note. X = yes.

figure 7 in Öğmen, 2003). V1 is essentially involved in later interactions, but there is no feedback into V1.

The integration area can be thought of as a form of *iconic memory*, a high-capacity, rapidly decaying form of storage, lasting for at least a few hundred milliseconds (Coltheart, 1983, 1999). That does not mean that we think of iconic memory as instantiated in a single area. This role of the integration area is consistent with the claim that iconic memory is essential for visual awareness (Koch, 2004): It is as if enough evidence has to be collected before one can become aware of a stimulus.

Because we only consider orientation space at one location in physical space, our model is rather limited in scope. A next step would be to combine it with a detailed model of lateral interactions in space (e.g., Herzog et al., 2003a, or Li, 2004) in order to arrive at a more complete explanation of feature inheritance. It might then be possible to explain the spreading of the feature over the whole grating. Moreover, feature inheritance is a form of incomplete backward masking. In describing the phenomenology of backward masking, the multiplicative interaction would implement hypothesis testing in the sense of DiLollo et al. (2000). Both the transition from temporal integration to masking and the transition from temporal integration to normal vision can be seen in our model. The former is determined by the duration of the mask, the latter by the duration of the target.

Another shortcoming of our model is the absence of stochastic noise in the cells. Including it ought to explain variability of human performance in feature inheritance and thus allow a fit of the psychometric curves of Herzog and Koch (2001). Such a model would likely also allow the application of a more fundamental decision rule, such as a maximum-likelihood one (instead of "sufficiently high local maxima"). Noise is also the reason that for very short stimulus durations, seeing becomes a signal-detection task.

A general issue that requires further study is the implementation of Bayesian mechanisms in neural circuitry. While many instances of multiplication have been found in the brain, Gabbiani et al. (2002) remains the only study of the local biophysical mechanisms involved. One proposal to perform Bayesian inference without coding multiplication in neurons has been put forward by Rao (2004). By representing probabilities in the logarithmic domain, multiplication is turned into addition, which is more easily implemented in the neural circuitry. He has shown that feedforward and recurrent connections perform Bayesian inference for arbitrary hidden Markov models; however, some strong mathematical assumptions are made in the process.

In conclusion, we have implemented the simple idea that the contents of perception are the result of a continuous comparison of sensory input with a template updated with some inertia, an integration stage, and a dynamic threshold.

16.8   Appendix: Model Details

All areas are modeled as populations of analogue, noiseless neurons. Orientation filtering in "V1" occurs through convolutions with Gabors. The horizontally oriented one is

$$G(x, y) = \frac{2\cos\alpha y}{\sqrt{\sigma_x \sigma_y}} e^{-\left(\frac{x^2}{2\sigma_x} + \frac{y^2}{2\sigma_y}\right)},$$

with $\alpha = 0.5$, $\sigma_x = 5$, and $\sigma_y = 30$. The time constants of the different areas are as follows: $\tau_{v1} = 20$ ms, $\tau_S = 40$ ms, $\tau_{PT} = 60$ ms, $\tau_{PT}^1 = 10$ ms, $\tau_T = 200$ ms, $\tau_O = 20$ ms, $\tau_I = 200$ ms, and $\tau_P = 20$ ms. The time constants of some of these areas are very long, but they can be effective time constants due to a positive feedback loop or attractor dynamics. The synaptic delay ε between pretemplate and template areas is taken to be 3 ms; between other areas, synaptic delay is irrelevant for our model. The pretemplate–template subsystem with global feedback inhibition (see equations 16.4–16.6) implements the fact that a candidate hypothesis, sent from V1 into the pretemplate area, has to compete with the stored hypothesis. A threshold proportional to the total activity in the template area is equivalent to an inhibitory term in the pretemplate activity.

Weights are as follows: $\alpha_{V1} = 1$, $\alpha_{PT} = 1$, $\alpha_{PT}^1 = 4/180$, $\alpha_T = 15$, $\alpha_T^1 = 3$, $\alpha_O = 0.5$, $\alpha_O^1 = 20$, $\alpha_1 = 20$, $\alpha_P = 1$, and $\alpha_{thr} = 0.26$. Synaptic depression in V1 has weight $\alpha_d = 0.8$. These have been tuned to reproduce the experimental results; this tuning is not necessarily unique. The baseline threshold is $T_0 = 0.05$. The minimum value that a local maximum in the perception area has to exceed at a certain time in order to "be perceived" is taken to be 50% of the overall maximum until that time.

The differential equations were integrated using the Euler method in MATLAB (MathWorks, Inc.). All initial activities were zero.

Acknowledgments

We thank Michael Herzog for countless valuable discussions, for comments on the manuscript, and for conducting many pilot experiments for us. We also thank Haluk Öğmen for many pleasant and useful discussions. Wei Ji Ma is supported by the Netherlands Organisation for Scientific Research and the Swartz Foundation. We are grateful to both. We thank the organizers and the other participants of the "First Half Second" workshop.

Notes

1. An alternative approach, making use of the noise distribution of neuronal responses, can be found in Pouget et al. (2003).

2. In the offset paradigm (i.e., when the target is a pair of offset lines, a vernier), the offset is also bequeathed to the entire grating, but the observer's attention is always on one of its edges (Herzog & Koch, 2001). It is unknown whether this holds for the orientation paradigm as well.

VI THE DYNAMIC RELATION OF UNCONSCIOUS AND CONSCIOUS PROCESSES IN VISION

17 Response Priming With and Without Awareness

Jens Schwarzbach and Dirk Vorberg

17.1 Introduction

Our perceptual system copes with a highly dynamic environment. Visual stimulation changes as objects move, as objects become occluded, or because we move ourselves. This poses intriguing problems not only for perception but also for our action system. We constantly update and sometimes radically change our action goals in a dynamic environment. Do previous and current states affect the upcoming actions, or do we press an internal "reset button" each time an action has to change? In this chapter we report findings on the dynamics of how we build up our actions on the existing representations of motor plans and compare them with the dynamics of perception.

17.1.1 Perceptual Changes

Many perceptual studies indicate that our perceptual system can be amazingly blind to the above-mentioned perceptual changes (O'Regan et al., 1999; Rensink, 2002). We typically study the perceptual aspect in visual masking studies by presenting two or more stimuli in rapid succession (Breitmeyer, 1984). If the presentation of the first stimulus, affects perception of the second stimulus, we speak of *forward masking*; if the later presented stimulus affects visibility of the first stimulus, we speak of *backward masking*. A special kind of backward masking is *metacontrast masking* (Fehrer & Raab, 1962; Stigler, 1910; Werner, 1935) in which test stimulus and mask overlap neither in time nor in space.

Metacontrast masking is a rich experimental tool for studying visual awareness. The temporal dynamics of the conscious percept and its dependence on stimulus conditions are well known. Strength of masking depends on three factors: stimulus onset asynchrony (SOA), the relation of light energy, and the spatial separation between prime and mask (Breitmeyer, 1984).

17.1.2   Motor Changes

In response priming paradigms, one also presents two stimuli in rapid succession in a choice task; however, these stimuli do not necessarily mask each other. A target stimulus is presented on which subjects are required to perform a speeded choice reaction. Another stimulus (the prime), briefly shown before the target, can speed up or slow down responses to the target depending of the congruence of their response mappings. Priming effects are computed as the reaction time difference between incongruent and congruent trials. When measuring priming effects separately for each SOA, we can describe the amount of priming as a function of temporal separation between prime and target, a so-called priming function. Several studies from our lab report that response priming effects typically increase with SOA (Vorberg et al., 2004).

17.1.3   Perception and Action

Interestingly, one can combine these two approaches and present two stimuli, each having an established stimulus–response mapping, in rapid succession where the first stimulus (the prime) is masked by the second stimulus (the mask). Such masked priming paradigms allow study of how primes of different visibility influence speeded choice reactions to the mask. Thus, masked priming is a means of studying perception and action simultaneously.

Perceptual questions can be related, for example, to the apparent brightness or identity of the prime, whereas action-related questions can be addressed by speeded choice reactions to the mask. An intriguing aspect of studies in masked priming is that we might be able to use them to learn about how visual awareness of a stimulus is related to its impact on the motor system.

Studies in masked priming have provided compelling evidence that invisible primes influence manual choice response time to the mask with different types of backward masking procedures (Dehaene et al., 1998; Eimer & Schlaghecken, 1998; Klotz & Wolff, 1995; Naccache & Dehaene, 2001; Schmidt, 2002). While these studies have focused on demonstrating preserved priming in the absence of visual awareness, we will emphasize the process of response priming itself in the current chapter.

17.2   The Dynamics of Response Priming: What Happens in the First Half Second?

When we overtly react to a stimulus, we have passed the stages of detection, identification, stimulus–response mapping, and motor preparation, without implying that these stages are fully sequential. In this section we first review our previously published data and a model of the dynamics of manual response priming in a two-choice task (Vorberg et al., 2003). Then, we test the generality of the model by increasing the number of response alternatives. We conclude the section with a revised model that accounts for the dynamics of response priming in *n*-choice tasks.

17.2.1 Response Priming in a Two-Choice Task

We used left- and right-arrow-shaped stimuli as primes and targets in a masked priming procedure with two-choice reactions. The prime arrow was briefly presented above or below fixation and was followed by the target arrow after a variable SOA at the same location (figure 17.1A). Size and contours of prime and mask were designed such that the outer contours of the prime fit exactly in the inner cutout of the mask. When shown in short succession, such stimuli produce a strong backward masking effect. In fact, the primes were invisible over the entire range of SOAs (see the section on awareness). Subjects were asked to press a button with their left or right index finger, respectively, depending on the orientation of the mask. The time course of priming was studied in a speeded choice reaction task to the orientation of the mask. Prime and mask were called *congruent* if they had the same orientation, and *incongruent* otherwise. The speed of manual choice responses depended on prime–mask congruence (figure 17.1B): Reaction times were shorter with congruent primes than with incongruent primes, replicating previous results (e.g., Neumann & Klotz, 1994). In addition, the experiment revealed that priming increased with temporal separation between prime and target. The net priming function ($RT_{incongruent} - RT_{congruent}$) was computed separately for each SOA. Priming effects increased almost linearly with SOA (figure 17.1C) and can be almost perfectly predicted by a simple equation $RT_{incongruent} - RT_{congruent} = SOA + b$, with the intercept b being equal to zero.

17.2.2 An Accumulator Model of Priming

To account for the temporal dynamics of the priming effect, we proposed an accumulator model of response priming (Vorberg et al., 2003). The model (figure 17.2) assumes separate accumulators collecting sensory evidence for stimuli mapped to left or right responses. A response is initiated as soon as the accumulated neural evidence for one versus the opposite response exceeds threshold. The model predicts response priming because primes bias the accumulators, driving their difference toward the target threshold on congruent trials and away from it on incongruent trials. Our model accounts well for response times, especially the linear dependence of priming effects with unit slope, as well as the probability of errors in two-response choice tasks.

It has been shown recently that the unit-slope prediction of the accumulator model also holds for other stimulus modalities (shape, color, semantic features) and response types (arm, leg, finger pointing, vocal responses); for a summary, see

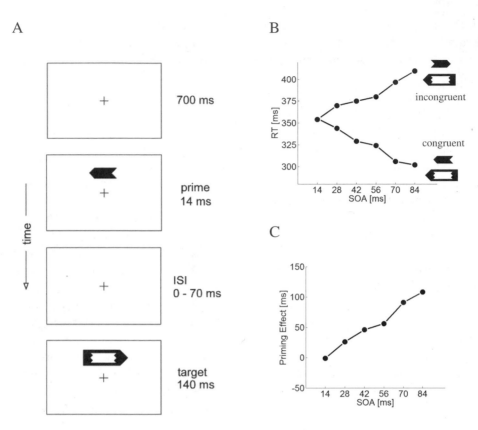

Figure 17.1
(*A*) Temporal sequence of a typical priming trial in the Vorberg et al. (2003) study. Left- and right-oriented arrows served as prime and target stimuli. Primes fitted exactly into the center cutout of targets. Orientation of prime and target varied unpredictably from trial to trial. Congruent and incongruent trials occurred equally often. ISI, interstimulus interval. (*B*) Effects of congruent and incongruent primes on choice reaction time (RT) as a function of stimulus onset asynchrony (SOA) in the first session of experiment 1. Error bars indicate ±1 *SD* around means. (*C*) The priming effect increased almost linearly with SOA. (After Vorberg et al., 2003)

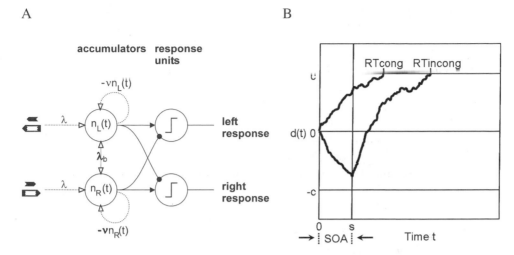

Figure 17.2
(*A*) Accumulator model of priming. Input spike trains are modeled as inhomogeneous Poisson processes by which spikes with rate λ increment state n of two accumulator units for left and right responses, respectively. Primes and targets are processed identically. Accumulators show saturation due to random decay of spike effects (rate v). Responses are initiated when the difference $d(t)$ between the accumulator states crosses threshold. (From Vorberg et al., 2003) (*B*) Sample time courses of $d(t)$ when a prime is followed by a congruent or incongruent mask with stimulus onset asynchrony (SOA) = s. Responses on incongruent trials are delayed by s ms on average, as compared with congruent trials. RTcong, reaction time–congruent; RTincong, reaction time–incongruent.

Vorberg et al. (2004). In spite of such variations in stimulus and response characteristics, experimental conditions in these studies agreed in one aspect: They all used two-choice tasks for assessing response priming. One question that motivated the study described here concerns the number of response alternatives.

17.2.3 Response Priming in *n*-Choice Tasks

Is response priming restricted to two-choice tasks? Recently, Wolff (1997) compared masked priming across different choice tasks and reported diminished priming effects when the task involved more than two response alternatives. This finding is puzzling and has implications for understanding the limits of priming without awareness. A problem we see with Wolff's study, however, is that by increasing the number of response alternatives, stimulus set size also varied such that large stimulus sets were more heterogeneous in stimulus shape than small sets. Because this applied to both the target and prime stimuli, the observed priming reduction might have been due to reduced prime–mask similarity rather than to number of response alternatives. Increasing the response set also affects the heterogeneity between responses, as is obvious when the spatial distances between finger positions are compared for two- and four-choice tasks. We chose eye movements as responses because they can be carried out in different directions while keeping stimulus–response mappings easy for participants and help solve stimulus and response heterogeneity problems.

Similarity Effects in Response Priming

In most of the studies summarized above, the effects of congruent primes on responding to a subsequent imperative stimulus were contrasted with those of incongruent primes. However, congruency is not necessarily all-or-none when there are multiple response alternatives that can be ordered by similarity. Do response-time benefits from congruent prime stimuli diminish in a graded fashion, as their similarity to the imperative stimulus decreases? Studying this question in detail seemed crucial also for understanding neural accumulation models, because how the degree of congruency affects priming should reveal something about the presumed accumulators' tuning for stimulus features.

Priming of Eye Movements: Experimental Procedures

To study how masked primes affect the latency and the kinetic parameters of saccadic responses, we conducted experimental studies that probed the time course of prime-congruency effects at varying degrees of similarity between primes and masks. Participants performed center–out saccadic eye movements to one of eight locations equally spaced on a circle around fixation. Pointer-shaped stimuli (figure 17.3) served as primes and masks; they were both presented centrally and pointed to one of the target positions (figure 17.4). As in the studies sketched above, mask stimuli contained a central cutout that strongly reduced the visibility of the preceding prime by metacontrast. Let us define prime–mask congruency by the difference in their orientations: Prime and mask are fully congruent if oriented identically, and maximally incongruent if they point in opposite directions. More generally, define congruency level by the angular difference $|\phi_{mask} - \phi_{prime}|$. We used the congruency levels 0°, 45°, 90°, 135°, and 180°, plus a neutral-prime control condition.

Participants   Eight participants (six female; mean age = 26.6, with a range from 21 to 44 years) with normal or corrected-to-normal vision participated in eight 1-hr sessions spread across 2 weeks. Four participants received course credits; the others were paid 5€ per hour. Except for participant J.S. (the first author) and his research assistant, participants were naive to the purpose of the experiment.

Stimuli   Stimuli were presented centrally black on white on a 20-in. SONY VGA color monitor with a 60-Hz refresh rate. Primes and masks varied in orientation, with their arrowhead pointing to one of eight peripheral target marks, 0.5° in size at 5° eccentricity. Mask stimuli subtended 1.3° in width and 1° in height. Prime stimuli had half the size of masks and fitted exactly into their central cutout. Neutral

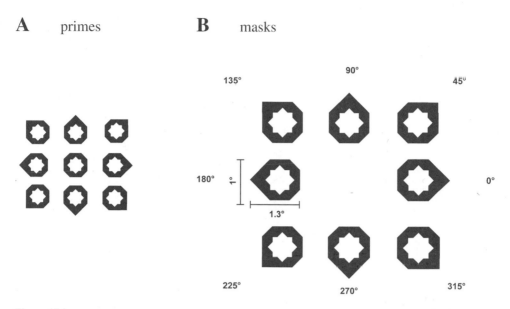

Figure 17.3
Oriented primes (*A*) and masks (*B*) pointing to one of eight peripheral locations as indicated by the direction of the arrowhead. Neutral primes (panel *A*, center) did not contain directional information. Primes fitted exactly into the mask central cutout.

primes without directional features were used for estimating the baselines for priming effects.

Task   The task was to perform a speeded saccade to the target indicated by the mask stimulus. A trial began with the simultaneous presentation of the fixation cross and the eight position marks (see figure 17.4). On each trial, participants started the event sequence by making a key press. After a variable delay, the prime appeared for 17 ms at the center of the screen and was followed by a central mask after an unpredictable SOA between 17 and 83 ms. Exposure duration of the mask was 50 ms; it always followed with fixed delay of 600 ms from trial start. Participants responded by directing their gaze as fast as possible to the peripheral target indicated by the mask. They could start the next trial 500 ms after fixating a peripheral target.

Design   SOA (17, 33, 50, 67, and 83 ms) and congruency (neutral, 0°, 45°, 90°, 135°, and 180°) were varied orthogonally in a repeated-measures design. Dependent variables were saccadic response time and gaze position (see the section on eye movement recording below). Each participant completed eight sessions with 16 replications per SOA–congruency combination, which led to 640 trials per congruency level, and a total of 3840 trials per participant.

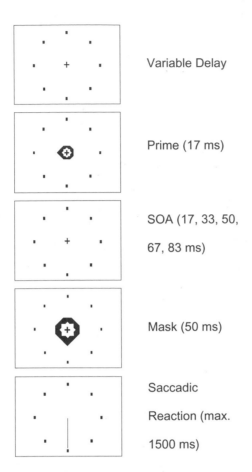

Variable Delay

Prime (17 ms)

SOA (17, 33, 50,

67, 83 ms)

Mask (50 ms)

Saccadic

Reaction (max.

1500 ms)

Figure 17.4
Event sequence on a typical trial. Participants started the trial by making a key press. After a delay, a prime stimulus appeared for 17 ms, followed by a mask stimulus presented for 50 ms. The prime–mask stimulus onset asynchrony (SOA) varied between 17 and 83 ms. The task was to direct gaze to the target position indicated by the mask. The angle between prime and mask direction varied unpredictably between 0° and 360°, in steps of 45°.

Procedure   Each session began with written instructions describing the task, with masks in all orientations shown on paper. Participants were instructed to fixate the central cross and to saccade as fast as possible to the peripheral location to which the large stimulus (i.e., the mask) pointed. Participants were not informed about the occurrence of primes. Each session consisted of 480 trials with a 10-min break midway.

Eye Movement Recording   Eye movements were measured with a video-based eye-tracking system (SMI Eye Link I), with temporal resolution of 250 Hz and spatial resolution of 0.2°. Participants viewed the screen from 90 cm, with their heads on a chin rest. For calibration, participants fixated a sequence of nine calibration targets (size 0.5°), which were presented in an unpredictable order on a 3×3 grid (width $= 24°$, height $= 18°$). Drift correction was performed at the beginning of each trial, when participants simultaneously fixated the central fixation cross and pressed a key. The actual fixation position served as the reference for the center of the screen throughout the remainder of a trial. Gaze position was available online. If, during a trial, a saccade end position fell within a radius of 1° of a saccade target mark, the corresponding target was counted as the participant's response, and the trial was terminated. Whenever participants fixated a position different from that indicated by the mask, or when an eye blink occurred, the trial was terminated with a warning tone.

Data Processing and Error Handling   Saccade onset was defined as the first sample in a series of at least three samples (12 ms) at which gaze velocity exceeded 30°/s. Similarly, the end of a saccade was the sample at which gaze velocity dropped below 30°/s. Saccade-onset and saccade-contingent gaze position (from 80 ms before to 80 ms after saccade onset) of the first saccade following presentation of the mask (the primary saccade) were included in the offline data analysis. Saccadic response time was determined by measuring the onset of the primary saccade with respect to the presentation of the mask. Trials were included in the analysis only when the target position was fixated correctly; otherwise they were considered fixation errors. Further reasons for excluding trials were (1) saccadic response time below 80 ms after onset of the prime (*anticipation*), (2) eye blink throughout the trial (*blink*), or (3) low-velocity *eye drift* (5°/s < velocity < 30°/s).

For each prime-congruency condition, all eight target positions were probed equally often. To reduce the number of conditions, we averaged across mask orientation. Furthermore, trials were classified by prime congruence, disregarding the sign of the orientation difference. For example, trials with mask pointing up and prime right (45°) were combined with corresponding trials with prime pointing left (315° $= -45°$).

Effects of Primes on Saccadic Response Times

As shown in figure 17.5, prime–mask congruency and SOA strongly affected saccadic response time (mean overall response time was 244 ms, with a standard deviation of 9.8 ms). Saccades were fastest when the prime's orientation coincided with that of the mask, and the more the prime's orientation deviated, the slower the saccades became. As compared to the neutral condition, response-time benefits were observed for congruent primes (congruency 0° or 45°), and response-time costs were observed for incongruent primes (90°, 135°, and 180°). Importantly, these effects were amplified by SOA: The longer the mask was delayed from the prime, the larger the benefits and costs, with relative ordering of congruency effects preserved. This visual impression was backed by the statistical results, which revealed a highly reliable SOA × Congruency interaction ($p < .0005$).

The reader may have noted an oddity in the relative impact of incongruent primes: Unexpectedly, saccades were initiated faster when primes and masks pointed in opposite directions than when their orientation difference was only 135°.

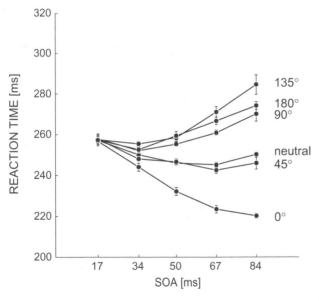

Figure 17.5
Mean saccadic response times, as a function of prime–mask congruence and stimulus onset asynchrony (SOA). Error bars show a within-subject confidence interval (Loftus & Masson, 1994). Reaction times are normalized by subtracting a subject-deviation score from each single data point (here, reaction time). The subject-deviation score is the difference of the grand mean (average across conditions and subjects) and the corresponding subject's mean. The standard error of the mean is computed with those normalized scores. The confidence interval CI for a condition j with mean M and standard error SE is: $CI = M_j \pm 2SE_j$.

This finding held for most individual participants, and was the same for saccades along the main versus diagonal axes (data not reported here), which makes an account in terms of oculomotor particulars unlikely.

To quantitatively compare the priming effects with our finding in the manual two-choice task, we estimated net priming by calculating the difference between the 180° and the 0° conditions for each participant. This should correspond to the net amount of priming in the two-choice task with arrows pointing in opposite directions, and, in fact, saccade latencies show priming dynamics similar to those for manual response times: As in Vorberg et al. (2003), net priming of saccade latencies also increases linearly with SOA, with slope approximately equal to one (figure 17.6). This observed priming time course agrees surprisingly well with the theoretical time course predicted by our accumulator model for the two-choice situation.

Discussion

Congruent primes lead to shorter response times than do incongruent primes (Klotz & Wolff, 1995; Leuthold & Kopp, 1998; Neumann & Klotz, 1994; Vorberg et al., 2003, 2004). This consistent finding in masked priming is not confined to manual

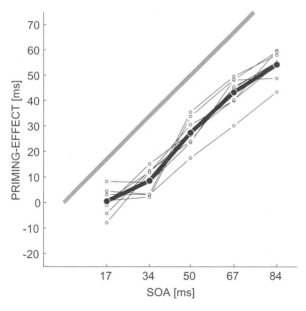

Figure 17.6
Net priming effect (PE; thick solid line) increases linearly with stimulus onset asynchrony (SOA) (PE = .858 × SOA − 16.1). Net priming effect is defined by the response-time advantage on maximally congruent (0°) trials versus maximally incongruent trials (180°). Thin lines with open circles show the data for individual participants. The gray diagonals show the slope-one prediction of the accumulator model.

two-choice tasks, as our results show, but extends to eye movements in a task with more than two response alternatives and with prime–mask congruency varied in a graded fashion. The present findings can be summarized as follows:

1. Priming effects on response time are ordered by congruency, with higher congruency leading to faster responses. These effects fan out with increasing delay between mask and prime ("fan effect").

2. There is an exception to the rule: 180° primes produce less response time slowing than 135° primes.

3. The response-time advantage by fully congruent (0°) versus maximally incongruent primes (180°) increases linearly with SOA, with a slope close to one.

Finding 3 is predicted by the accumulator model. But can the model also account for the fan effect and the 180° versus 135° reversal? In the original model, we assumed two accumulators that collect sensory evidence for stimuli mapped to left or right responses. Accumulators had excitatory and inhibitory connections to their corresponding and complementary response unit, respectively. To extend the model to the eight-choice saccade task, with stimuli and responses representing directions and target locations in two-dimensional space, we assumed accumulators that are tuned to directional information. Neurons in the motor cortex, as well as in visual areas, have been shown to be sensitive to motion direction and stimulus orientation, with cosine tuning functions (Georgopoulos et al., 1982; Georgopoulos et al., 1986; Maunsell & Van Essen, 1983). A cell's response to a stimulus is equivalent to the dot product of the two vectors representing the cell's preferred direction and the directional information contained in the stimulus, respectively. Unless accumulators are allowed to take negative values, four or more spatially tuned accumulators are needed to represent two-dimensional space adequately. More crucial than the number of accumulators in the model is the shape of tuning functions, however. The canonical cosine tuning function produces maximal excitation for the preferred stimulus, and maximal inhibition for the stimulus pointing in the opposite direction.

Computer simulation of the extended model with eight accumulators endowed with cosine tuning has shown that the model easily predicts finding 1, the fan effect, that is, response priming effects ordered by congruence and spreading out with SOA, and finding 3, the linear increase of net priming with SOA, with a slope close to one. However, the model cannot predict finding 2, the 180° versus 135° reversal. More detailed analysis revealed that this failure is due to two assumptions: the shape of the tuning function and the single-decision rule. Replacing cosine tuning (with minimum rigidly fixed at 180°) with a more flexible tuning function admitting more finely tuned accumulators solves part of the problem. We used Mexican-hat tuning functions, characterized by strong "center" excitation flanked by strong "surround" inhibition, which are commonly found in neurons of the visual (Kang et al., 2003; Pugh et al., 2000; Ringach, 1998; Ringach et al., 2003) and oculomotor (Schall et al., 1995) system. It seemed that with sharper tuning functions of this type, which produce stronger inhibition for more similar stimuli than those opposite to the preferred direction, the model could do the job and correctly predict the 135° versus 180° reversal of congruency effects. However, simulations show that even with tuning function minima at ±135°, that model does not predict the reversal unless we give up the single-decision rule, which worked well in the two-accumulator model. There, we assumed that the decision to initiate a response is given when the difference between accumulator activations exceeds some critical value. The natural extension of this rule to the n-accumulator case is to initiate a response when the *population vector*, that is, the summed accumulator activations weighted by their preferred orientation, exceeds some threshold value. With the population-vector decision rule, the 135° versus 180° reversal is not predicted, however, even with appropriate Mexican-hat tuning functions, because the large excitatory contributions to the population vector tend to swamp the smaller inhibitory contributions. Replacing the population-vector rule by a *separate-decisions* assumption can solve the problem: Here, the assumption is that each response unit separately monitors its accumulator inputs, and the decision is determined by the unit that first exceeds its threshold activation.

With these modifications, the extended accumulator model provides an account of the effects of masked primes on the time to decide on and to initiate a saccade towards one of n target locations.

17.3 Priming With and Without Awareness

Finally let us consider the *perceptual* aspects of masked primes, which we have neglected so far. In line with the current research on priming without awareness discussed before, we have tacitly assumed that the effects described here arise without any causal role of the phenomenological aspects of the primes. Our stance in this issue is closely related to the theoretical position put forward recently by Lamme and his colleagues (Lamme, 2000; Lamme & Roelfsema, 2000; Lamme et al., 2000; Lamme et al., 2002). On the basis of a wealth of neurobiological evidence, Lamme has argued that the feedforward activation of cells in the brain is not sufficient for generating awareness, which will not arise unless there is recurrent processing mediated by horizontal and feedback connections. The absence of recurrent processing does not preclude other effects of stimuli, however. On the contrary, "the whole feedforward path of processing may be activated by an unperceived stimulus" (Lamme, 2000, p. 395). Strong evidence for this position has been obtained in

single-cell recordings in backward masking of figure–ground signals, which were
selectively suppressed by the mask, whereas the initial response transients that represent primitive features were unaffected (Lamme et al., 2002). By this account, it
should be possible to find dissociations between masking and priming for stimuli in
close temporal succession. Therefore, in the next section, we look for experimental
evidence of such dissociations.

17.3.1 Prime Visibility in the *n*-Choice Task

After the conclusion of the choice sessions described above, we tested in a separate
session how well our participants were able to see and recognize the masked primes,
that is, to report on their identity. Experimental conditions were identical except for
the following details.

Task.   Participants were instructed to focus attention on the prime stimulus, and to
report on its orientation by saccading to the corresponding peripheral mark, trying
to ignore the orientation of the mask. To prevent contamination of conscious
perception with unconscious effects of primes, participants were to withhold their
response until the fixation cross disappeared from the screen 500 ms after prime
onset. Premature responses were signaled as errors. Instructions stressed the importance of not confusing prime and mask orientation. Slow-motion demonstration of
the stimulus events and practice trials preceded the experimental session.

Design.   All prime orientations occurred equally often; neutral primes were
omitted. Mask orientation differed from prime orientation by 0°, 90°, 180°, or 270°.
Note that prime and oriented masks were always congruent with respect to axis type
(main, diagonal). On one fifth of the trials, mask shape was neutral. SOA varied
from 17 to 100 ms, in steps of 16.7 ms. The order of conditions was randomized within
blocks. There were 2,080 trials per participant, organized in eight blocks of 260 trials
each.

Data analysis.   Confusion matrices were constructed for each combination of SOA
and mask type. Since mask orientation may bias the reported orientation of the
prime, we adapted methods of signal detection to separate sensory from bias effects
(for discussion of the issue, see Vorberg et al., 2004). We estimated the discriminability index d' for each particular prime orientation with mask type fixed and
then averaged the resulting d' measures across prime and mask orientations.

Results and Discussion
The results are shown in table 17.1 and figure 17.7, separated according to mask
type (oriented vs. neutral). Obviously, recognition of prime orientation was above
chance for all SOAs. Moreover, performance level increased with SOA and, thus,
was highly correlated with priming effects.

Table 17.1
Recognition performance of masked prime, in terms of TSD index d', as a function of prime–mask SOA and mask type

SOA (ms)											
1/		34		50		67		84		100	
Or mask	Nt mask	Or mask	Nt mask	Or mask	Nt mask	Or mask	Nt mask	Or mask	Nt mask	Or mask	Nt mask
d' 0.53	0.875	0.58	1.15	0.96	1.41	1.19	1.62	1.56	1.76	2.05	2.20

Or, oriented; Nt, neutral; TSD, theory of signal detection.
Prime and mask exposure duration was 17 and 50 ms, respectively.

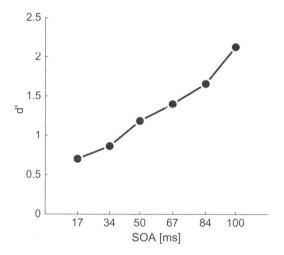

Figure 17.7
Prime recognition across all prime orientations was above chance and increased linearly with SOA.

With constant stimulus intensity, complete metacontrast masking requires exposure durations much larger for the mask than for the prime. With the mask serving as imperative stimulus in eye movement studies, long mask duration is problematic, however, because it tends to "glue" the gaze to the mask and to prevent express saccades to the target locations (Fischer & Ramsperger, 1984). For these reasons, we used a 50-ms mask as a compromise, which inevitably leads to rather inefficient type A masking of the 17-ms primes, as evidenced by the recognition data presented here.

Better-than-chance recognition of the masked prime stimuli seems to create problems for the position that priming effects were dissociated from conscious perception of primes. In fact, since net priming and recognition performance were both strictly increasing with SOA, our recognition data cannot be used to reject the traditional account of claims for subliminal perception. Such accounts hold that effects presumed to be unconscious reflect some uncontrolled conscious awareness of the inducing stimulus, an argument that seems even more compelling if both measures covary across conditions. However, failure to demonstrate a dissociation does not imply that none exists, since covariation does not imply causation, as we will now argue. In fact, we prefer to account for the present priming results in terms of processing mechanisms that operate prior to conscious perception of prime stimuli.

17.3.2   Prime Visibility in the Two-Choice Task and Its Relation to Response Priming

It is well-known (Breitmeyer, 1984) that the shape of the masking function depends on the physical parameters of prime and mask. Exceedingly long mask durations can lead to perfect masking over a large range of SOAs. Monotonic reduction in masking with SOA (type A masking function) is typically found when mask duration and/or energy exceeds that of the prime, whereas nonmonotonic inverted U-shaped masking functions (type B) often arise for the reverse ordering. In the two-choice task, we used these known relations between prime and mask duration to study response priming under qualitatively different masking conditions (perfect, type A, and type B masking).

Masking and corresponding priming functions of the two-choice task (Vorberg et al., 2003) are summarized in figure 17.8. The shape of the masking function changed from flat (i.e., perfect masking over the entire SOA range), to linearly decreasing (i.e., less masking with longer SOA), or inversely U-shaped (i.e., higher stimulus visibility at short and long SOAs as compared to intermediate SOAs) when the exposure durations of prime and mask stimuli were varied. Under all these qualitatively different time courses for visibility, priming remained invariant following the SOA rule: $RT_{incongruent} - RT_{congruent} \approx SOA$. Note that *increasing* priming effects within an SOA range where prime recognition is *decreasing* (i.e., type B masking) cannot be reconciled with the notion that conscious perception is causal for priming. Thus, type B masking offers ideal opportunities for revealing dissociations when the priming time course is increasing. In contrast, type A masking inevitably leads to correlated effects of priming and conscious perception when the priming time course is increasing and thus offers no chance for dissociations even if separate mechanisms underlie priming and perceptual masking.

Thus, priming–recognition covariations are inconclusive under type A masking conditions. Therefore, above-zero visibility of the prime stimuli in the *n*-choice experiment does not conflict with our earlier findings of priming–masking dissociations and does not establish that phenomenological awareness played any causal role in priming. By the close correspondence of their temporal dynamics, we infer

A

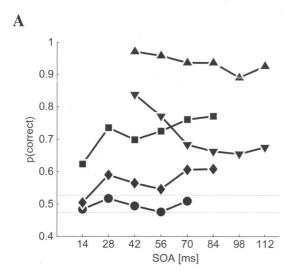

B

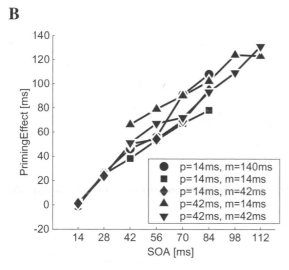

Figure 17.8
Replotted masking and priming functions from the two-choice task (Vorberg et al., 2003). Symbols refer to different combinations of prime and mask durations, denoted with letters p and m, respectively. SOA, stimulus onset asynchrony. (*A*) Masking functions dramatically changed from perfect masking (prime duration, 14 ms; mask duration, 140 ms) to type A masking (prime duration 14 ms; mask duration 14/42 ms) or to type B masking (prime duration, 42 ms, mask duration, 14/42 ms). (*B*) Under identical stimulus conditions, priming functions invariantly followed the SOA law ($RT_{incongruent} - RT_{congruent} \approx SOA$, where RT denotes reaction time)

instead that the same mechanism that underlies priming of manual RTs also underlies the priming of saccade latencies. This argument is also in line with Lamme's (2000) theoretical position sketched above.

17.4 Summary

A consistent finding in the literature on masked priming is that in manual two-choice tasks, congruent primes lead to shorter response times than do incongruent primes (Klotz & Wolff, 1995; Leuthold & Kopp, 1998; Neumann & Klotz, 1994; Vorberg et al., 2003, 2004). Here we extended these findings to eye movements, in a task with more than two response alternatives and with prime–mask congruency varied in a graded fashion. Priming effects on response time were ordered by congruency, with higher congruency leading to faster responses. These effects fan out with increasing delay between prime and mask. However, 180° primes produced faster response times than 135° primes. The response-time advantage by fully congruent (0°) versus maximally incongruent primes (180°) increased linearly with SOA, with a slope close to one, and was comparable to priming effects obtained in manual two-choice tasks.

To account for priming ordered by similarity and the observed reversal in priming effects for 135° and 180° congruency, we modified our previously published accumulator model (Vorberg et al., 2003) to include center–surround (Mexican-hat-shaped) tuning functions for saccade direction and by replacing a population vector decision rule with a decision rule that monitors each response separately for a threshold crossing.

Although priming effects in our *n*-choice task were clearly correlated with recognition performance, we prefer to account for the priming results in terms of processing mechanisms that operate prior to conscious perception of prime stimuli. We argue that priming-recognition covariations are inconclusive under type A masking conditions. Comparisons under qualitatively different masking conditions (perfect, type A, type B masking) have shown invariant priming. The finding of *increasing* priming effects within an SOA range where prime recognition is *decreasing* (i.e., type B masking) cannot be reconciled with the notion that conscious perception is causal for priming.

Acknowledgments

The authors wish to thank Angelika Lingnau for numerous helpful comments and suggestions.

18 Visual Masking Reveals Differences Between the Nonconscious and Conscious Processing of Form and Surface Attributes

Bruno G. Breitmeyer and Haluk Öğmen

18.1 The Existence of Nonconscious Visual Processing

Perception can be defined as the registration of sensory information in consciousness. However, in vision not all processed information attains a state of perceptual awareness. This is trivially true, for instance, of retinal processing of chromatic and luminance information. This information must be transmitted to, and transformed at, higher visual centers before attaining consciousness. However, even at later, cortical levels much information processing proceeds without visual awareness. A number of empirical observations support this view. The observations are based on neurological case studies of selective loss of visual capacities and on studies of normal observers under experimental conditions that render a relevant stimulus inaccessible to consciousness.

For example, localized lesions of cortical area V4 produce achromatopsia (cortical color blindness) while leaving intact discriminations among wavelengths, an ability presumably depending on intact earlier levels of cortical processing such as V1 (Zeki, 1997; Zeki & Marini, 1998). Conversely, the phenomenon of blindsight in humans illustrates that even when area V1 is severely compromised, patients can nonetheless respond to aftereffects and to attributes of stimuli such as motion and coarse form (Weiskrantz, 1997; Weiskrantz et al., 2003) as well as their wavelength composition (Stoerig & Cowey, 1992), even though they report not seeing the stimuli. These among many other neurological case studies indicate that chromatic, form, and motion information can be processed at conscious as well as nonconscious levels in humans.

Recently Milner and Goodale (1995; Goodale et al., this volume) reviewed extensive neuropsychological, behavioral, and psychophysical findings supporting their proposal that the visual system consists of at least two quasi-independent subsystems. One subsystem constructs a representation of the world for higher cognition; the other is responsible for rapid control of action. The former, relying mainly on the ventral cortical pathway, is thus tied to perception and "offline" control of behavior mediated by cognitive processes associated with consciousness, memory, planning, and other executive functioning. The latter, relying mainly on the dorsal cortical stream of processing that contributes to spatial vision (Ungerleider, 1985), primarily performs immediate "online" control of behavior that can proceed without consciousness. Insofar as emotions prepare and motivate organisms for specific behaviors, one also can make the distinction between vision for perception and vision for emotion. As with vision for action, vision for emotion can proceed without awareness of stimuli (Ladavas et al., 1993a).

Investigations of human observers with intact visual systems also support the existence of high-level information processing that proceeds without conscious awareness. Phenomena such as the attentional blink (Raymond et al., 1992; Shapiro, 2001; Potter, this volume) indicate that directed attention is a necessary condition for conscious report of visual information. Absent such attention, there is no awareness of the information. Nonetheless, some information remains available to the visual system and can produce priming (Shapiro et al., 1997). Although problematic (Duncan, 1985; Merikle & Daneman, 1998), the phenomena of "subliminal perception" and, more generally, "subliminal cognition" (Kihlstrom, 1996) indicate nonconscious information processing. Here, visual input is unavailable to consciousness as indicated by subjective or objective criteria. Nonetheless, it is processed at sufficiently high levels to affect various cognitive and motor processes (Dolan, 2002; Kinoshita & Lupker, 2003; Taylor & McCloskey, 1990).

A phenomenon and experimental paradigm that has been particularly useful in studying nonconscious visual processing is *masked priming*. Typically, such priming consists of a brief presentation of a target or priming stimulus that is followed at short intervals by a mask stimulus that prevents conscious report of the prime. Despite the prime's not being seen, it can nevertheless have effects on the processing of semantic (Kinoshita & Lupker, 2003), emotional (Wong & Root, 2003), and figural (Klotz & Wolff, 1995; Neumann & Klotz, 1994) aspects of a subsequent visual stimulus. *Metacontrast* is a specific type of visual backward masking in which the visibility of one briefly presented stimulus, called the *target*, is suppressed by a spatially contiguous stimulus, called the *mask*, presented shortly after the target. Typically, the suppression of the target's visibility is strongest when the onset of the mask follows that of the target by 30–80 ms. Despite the profound metacontrast suppression of the target's visibility, Neumann and coworkers (Ansorge et al., 1998; Klotz & Wolff, 1995; Neumann & Klotz, 1994) found that the target nonetheless can prime discriminative motor responses to the subsequently presented mask stimulus. Such nonconscious or direct parameter specification of motor responses (Neumann & Klotz, 1994) renders metacontrast, in conjunction with other masking paradigms, as useful tools for investigating the types and levels of conscious and nonconscious information processing in vision of normal human observers.

18.2   Processing of Form and Surface Properties in Object Perception

A visual object is spatially delimited by discontinuities between the reflectance properties of its surface and those of the surround. The resulting visual contours are thus important for image segmentation and the perception of an object's shape or form; and the reflectance properties of the area bounded within the contours give rise to surface attributes such as luminance, color, and texture. Surface as well as form properties are important aspects of spatial perception and object recognition (Cutting & Millard, 1984; Ramachandran, 1988). Differences between the processing of contour and surface or area properties have played key roles in recent as well as past computational theories of vision. Marr (1982), in his description of the full primal sketch, makes the distinction between processes that detect boundaries and processes that specify large-scale surface properties. More recently Grossberg (1994; Cohen & Grossberg, 1984) introduced two distinct computational strategies involved in object recognition, the boundary contour system (BCS) and the feature contour system (FCS). The BCS specifies the locations and orientations of an object's contours whereas the FCS specifies the surface attributes, such as luminance contrast and color, bounded by the contours.

Psychophysical findings also support the distinctions between contour and surface processing. The importance of surface-area processing, as distinct from contour processing, to the perception of area brightness and perceptual filling in has been noted in several past and recent studies (Paradiso & Nakayama, 1991; Pessoa & De Weerd, 2003; Stoper & Mansfield, 1978). As shown by Arrington (1994), in the context of Grossberg's (1994) FAÇADE (*Form-and-color-and-depth*) theory, the FCS is particularly important in modeling of area brightness and filling in.

Distinct boundary and surface processing mechanisms also correlate with neurophysiological findings (Lee et al., 1995). In this connection, Grossberg's (1994) FAÇADE theory associates the FCS and BCS with the cortical parvocellular (P) blob and interblob pathways, respectively. The former stream processes predominantly wavelength or chromatic information, and the latter, mostly form information (DeYoe & Van Essen, 1988; Livingstone & Hubel, 1988), although V1 cells have been found that show concomitant sensitivity to orientation (form) and color (Leventhal et al., 1995). Recent work by Felleman and coworkers demonstrates that within the P thin-stripe regions in cortical area V2, which receive input from the P blob areas of V1, color variations are mapped in distinct spatial areas (Xiao et al., 2003), which in turn are surrounded by areas devoted to the processing of luminance contrast (i.e., luminance increments or decrements relative to a uniform background luminance; Felleman, personal communication). Thus the P thin-stripe pathway, processing both color and luminance contrast, appears to be part of a more inclusive system responsible for processing additional surface attributes such as texture, shading, and so on.

18.3   Differences between Visual Masking of Form and Surface Features

It is well established that different attributes of a target stimulus such as form, contour, contrast, and color are subject to visual masking and that visual masking performance depends on the task required of, and therefore on the criterion content adopted by, a psychophysical observer (Breitmeyer, 1984; Breitmeyer & Öğmen, 2000). Thus, if one requires observers to discriminate between form or contour clarity of the target, one might expect to obtain masking functions (level of target visibility as a function of stimulus onset asynchrony; SOA) that differ from those obtained when observers are asked to respond on the basis of a surface attribute such as luminance contrast (Petry, 1978; Stober et al., 1978).

In recent research (Breitmeyer et al., in press) we have been investigating the changes produced by visual masking in the perception of a target's contour and contrast. Besides metacontrast (described above), we also employed paracontrast masking. Relative to metacontrast, *paracontrast* uses the same target and mask stimuli; however, their temporal order is reversed so that the mask's onset precedes, rather than follows, that of the target. The stimuli used in these studies (figure 18.1a) consisted of a dark, disklike target and a surrounding annular mask presented on a light background. The target and the mask were presented for 10 ms each at SOAs ranging from −750 ms (paracontrast: mask precedes target) to 500 ms (metacontrast: mask follows target). When measuring the effects of para- and metacontrast masking at any given SOA on the perceived contrast of the target, we presented, along with and to the right of the masked target, an unmasked comparison disk whose luminance contrast could be adjusted over successive trials until its apparent contrast matched that of the target. Thus, lower luminance-contrast matches correspond to lower visibility (greater masking) of the target's apparent contrast. When measuring the effects of masking on the perception of contour at a given SOA, the target could consist of a complete disk as shown in figure 18.1a or a disk with a contour truncation at either its top or bottom. Here, using a three-alternative forced-choice procedure, the observer was required to indicate on each trial which of the three possible targets was presented. Lower proportions of correct responses corresponded to lower visibility (greater masking) of the target's contour. For both tasks the target stimulus was always presented to the left of fixation, and over several trials its visibility was measured at one SOA at a time, with random order of SOAs across blocks of trials. This procedure minimized the effects of temporal and spatial uncertainty.

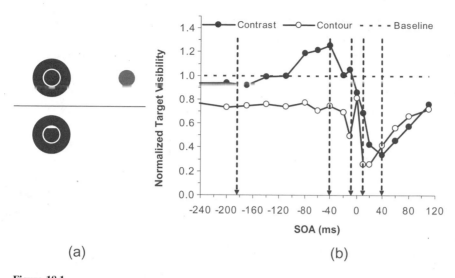

(a)   (b)

Figure 18.1
(*a*) Schematic examples of stimuli used in the contrast matching task (upper panel) and the contour discrimination task (lower panel). In the contrast match task, the left disk, always at a fixed contrast, was the target, which was preceded or followed by the surrounding ring mask at variable stimulus onset asynchronies (SOAs). The contrast of the right disk, which was presented simultaneously with the target, could be adaptively varied until it appeared equal in contrast to that of the masked target. In the contour discrimination task, the target and mask were presented randomly to the left or right of fixation. The target could be a disk with an upper contour deletion as shown, a similar lower contour deletion, or a full disk. (*b*) Normalized target visibilities for contrast matching and contour discrimination tasks as a function of SOA. Lower visibilities indicate stronger masking.

Figure 18.1b shows normalized target visibilities for the two tasks, averaged across three practiced observers. In the figure, we have excluded performances at paracontrast SOAs beyond −240 ms and at metacontrast SOAs beyond 120 ms. Baseline performance (visibility = 1.0) corresponds to the luminance match in the contrast matching task, and the accuracy in the contour discrimination task, for unmasked targets. At the respective longest paracontrast and metacontrast SOAs of −750 ms and 500 ms (not shown in figure 18.1b), where masking is very weak or nonexistent (Breitmeyer, 1984), the normalized target visibility approached 1.0, as expected. More informative are the changes of target-contrast and target-contour visibilities that occurred between the SOAs of −350 and 200 ms. Both tasks tend to yield non-monotonic U-shaped masking functions for paracontrast (when including the more extreme SOA values of −500 and −750 ms) as well as metacontrast. These results are expected, since they have been reported repeatedly in past visual masking studies (Breitmeyer, 1984). With paracontrast masking, both tasks yield a local minimum in the target-visibility function at SOAs between −200 and −150 ms, a large value compared to some prior findings of 30–70 ms (Kolers & Rosner, 1960) but comparable to results reported by others (Cavonius & Reeves, 1983; Scharf & Lefton, 1970). The correlated reductions of contour and contrast visibilities between −200 and −150 ms most likely are related to the well-established finding that performance in contour discrimination and other spatial resolution tasks generally worsens as stimulus contrast is reduced. Although the physical contrast of the target did not vary in our masking studies, reductions of its apparent contrast due to masking thus would be expected to lead also to reductions of contour visibility.

However, as shown in figure 18.1b, this direct coupling of contour and contrast visibilities breaks down at shorter paracontrast SOAs. Note that at an SOA of −40 ms the target's contrast visibility attains a local *maximum* whereas its contour visibility remains low and actually attains a local *minimum* at an SOA of −10 ms. Several aspects of this unexpected dissociation between contrast and contour visibility are important. As observers in this study, the author and the two naive subjects noted that at short paracontrast SOAs, the inside of the disk appeared very dark whereas its contours appeared fuzzy or blurred. Thus, consistent with theoretical and empirical results reviewed above, both the phenomenology and our experimentally measured findings indicate that visual mechanisms processing stimulus contours or boundaries are distinct from those processing the contrast in the area bounded within the contours. Second, consistent with Bachmann's (1994, this volume) repeated findings, the enhancement of area-contrast visibility at short paracontrast SOAs may be related to enhancing effects that a prior stimulus can have on the visibility of a stimulus following closely in time. Our results also indicate that the enhancement is specific to contrast-processing mechanisms, since suppression is produced in the contour-processing mechanisms. The optimal contour suppression found at short paracontrast SOAs and the optimal contrast suppression found at long ones also might explain the discrepancies between the short optimal paracontrast masking SOAs reported by Kolers and Rosner (1960) and the longer ones reported by other investigators (Cavonius & Reeves, 1983; Scharf & Lefton, 1970). It is possible that in Kolers and Rosner's (1960) study reports of target visibility depended largely on high-resolution form information, whereas in the other experiments they depended more on the low-resolution, area-contrast information.

The metacontrast portions of the masking functions illustrated in figure 18.1b show that the minima in the target-contour and target-contrast visibility functions occur at 10 and 40 ms, respectively. This difference again indicates that contour and area-contrast attributes are processed by distinct visual mechanisms, and interestingly, these findings indicate that the processing of surface contrast is slower by 30 ms than that of contour. This time difference approximates recent psychophysical (Caputo, 1998) and neurophysiological (Lamme et al., 1999; Scholte et al., this volume) results showing that processing of area contrast requires several tens of milliseconds longer than processing of contour. These results indicate that form boundaries are processed by fast intra-area (e.g., V1 or V2) activity not requiring feedback from higher areas (Zhou et al., 2000). By contrast, the processing of area or surface properties requires the additional activation of reentrant pathways originating from higher cortical areas (Super et al., 2001). Relative to the feedforward processing of contour, these additional reentrant activations prolong the time required to process the surface attributes. Thus, for optimal suppression of surface attributes such as area contrast, the onset of a metacontrast mask accordingly can be delayed by a longer time interval than that required for optimal suppression of contour attributes.

18.4   Nonconscious Processing of Stimulus Color and Form

The rationale of nonconscious processing studies runs as follows. Any effect a masked target has on the processing of, or response to, subsequently presented stimuli, for example, the mask, must occur at an invisible—hence nonconscious—level of processing. The results of such studies must demonstrate the following two conditions: (1) that the target has had the expected effect on the subsequent stimulus and (2) that the target was invisible. Clear examples of such metacontrast studies were reported by Klotz and coworkers (Ansorge et al., 1998; Klotz & Wolff, 1995). These investigators used outline diamonds and squares as targets and larger outline diamonds and squares as surrounding masks. They found that a target whose form the observers were unable to discriminate could nonetheless prime responses to the form of the after-coming mask. Recently, a similar rationale has been used to study nonconscious priming by color (Ro et al., in preparation; Schmidt, 2002). These studies also demonstrated that a target whose color visibility was suppressed could nonetheless prime discriminative responses to the color of the subsequent mask.

Similar rationales were adopted in the studies discussed below. In all of these studies, initial experiments determined the target–mask SOA at which maximal suppression of a target's attribute, color or form, was most likely to occur. This SOA was subsequently used in all other phases of each study, which included (1) determining the effects of a target attribute on the response to the related attribute of the following mask and (2) determining the visibility of the target's attribute through use of a multi-alternative, forced-choice procedure. Results from the former phase(s) were included in the data analysis only if an observer's target discriminability obtained in the latter phase(s) was statistically at the chance level. Such a level is consistent with the suppression of the visibility of the target attribute, thus forcing an observer to adopt a pure guessing strategy.

18.4.1   Nonconscious Priming by Color

In one set of experiments (Breitmeyer et al., 2004c) all stimuli were centered foveally on a white background of a color video screen. Small disks whose color was either a desaturated blue, a desaturated green, or a white served as target primes, and surrounding rings whose color was either a desaturated blue or a desaturated green served as metacontrast masks[1] (figure 18.2a). We chose white as one of the prime colors, believing that, as a "neutral" color, it would have neutral (equal) priming effects on the subsequently presented blue or green masks. The target and mask durations were 14.3 and 28.7 ms, respectively, and the metacontrast SOA was 43 ms. For each trial the task of the observers was to determine as quickly and accurately as possible, by depressing one of two response buttons, which of the two mask colors was presented. On the basis of the assumption of nonconscious color priming, we expected choice reaction times (RTs) to the mask color to be fastest when the target–mask color pairing was congruent (e.g., blue target, blue mask), slowest when the color pairing was incongruent (e.g., green target, blue mask), and intermediate when a neutral white target prime was used.

In line with prior findings (Ro et al., in preparation; Schmidt, 2002), the results, collapsed over mask colors, supported these expectations: Congruent trials yielded the fastest RTs; incongruent trials, the slowest RTs; and white-prime trials, intermediate RTs.[2] However, when we compared the results obtained with the blue mask to those obtained with the green mask, an unexpected finding was observed for the

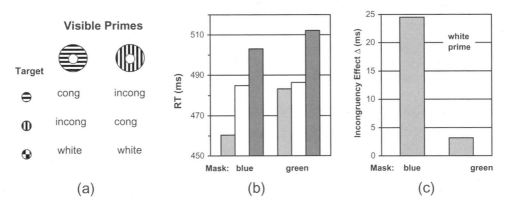

(a)   (b)   (c)

Figure 18.2
(*a*) Schematic representation of the disk primes and annulus masks. Horizontal, vertical, and cross-hatched patterns designate blue, green, and white colors, respectively. Congruent (cong), incongruent (incong), and white prime–annulus pairings are indicated. (*b*) Mean choice reaction times (RTs) to blue and green annuli as a function of congruent-, white-, and incongruent-prime conditions. Results are presented separately for blue and green annuli. (*c*) Incongruency effects (increases in choice RT relative to the congruent condition) produced by the white prime.

white-prime condition. As figure 18.2b shows, the white prime was far from neutral; it tended to act more like a green prime than a blue one in that, relative to the congruent condition, it acted like an incongruent prime for the blue masks by increasing RTs significantly and like a congruent prime for the green mask by not increasing RTs. The significant difference between these "incongruency effects" of the white prime is shown in figure 18.2c.

Subsequently, we wondered if the nonconscious priming effects of the white disk, mimicking those of the green disk, were explainable by the white disk's generating responses at a *percept-dependent* level of processing that were more similar to the corresponding percept-dependent responses generated by the green disk than those generated by the blue disk. To test this hypothesis of percept-dependent similarity, the three disks were presented without a subsequent mask, so as to render them clearly perceivable. After each trial, observers were required to name the color of the disk they perceived. Although observers were correct in their perceptual color naming on a majority of the trials, unexpectedly the proportion of perceptual blue–white confusions (23.3%) was significantly higher than that of green–white confusions (6.45%). Thus, a similarity between white and green primes at the level of a percept-dependent nonconscious processing cannot explain the RT findings.[3] The similarity between white and green primes must lie at another level of processing. We suggest that this level is *stimulus-dependent*—that is, a level of processing where responses are selective for a prime's physical property of wavelength rather than its perceptual attribute of color. Indeed, photometric analyses of the red, green, and blue phosphors excited when the white disk was present revealed that the majority of the luminance energy contributing to the white prime derives from the middle-wavelength green phosphor (68%) whereas a minority derives from the short-wavelength blue phosphor (12%).

18.4.2   Comparison of Nonconscious to Conscious Priming by Color

Following the above line of reasoning, it seems reasonable to expect that consciously perceived primes yield very different results. This follows from the fact that perceived primes, by definition, must activate percept-dependent levels of cortical processing. We tested this expectation by using stimuli very similar to those shown in figure 18.2a but with the following crucial exception. It is well-known that the strength of metacontrast, particularly for stimuli centered at the fovea, decreases significantly as the spatial separation between the outer contour of the target and the inner contour of the surrounding mask increases (Bridgeman & Leff, 1979; Kolers & Rosner, 1960). Hence, one way of rendering the target visible is to increase the target–mask contour separation. Using methods and stimuli very similar to those used in the experiments described above, we compared the priming effects of desaturated blue, desaturated green, and white target disks on choice RTs to desaturated

blue and desaturated green surrounding masks under two target–mask contour sep-
arations, 0 and 3.4 minarc. An optimal target–mask metacontrast SOA of 50 ms was
used throughout. While the former contour separation rendered the target invisible, the latter rendered it visible on all but a few of the trials.

Inspection of figure 18.3a reveals that the expected congruency effects were
obtained. It is clear that under both target-visibility conditions, congruent trials produced the fastest RTs; incongruent trials, the slowest RTs; and white trials, intermediate RTs. Equally evident is the fact that, as in the previous experiments, the
white prime acted more like a green than a blue prime when the target primes were
rendered invisible by the immediately adjoining mask. In contrast, it acted more
like a neutral prime when the target primes were rendered visible by a contour-
separated mask. This latter result suggests that the white disks, being visible, produce
percept-dependent priming effects that are equal for the blue and green masks. If
so, then the perceived similarity of white and green primes should be equal to that
of white and blue primes. To test this hypothesis of percept-dependent similarity,
the observers were required to name, at the end of each trial, the perceived color
of the visible target disk (here also followed by contour-separated masks). Although
observers were correct in their perceptual color naming on a majority (52%) of the
trials, the perceptual blue–white confusions, at 14.8%, did not differ significantly
from the 18.9% of green–white confusions ($p > .07$). This indicates that at the level
of percept-dependent processing, the white prime's similarity to the green prime
equals similarity to the blue prime. Thus, given the same temporal parameters, a
change in the perceptual status of the primes from invisible to visible changed their
nonconscious, stimulus-dependent priming effect to a conscious and, perforce,
percept-dependent one.

18.4.3   Conclusions and Discussion

The above results shown in figures 18.2 and 18.3 indicate that the white prime and,
by extension, the blue and the green ones, when visually suppressed, act at a level
of processing that is stimulus dependent; however, when not suppressed, they act at
a percept-dependent level of processing. Several investigators (Lamme et al., 2000;
Leopold & Logothetis, 1996; Super et al., 2001) have made the distinction between
early stimulus- and later percept-dependent cortical activity. The suppression of the
later response components in V1 of the monkey and in early visual cortex in humans
has been implicated in metacontrast masking (Bridgeman, 1980). Moreover,
Leopold and Logothetis (1996) argued that a majority of neurons in later stages
of cortical processing (e.g., V4), but only a minority of neurons at earlier levels
(e.g., V1), tend to respond in a percept-dependent manner. Thus reentrant activity
originating from higher percept-dependent visual areas could modulate the late
response component of those V1 neurons showing percept dependency (Lamme

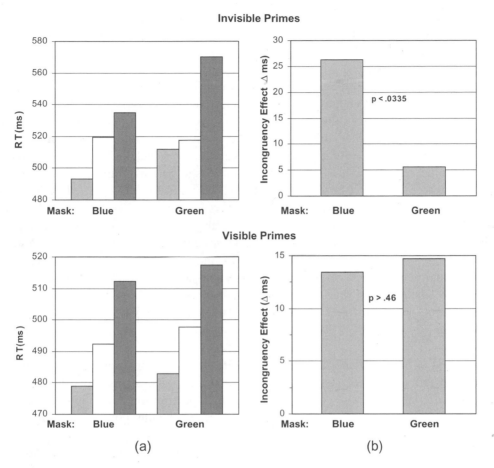

Figure 18.3
(*a*) Mean choice reaction times (RTs) to blue and green annuli as a function of congruent-, white-, and incongruent-prime conditions. Results are presented separately for blue and green annuli. (*b*) Incongruency effects (increases in choice RT relative to the congruent condition) produced by the white prime. Upper panel: invisible prime; lower panel: visible prime.

et al., 2000; Super et al., 2001). Based on these distinctions, the present results suggest that stimulus-dependent color priming occurs at cortical levels as early as area V1, consistent with claims that we are unaware of activity in this visual cortical area (Crick & Koch, 1995).

This interpretation also agrees with Zeki's (1997; Zeki & Marini, 1998) conclusion that the response magnitudes of color-selective cells at early (e.g., V1 and V2) levels of processing vary substantially with the wavelength of a color-constant stimulus whereas those at the V4 level show color constancy by not varying their magnitudes appreciably despite appreciable changes in the wavelength composition of the stimulus. There currently is some uncertainty as to where in humans the homologue of the monkey "color center" is located. While Zeki (1997; Bartels & Zeki, 1999) has argued that the human color center consists of areas V4 and V4α, others (Hadjikhani, 1998; Heywood et al., 2001) have argued that in humans it instead is area V8, located anterior to human area V4. Despite this uncertainty, it is clear from our findings that the nonconscious response priming by colored stimuli can result from visual activation at relatively early, stimulus-dependent levels of processing such as V1 and V2 and that conscious priming by colored stimuli requires activation of later, percept-dependent levels of processing such as V4.

18.4.4 Comparison of Nonconscious Priming by Color and Form

According to Lamme et al. (2000) and Super et al. (2001), the early response component of V1 cells, reflecting afferent feedforward activity, is stimulus dependent, whereas the later response component, reflecting reentrant feedback activity from higher cortical areas, is percept dependent. Since our results point to a stimulus-dependent process responsible for nonconscious color priming, it is reasonable to hypothesize that the early cortical response component is implicated in nonconscious priming by color. By extension, it is reasonable to assume that a similar component is implicated in nonconscious priming by form. These hypotheses were recently investigated by Breitmeyer et al. (2004a).

Recent neurophysiological investigations of visual masking reported by Macknik and Livingstone (1998) indicate that in V1, paracontrast specifically suppresses the early neural response component. Hence, if these early stimulus-dependent responses, as assumed, are involved in nonconscious color and form priming when a prime–metacontrast mask sequence is used, an additional paracontrast mask should reduce the strength of the early response component to the prime and thus also the nonconscious color priming effect. To test these specific hypotheses, we designed experiments whose stimuli and temporal parameters are schematized in figure 18.4. In one experiment we tested the effects of a neutral paracontrast mask on nonconscious color priming, and, in the other, its effects on nonconscious form priming. In the color priming experiments (see figure 18.4, upper panel), we used

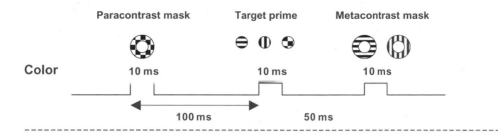

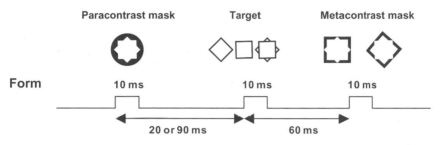

Figure 18.4
Upper panel: Schematic representation of the temporal parameters specifying the presentation sequence of the paracontrast mask, disk target primes, and metacontrast mask used in the color priming experiment. Horizontal, vertical, and crosshatched patterns designate blue, green, and cyan colors, respectively. Lower panel: Schematic representation of the temporal parameters specifying the presentation sequence of the paracontrast mask, targets, and metacontrast masks used in the form priming experiment.

optimal paracontrast and metacontrast SOAs of −100 and 50 ms, respectively, as determined by preliminary experiments. Since there are differences between optimal paracontrast masking of form and surface properties (see figure 18.2 above), in the form priming experiment (see figure 18.4, lower panel) we used an optimal metacontrast SOA of 60 and paracontrast SOAs of either −90 or −20 ms. In all of these experiments, we compared nonconscious priming in the absence of a paracontrast mask (no-para condition) to condition(s) in which a paracontrast mask was used (para condition[s]). Para and no-para trials were run in separate blocks counterbalanced for order across observers. The results for the color priming experiment are shown in figure 18.5. Note in figure 18.5a that a typical priming effect is obtained for both the no-para and para conditions, with congruent trials (e.g., blue prime followed by blue mask) yielding the shortest RTs, incongruent trials (e.g., blue prime followed by green mask) yielding the longest RTs, and neutral trials (e.g., cyan prime followed by blue mask) yielding intermediate RTs. However, equally noticeable is that there is a significant difference between the magnitude of the priming effects obtained for the no-para and para conditions. As expected, the effect is much weaker in the para than in the no-para condition.[4] Figure 18.5b shows

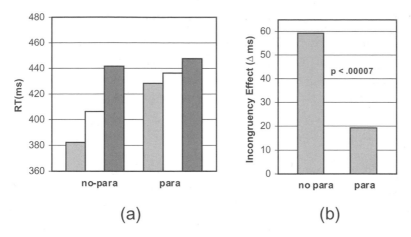

(a)   (b)

Figure 18.5
(*a*) Mean choice reaction times (RTs) to the colors of the metacontrast mask rings for the no-paracontrast (no-para) and paracontrast (para) conditions. Results for the congruent, neutral, and incongruent pairings of disk and mask colors proceed from left to right. (*b*) The results shown separately for the no-para and para conditions in terms of incongruency effects (reaction time differences between the incongruent and the congruent target–mask color pairings).

this difference in terms of the *incongruency effect*, defined as the difference between the congruent and the incongruent priming effects. Since they are suppressed by paracontrast, the stimulus-dependent processes responsible for nonconscious color priming may involve activity as early as the initial response component of V1 wavelength-selective neurons.

A quite different picture emerges when we inspect the results of the nonconscious form priming experiments, shown in figure 18.6. The results, depicted in figure 18.6a, again show the typically reported form priming effects (Ansorge et al., 1998; Klotz & Wolff, 1995), with congruent trials (e.g., diamond prime followed by diamond mask) yielding the shortest RTs, incongruent trials (e.g., square prime followed by diamond mask) yielding the longest RTs, and neutral trials (e.g., star prime followed by diamond mask) yielding intermediate RTs. However, in contrast to the color priming experiment, in this experiment paracontrast did not reduce the predicted priming effects. In fact, as shown in the upper panel of figure 18.6b, the incongruency effects were slightly, but not significantly, larger in the para than in the no-para condition. These trends held for paracontrast SOAs of both −90 and −20 ms (see the upper and lower panels of figure 18.6). Hence, these results indicate that nonconscious form priming is not produced as early as the initial response components of neurons in V1. Instead, they implicate neural activity, either stimulus dependent or percept dependent, occurring at some later level of processing.

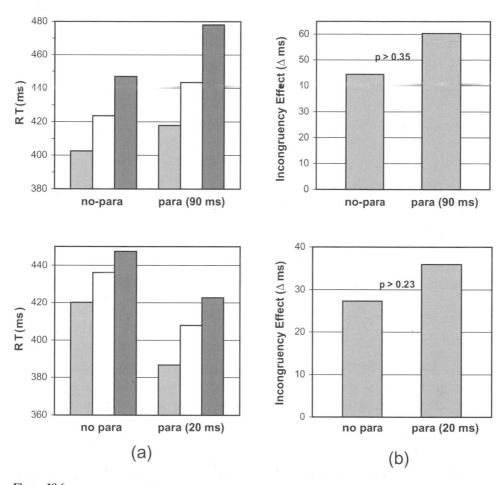

Figure 18.6
(*a*) Choice reaction times (RTs) to the metacontrast mask forms for the no-paracontrast (no-para) and paracontrast (para) conditions. Results for the congruent, neutral, and incongruent pairings of target and mask forms proceed from left to right. (*b*) The results shown separately for the no-para and para conditions in terms of incongruency effects (reaction time differences between the incongruent and the congruent target–mask color pairings). Upper panels show the results for the paracontrast stimulus onset asynchony (SOA) of −90 ms; lower panels for the paracontrast SOA of −20 ms.

18.5   Summary and Discussion

The existence of visual information processing that is not accessible to conscious report has been reported repeatedly in investigations of neurological patients and of normal human observers. What is still in question and thus open to further investigation is to what extent nonconscious and conscious vision are similar or distinct in terms of what information is being processed and of where in the visual system it is being processed. The above findings and analyses shed some light on these questions.

18.5.1   Types and Levels of Information Processing

The two issues, the what and where of information processing, are closely related. For instance, color and motion are processed in separate cortical visual areas (Zeki, 1997), and surface information (e.g., luminance contrast, color) and form or contour information (e.g., orientation) are processed in separate cortical P-thin stripe and P-interstripe pathways, respectively (DeYoe & Van Essen, 1988; Felleman, personal communication; Livingstone & Hubel, 1988; Xiao et al., 2003). Besides these differences *among* cortical area- or pathway-specific types of information processing, our results also indicate that nonconscious and conscious information processing can be hierarchically specific *within* a pathway. For instance, in the chromatic pathway, neural responses correlate progressively less with the physical wavelength composition and more with the perceptual color qualities of a stimulus as one progresses along the geniculocortical color processing hierarchy (Gegenfurter, 2003; Wachtler et al., 2003; Zeki, 1997; Zeki & Marini, 1998). Moreover, the fact that words that are not consciously perceived can produce semantic priming (Kinoshita & Lupker, 2003) suggests that the visually nonconscious form information can be available at relatively high levels of processing. The differences between unconscious semantic priming effects of words like *part* and *trap* appear to involve form-specific levels of word-form processing that are sufficiently sophisticated and informative so as to share properties with the level that allows us to read and thus perceive the words (Dehaene et al., 2001). It is likely, therefore, that the form of words and, by extension, other visual stimuli can be processed nonconsciously at a percept-dependent level.

This inference, in need of further testing, is consistent with the psychophysical results reported above and with results found by Breitmeyer et al. (2005). Their study investigated the effectiveness of parts—that is, vertices/corners and sides of an outlined diamond or square compared to a whole diamond or square—in nonconsciously priming responses to a larger surrounding diamond or square mask. They found that while the form parts produced weaker nonconscious priming than did the whole forms, the vertices or corners, which perceptually group more strongly to resemble the whole forms, in turn acted as stronger nonconscious primes than the sides, whose perceptually grouped resemblance to the whole forms is weaker (Humphreys et al., 1994). Most neurophysiologically plausible models of visual object recognition assume that the earliest cortical form-selective representations of a visual object are in terms of form primitives, namely, line or edge orientation (Marr, 1982; Treisman, 1988). Conjunctions of these form primitives (and other feature primitives like curvature, size, color, and contrast), necessary to construct a representation of the whole form, are assumed to occur at subsequent processing levels (Treisman, 1988). These hierarchical models are consistent with findings showing that extraction of angle features begins no earlier than V2 (Ito & Komatsu, 2004), whereas at later levels, such as V4 and inferotemporal cortex, neural responses are selective for progressively more complex conjunctions of simple features and thus lend themselves to more holistic constructions of a particular form (Pasupathy & Connor, 2002a, 2002b; Tsunoda et al., 2001). Since a majority of neural activity in V4 and inferotemporal cortex tends to be percept dependent rather than stimulus dependent (Leopold & Logothetis, 1996), one would expect the late nonconscious processing of high-level feature conjunctions and whole forms, in turn, to be percept dependent rather than stimulus dependent.

The question arises as to how a percept-dependent processing of form can be nonconscious, if a percept, by our definition, implies awareness or conscious registration of sensory information. One way to think of nonconscious percept-dependent processing is to note that although neural activity at successively higher levels of the ventral object-processing pathway becomes progressively more percept dependent (Leopold & Logothetis, 1996), such activity is insufficient for conscious report (Beck et al., 2001; Dehaene et al., 2001; Lumer et al., 1998). More specifically, one can define nonconscious percept-dependent processing of form in terms of hierarchical cortical activities that represent not only the location and orientation of contours but also their conjunctions forming higher order attributes such as corners, angles, and so forth, and ultimately their entire integrated structure. In effect, the entire form is initially represented as a "skeletal" contour structure, without, as yet, any filling in by a subsequent integration of surface attributes within its boundaries. This implies (1) that the *entire contour outline (form)* of the visual object attain a representation that *in itself is invisible* and (2) that the *filling in of surface attributes (within the contours) is necessary for perceptual awareness* of the object. Not only do the findings of the experiments reported in this chapter point to such a view but so does Grossberg's (1994) FAÇADE theory of vision. In this theory the BCS on its own does not generate visible contrast. Consequently, cortical coding of contour boundaries as such is invisible and becomes visible only when the FCS fills in the surface bounded by the contours (Grossberg, 1994). Applied to the masking results reported in this chapter, an invisible BCS representation of the entire form of a masked prime can improve (impair) object recognition of the subsequently presented form-congruent (form-incongruent) mask.

With regard to color, we have suggested that the wavelength-dependent nonconscious processing found in our color priming studies occurs at the earliest levels of visual cortex. However, an alternative interpretation of low-level chromatic processing relies on the fact that nonconscious chromatic processing occurs not only in normal observers, when the visibility of a stimulus is suppressed by a metacontrast mask, but also in blindsight patients, whose chromatic processing could occur at subcortical sites such as the pulvinar (Breitmeyer & Stoerig, this volume; Stoerig & Cowey, 1992). Since pulvinar activity is precortical, one might expect that the unconscious chromatic processing in blindsight also provides the means of wavelength-dependent chromatic processing in intact observers.

Finally, it is possible that a surface processing system, akin to the FCS proposed by Grossberg (1994), fills in not only color and luminance contrast but also texture contrast and other surface attributes. Since discrimination of the luminance contrast of a surface (Breitmeyer, 1984) as well as of its texture (Caputo, 1998) can be suppressed by metacontrast, the existence of nonconscious priming by surface attributes other than color is readily testable. Investigations of texture attributes would be particularly interesting in view of the recent work on masking with texture-defined patterns (Lamme et al., 2002).

Acknowledgments

Preparation of this chapter was supported by National Science Foundation Grant BCS-0114533 and National Institutes of Health Grant R01-MH49892.

Notes

1. Desaturated blue and green stimuli were used because preliminary studies showed them to be optimal for producing the strongest metacontrast masking, particularly when the target and mask were not the same color.

2. In this and all subsequently described experiments, response error rates were at most 3% for any congruency condition. Hence, speed–accuracy trade-offs cannot explain the RT differences among the congruency conditions.

3. In a separate condition, color-name responses for masked disks were also obtained. Here, the frequency of correct color naming of the disks was nearly at a chance level of 33.3%. Moreover, for the remaining (approximate 66.7%) incorrect color-name responses, the white–blue, white–green, and blue–green confusions each also approached 33.3%, again confirming that the observers could not perceive the masked disks and simply guessed their color.

4. We used two colors for the paracontrast mask, cyan and red. Since cyan, a mixture of blue and green, serves as a neutral color relative to blue and green, a cyan paracontrast mask may have acted as a neutral prime (in addition to the cyan disk) preceding the metacontrast mask. Thus, the attenuation of the priming effects in the para condition shown in figure 18.5 may have been due to the priming effects of the paracontrast mask rather than to its masking effects. For that reason we also used a red paracontrast mask, since, in hue-saturation space, red is 180° out of phase (antipodal) with respect to cyan. The red paracontrast mask also produced a reduction of the nonconscious color priming effect (see figures 5 and 6 in Breitmeyer et al., 2004a). Hence, the paracontrast masks acted as masks rather than merely as primes.

19 The Cognitive Neuroscience of Unconscious and Conscious Vision

Tony Ro

Within the first half second of a stimulus's entry into our visual fields, our cognitive and neural systems are typically able to accurately code, perceive, identify, and even respond to events that occur in the external world. Sometimes, however, such stimuli never enter our conscious awareness (i.e., they are not phenomenally or subjectively experienced) and go completely unnoticed. In many of these cases when visual information eludes our awareness, however, there is ample evidence that this information is nonetheless processed to very sophisticated levels of analyses. Some recent work on the cognitive and neural bases of consciousness (i.e., the subjective awareness) in visual perception has provided some insight into the mechanisms and structures involved with subjective visual experience. This chapter mainly focuses on the neural bases for unconscious and conscious vision as suggested by studies in patients with neuropsychological deficits of visual awareness, as well as studies inducing unawareness of visual information with transcranial magnetic stimulation (TMS). The emphasis is placed on *what* exactly is "seen" with and without awareness, *when* and *where* in the brain unconscious and conscious vision occurs, *why* both unconscious and conscious visual processing occurs, and *how* unconscious and conscious information is processed and represented in the brain.

19.1   What Is Processed With and Without Awareness?

Numerous studies have demonstrated that different types of attributes and properties of visual stimuli are coded and processed without visual awareness. However, the extent of information processing of unconscious stimuli may be very different from that of conscious vision. For example, it may be that unconscious visual information is only coded to certain and perhaps more primitive (i.e., raw and basic) levels of neuronal and cognitive processing and is subject to little or no influence from memory or other higher order cognitive process, such as strategic control. Consistent with this idea, evidence that unconscious visual information is coded only in terms of physical, preconstancy levels, whereas conscious visual information is coded to levels of perceptual constancy, has recently been obtained in several psychophysical and neuropsychological studies. This chapter provides a selective review of some recent studies examining this difference between unconsciously and consciously represented visual information.

Reports in neurologically intact participants (e.g., see Breitmeyer & Öğmen, this volume), as well as neuropsychological studies in patients, converge in demonstrating that shape, wavelength, motion, and sometimes even semantic information can be processed without awareness. In recent studies examining the unconscious perception of colors in neurologically normal participants, Breitmeyer et al. (2004b) showed that individual wavelength (i.e., phosphor composition on a CRT screen) components of colored stimuli, rather than the perceived colors of such stimuli, are processed without awareness. For example, an unconscious light gray stimulus, which was composed mostly of green phosphor, acted more like a green stimulus than a blue one, despite being perceived more as a blue stimulus than a green one in a conscious perceptual report control task. In other studies, my colleagues and I have also shown that form as well as wavelength information is processed without awareness, but that these unconscious form priming effects in neurologically normal subjects also occur at very early levels of visual information processing, prior to the abstract coding of responses based on shape (Ro et al., in preparation). In one of the experiments examining the extent of unconscious form processing, we showed that a stimulus that is mapped to the same response as another physically different shape does not show any evidence of response channel activation without awareness (figure 19.1). In this study, we assessed whether there was an increase in response times for physically different, but response congruent stimuli when the preceding stimulus was unconscious, as assessed after each trial by subjective verbal report. No effects of response congruency were obtained, but an identical stimulus that was unconscious and that, of course, activates the same response as the subsequent mask did show influences in the form of faster response times to the mask. Thus, these results suggest that unconscious visual information is not subject to the same types of processes and influences as is conscious vision and that unconscious information may be coded to relatively primitive levels of visual processing, prior to the assignment of indirect, complex response mappings.

At first, it may seem that these results are inconsistent with some recent studies showing that unconscious stimuli may automatically influence actions (Klotz & Neumann, 1999; Schmidt, 2002; Schwarzbach & Vorberg, this volume; Vorberg et al., 2003), responses to categorical number stimuli with shared response mappings (Naccache et al., 2002), and responses to complex targets with more than one associated response (Mattler, 2003). Furthermore, it has been proposed, based on some of these results, that unconscious representations may directly affect activity

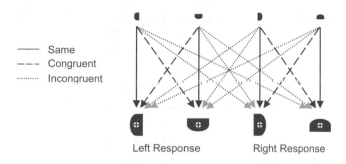

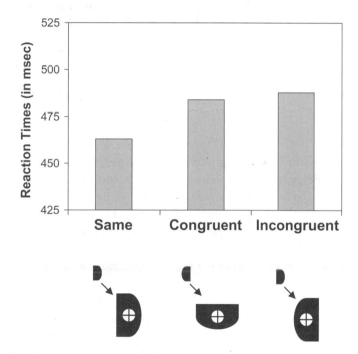

Figure 19.1
The results of an experiment examining whether a physically different, unconscious stimulus that shared a response with a subsequent mask would influence speeded responses to the identity of the mask. Top: Examples of some of the stimuli and response pairings used in this experiment. Bottom: Although unconscious identical stimuli speeded reaction times to subsequent masks, a physically different stimulus that nonetheless shared a response assignment (response congruent conditions) with the masks was noninfluential.

occurring in response-related (Klotz & Neumann, 1999; Schmidt, 2002; Vorberg et al., 2003) and higher mental operation processing (Mattler, 2003) regions of the brain. However, these interpretations are not in contrast to our recent results demonstrating a lack of influences on higher level motor processes, since our experiment used indirect and more complex and arbitrary stimulus–response mappings than have previous studies. In particular, more than one stimulus specified the same response in our studies, which is unlike the studies of Schmidt and Vorberg, Mattler, Schwarzbach, and colleagues, who showed influences of unconscious stimuli on stimulus–response mappings with a direct (one-to-one) mapping or spatial correspondence. The main difference, then, between our recent study and other investigations examining influences of unconscious stimuli on motor specifications is that these other studies always used stimuli that specified only one response and that always primed either the identical or the opposite response stimulus or directly specified the location of the response.

Furthermore, although studies by Naccache, Dehaene, and colleagues (Naccache & Dehaene, 2001; Naccache et al., 2002) have shown that unconscious numbers can influence the processing of different numbers that are assigned to the same response, these effects may have been due to automatic semantic extraction and spreading activation based on low-level processing of the unconscious number. For example, the unconscious processing of the number *4* might speed responses to the number *2* because they semantically belong to the same category as defined by the task: to respond with one hand for numbers less than 5 and the other hand for numbers greater than 5 (see below for a further discussion on the automatic and, as a result, perhaps low-level nature of semantic priming without awareness). Thus, our recent results extend the influential theory that visual processing for motor responses (i.e., directed actions) is separate from that involved in conscious perception (Milner & Goodale, 1995) by showing that these unconscious effects do not influence higher levels of response-related and motor activity.

Neuropsychological examples of visual processing without awareness come from patients with damage to the early areas of the primary visual pathway. Lesions of the primary visual cortex, for example, typically induce cortical blindness on the contralesional side, but patients with such damage may nonetheless be able to discriminate between basic shapes, locations, motion direction, and wavelengths despite being unaware of the visual information, a phenomenon referred to as *blindsight* (for reviews, see Stoerig & Cowey, 1997; Weiskrantz, 1996). In addition to preserved visual processing, patients with blindsight have preserved motor control, such as pointing or making saccadic eye movements to "unseen" targets (Blythe et al., 1987; Perenin & Rossetti, 1996; Poeppel et al., 1973; Weiskrantz et al., 1974). Higher forms of visual perceptual processing, such as that of color perception rather than wavelength discrimination (Stoerig & Cowey, 1989), as well as semantic information, however, have not been conclusively demonstrated in patients with blindsight, further suggesting only raw and physical coding of unconscious visual information up to only preconstancy levels.

Hemispatial neglect is another neuropsychological disorder that has provided insight into what type of visual information is processed without awareness (for reviews, see Driver & Mattingley, 1998; Rafal, 1994, 2000; Vallar, 1998). Neglect patients typically fail to perceive, respond to, and/or act upon events that occur on the side opposite their lesion (i.e., usually the left visual field with right-brain damage). Patients with neglect show striking dissociations between preserved visual information processing and unconsciousness. Unlike patients with blindsight, however, neglect patients seem to have much more extensive processing of visual stimuli in their "neglected" field. To name a few, patients with hemispatial neglect have been shown to have preserved figure–ground organization (Driver et al., 1992), location information of unconscious visual information as assessed through normal coding of geometric visual illusions (Daini et al., 2001; Mattingley et al., 1995; Olk et al., 2001; Ricci et al., 2004; Ro & Rafal, 1996; Vallar et al., 2000), and even preserved semantic priming from unconscious pictures (Berti & Rizzolatti, 1992; McGlinchey-Berroth et al., 1993) and words (Ladavas et al., 1993b).

The studies demonstrating preserved processing of visual illusions in neglect despite unawareness of the inducing features from the affected hemifield, such as when the inducing fins of the Müller–Lyer or Judd illusions are in neglected space (e.g., see Ro & Rafal, 1996), suggest that the unconscious visual information may be processed to stages beyond size constancy, a mechanism proposed to give rise to these illusions. However, because these types of visual illusions may be generated for reasons other than depth and size scaling factors (e.g., by a crude assimilation of features), no firm conclusions can be made with respect to exactly what levels unconscious visual information is processed to based on these types of studies in neglect. In other words, apart from demonstrating that position and feature information is coded without awareness in neglect, these neglect studies with visual illusions cannot determine whether unconscious visual information is processed to levels of, or beyond, size constancy. The finding that visual illusions also frequently affect actions in neurologically normal participants (Franz, 2001; Franz et al., 2000; Pavani et al., 1999; but see Aglioti et al., 1995; Haffenden & Goodale, 2000b; Haffenden et al., 2001) is consistent with the hypothesis that unconscious illusion information in neglected space may reflect a very crude and raw representation of visual information interpretation and suggests that these types of illusions may indeed be perceived by processes such as assimilation rather than depth and size constancy.

Demonstrations of semantic processing without awareness may also simply reflect semantic activations based on very raw and primitive forms of visual information prior to any higher level perceptual influences. Recent behavioral and electrophysiological work using event-related potentials to examine unconscious semantic priming (Kiefer, 2002; Ortells et al., 2003) and the attentional blink (Luck et al., 1996) suggests that these unconscious semantic activations do occur automatically and, in contrast to consciously perceived words, may not be used strategically (Cheesman & Merikle, 1986; Merikle & Joordens, 1997; Merikle et al., 1995; Ortells et al., 2003). Thus, these semantic activations without awareness most likely reflect basic automatic activations of words without any influences from higher order cognitive processes such as strategic control.

In contrast to these studies showing differential forms of unconscious visual information processing, we are typically able to *perceive* almost all visual stimuli consciously, but these conscious visual percepts are usually prone to heavy influences from top-down processes. Thus, although unconscious vision may be based on raw and primitive forms of visual representations, conscious visual perception may typically be derived from postconstancy (e.g., color rather than wavelength) forms of information and therefore may be sometimes even less accurate than unconscious vision. Context effects provide a classic demonstration of this inaccuracy of conscious vision, wherein identical stimuli are perceived as different due to differences in the surrounding stimuli, such as in simultaneous color contrast. Based on such evidence, a distinction can be made between conscious and unconscious vision: It may be that *unconscious vision* simply reflects primarily a bottom-up process operating on only the sensory, low-level, physical aspects of visual information subject to little influence from top-down processing; in contrast, *conscious visual perception* may operate on perceptually derived, high-level aspects of stimuli that are subject to top-down influences (see Goodale et al., this volume, for similar distinctions).

19.2   When Do Unconscious and Conscious Processing Take Place?

Because unconscious vision may rely upon raw and primitive forms of visual representations, one might argue that unconscious vision occurs faster than conscious visual perception. For example, Goodale has suggested that unconscious vision, or vision for action, as assessed through extensive studies on visual agnosic patient D.F. as well as on normal subjects (Goodale et al., this volume; Goodale & Milner, 1992; Milner & Goodale, 1995), is faster and online. In other words, much of vision may be processed unconsciously for producing and guiding actions. Because actions must be directed to visual events that are sometimes transient and abrupt, such as reaching out for a falling book, the proposal that unconscious perception for action occurs online and is relatively fast in comparison with conscious vision makes much sense

(Goodale et al., this volume; Hu & Goodale, 2000). Conversely, conscious vision may be slower than unconscious vision because the processing time required to generate awareness and postconstancy percepts very likely is greater than that required to code the basic primitive features of visual information.

Some more direct evidence that suggests that conscious percepts require longer intervals of time to generate as compared to unconscious vision has been provided by studies examining V1 cells of monkeys (Lamme & Roelfsema, 2000; Super et al., 2001). These neurophysiological studies suggest that activity lasting hundreds of milliseconds beyond the first responses to a visual stimulus may be involved with the coding for consciousness via feedback projections from higher visual areas. In a recent study, my colleagues and I have also demonstrated, using TMS, that feedback, reiterative activity is likely to play a large role in the strengthening of percepts for visual awareness.

By way of background, TMS is a noninvasive technique used for investigating brain function that entails transiently disrupting normal neural activity by administering a TMS pulse. A stimulating coil is held over the scalp, and a brief electrical current is passed through the stimulating coil. The magnetic field that is generated around the coil induces current in the brain (for reviews on TMS, see Hallett, 2000; Jahanshahi & Rothwell, 2000; Pascual-Leone et al., 2000; Robertson et al., 2003; Walsh & Cowey, 2000). Unlike other recent functional neuroimaging techniques (e.g., positron emission tomography, functional magnetic resonance imaging), which typically measure blood flow to determine whether activity in a given brain region is correlated with a given brain function, TMS is a technique that, like the lesion method, allows us to determine whether a given brain region is necessary for a given brain function. Thus, TMS affords a causal rather than correlative method of investigating brain function with very transient and focal brain disruption, without concerns regarding plasticity and reorganization of brain function typical in patient lesion studies.

In addition, the extent and, more important for the purposes of investigating visual processes within the first half second, the timing of the neural disruption can be controlled by different configurations of stimulating coils. Thus, when appropriately time-locked visual events occur with respect to a TMS pulse, visual suppression can be induced. The most commonly used coil for inducing visual suppression with TMS is the 9-cm circular coil, as many studies have failed to induce consistent and reliable suppression with more focal coils (e.g., see Kastner et al., 1998). When the base of the coil, at the junction between the handle and the coil itself, is placed approximately 2 cm above the inion, visual perception can be suppressed (i.e., a scotoma induced) for brief intervals when the TMS is appropriately time locked to visual events (figure 19.2; for more details, see Amassian et al., 1989; Corthout et al., 2000; Kammer, 1999; Kastner et al., 1998). The placement and movement of the

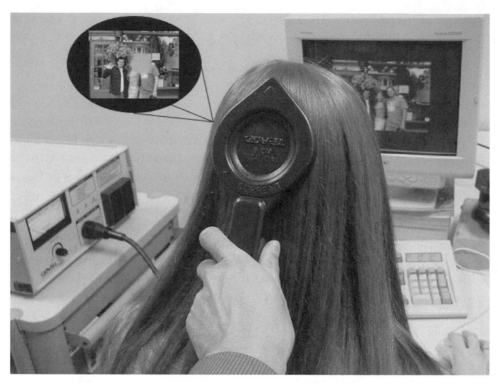

Figure 19.2
A typical setup for a transcranial magnetic stimulation experiment examining visual cortical function. A stimulating coil is held approximately 2 cm above the inion, and a pulse is delivered between approximately 60 and 120 ms after a visual stimulus is presented.

coil can systematically alter the location of the TMS-induced scotoma. For example, by slightly displacing the stimulating coil in different directions or, analogously, changing one's fixation with respect to a visual stimulus while maintaining the coil positioning, very systematic spatiotopic mappings of visual cortex can be revealed (figure 19.3). Using a single pulse, the disruption of neural tissue can last anywhere from tens of milliseconds to hundreds of milliseconds, depending on the location and intensity of the TMS pulse, thereby allowing for a distinction in the types of information processed without awareness.

Using TMS, we employed a metacontrast masking paradigm to evaluate the role of early human visual cortex in the occipital lobes in visual awareness (Ro et al., 2003). Our study had two main goals: to determine whether TMS-induced suppression of the metacontrast mask would induce recovery of the otherwise imperceptible preceding target disk and also to determine whether the preceding target disk had *later* influences on the perceptibility of the mask. To assess the latter, only half

Stimulus

Perception

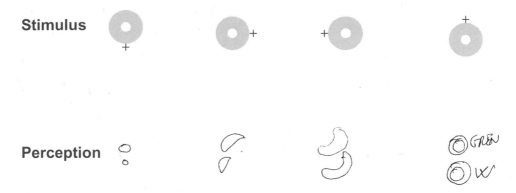

Figure 19.3
Insights into the nature of the transcranial magnetic stimulation (TMS) induced scotoma. These illustrations are from one neurologically normal observer viewing the annulus (top half) at different locations with respect to fixation. Each stimulus was presented approximately 80 ms before a TMS pulse. Note the systematic and foveally restricted extent of the induced scotoma, as well as the reproducibility across the two trials (each drawing in the bottom half), that alters the perception of the annulus as represented by the drawings from this observe. For the stimulus presented below the fixation, no effects on visibility of this stimulus were induced, but there was a reported change in color perception.

of the trials had a target disk, and comparisons of the magnitude of conscious mask perception were made between the disk-present versus disk-absent trials. TMS suppression of the disk and mask was assessed by having subjects verbally report after each trial first whether the target disk was perceived and then whether the annulus mask was perceived. Prior to the main experiment, the optimal location and intensity for inducing visual suppression was localized in each participant.

The data in figure 19.4 (top panel) illustrate that when TMS induced suppression of the annulus mask, disk recovery had occurred. That is, when the mask was suppressed from neuronal processing in occipital cortex, as a consequence of the induced current into visual cortex at the time of mask arrival via TMS, the otherwise imperceptible disk was now visible. This result parallels other findings demonstrating TMS's unmasking of visual stimuli when TMS interferes with the visual processing of patterned masks (Amassian et al., 1993). Unexpectedly, there was a reasonably high false-alarm rate in our study (see figure 19.4, top panel). Specifically, subjects frequently reported seeing a disk when in fact no disk was presented. This effect may have been due to frequent perceptions of TMS-induced phosphenes or partial, incomplete suppression of the mask that was then subsequently confused as being the disk.

More important, however, the results showed that there was a larger TMS suppression of the annulus mask when a disk preceded it in comparison to the no-disk trials (see figure 19.4, bottom panel). This result is particularly striking because it shows that a stimulus that was presented *prior* to the annulus, in conjunction with

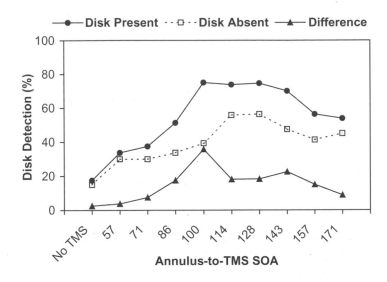

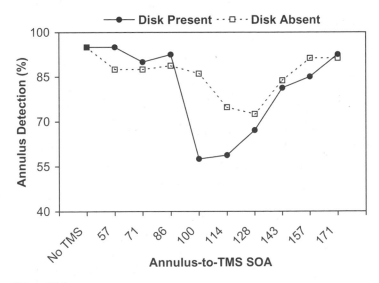

Figure 19.4
Data from a transcranial magnetic stimulation (TMS) study examining reiterative processing for conscious vision in occipital cortex. A metacontrast masking paradigm was used in conjunction with TMS to determine whether a previously presented stimulus could affect later processing and whether an otherwise imperceptible prior stimulus would be recovered by TMS suppression of the mask. Top: The percentage of disks (masked stimulus) reported to be seen by the participants as a function of the mask-to-TMS stimulus onset asynchrony (SOA; in milliseconds). Note the increase in disk report data at the same SOAs as when the mask was suppressed by the TMS. Bottom: The percentage of annuli (masks) seen as a function of the mask-to-TMS SOA. Note the larger magnitude of visual suppression of the mask when a preceding stimulus was presented.

a TMS pulse, affected the visibility of the later appearing annulus. There are two ways in which this result could be interpreted. Since the single-pulse occipital TMS that was administered was always restricted over a very specific region of visual cortex (i.e., the foveal representation of primary visual cortex), it might be that the disk was still being processed in visual cortex when the mask was later presented and that this ongoing processing of the disk further impaired perception of the mask with TMS suppression. This result seems unlikely, however, because this should have led to suppression of the visibility of the disk, which we did not observe (see figure 19.4, top panel). Alternatively and more likely, these results suggest that the disk was being reiteratively fed back into V1 to strengthen its percept for subsequent awareness. The disk recovery results with TMS suppression of the mask are consistent with this alternative interpretation and suggest that more lengthy feedback processing is required for generating conscious percepts of visual events. In other words, these TMS and metacontrast masking results suggest that conscious perception requires reiterative processing that is likely to take much longer than perhaps the more direct unconscious visual processes. This lengthier processing time via these feedback–reiterative loops may be a necessary and sufficient component for the strengthening and forcing of the neuronal representations of visual information into subjective awareness.

Other and much more indirect evidence suggesting faster unconscious vision is derived from the simple and repeated observations that reflexive saccades to visual events are typically made faster than voluntarily generated saccades to visual targets (e.g., see Henik et al., 1994; Ro et al., 1997). It has been suggested, based on these types of observations, that in humans, reflexive saccades are more directly mediated via an oculomotor reflex from the retina directly to the superior colliculus, which itself can generate an eye movement command (Bruce & Goldberg, 1985). Many of these reflexive types of eye movements may be generated without awareness, as recent studies demonstrating oculomotor capture without awareness have shown (Ladavas et al., 1997; Theeuwes et al., 1998). Voluntary saccades, on the other hand, involve cortical circuitry that likely involves longer processing times and, by definition, are conscious and volitional. Consistent with these eye movement differences, patients with blindsight can frequently generate reflexive saccades to peripheral events (see above) and demonstrate saccade inhibition from unconscious distractors that are presented in the blind hemifield (see the next section). Thus, the timing of differentially generated types of saccades may provide some further evidence that unconscious forms of vision may rely upon faster and more direct visual processing pathways.

19.3   Where Do Unconscious Vision and Conscious Visual Perception Occur?

As suggested by the findings of preserved saccades to "unseen" targets in blindsight, one hypothesis of the neural substrate for unconscious vision claims that unconscious visual processing in blindsight occurs due to spared visual input directly into the superior colliculus via extrageniculate retinal projections. Evolutionarily speaking, this makes sense, since this retinotectal pathway has been superseded by the primary visual pathway, which projects from the retina through the thalamus on up to primary visual cortex in the occipital lobes. Thus, the more primitive visual pathway via the superior colliculus may still be coding visual information, albeit unconsciously. Note, however, that this may not be the only source of an unconscious visual processing pathway, as direct projections from the occipital cortex to the dorsal stream may also be involved with unconscious vision or vision for action (Goodale et al., this volume; Goodale & Milner, 1992; Milner & Goodale, 1995). The superior colliculus also sends projections, albeit through the pulvinar, to the extrastriate cortex, in particular the dorsal stream (Kaas & Huerta, 1988; Robinson & McClurkin, 1989).

There is ample evidence for retinotectal contributions to unconscious vision in blindsight derived from investigations demonstrating superior colliculus involvement. For example, Rafal and his colleagues showed that patients with a visual cortex lesion resulting in a hemianopsia were affected under monocular viewing conditions by distractor stimuli in the blind fields when making saccadic eye movements to targets in the good hemifield, but not when making manual key-press responses under identical conditions (Rafal et al., 1990). Furthermore, they showed that the distractors influenced performance more when presented into the temporal visual hemifield, which has more direct projections into the superior colliculus than the nasal hemifield, of the cortically blind patients (but see Williams et al., 1995). In another study, Dodds and colleagues (Dodds et al., 2002) showed that a patient with cortical blindness on one side had a higher proportion of correct guesses of the location of visual targets (i.e., more blindsight) when the target stimuli to be discriminated were projected to the temporal hemifield under monocular viewing conditions, further implicating a role of the superior colliculus in blindsight.

More recently, however, Walker and his colleagues have failed to replicate these results suggesting collicular involvement in blindsight (Walker et al., 2000). In a larger group of patients, this saccade distractor effect reported by Rafal and colleagues was not apparent in the nasal or temporal hemifields of their patients, although it was measured in normal subjects. The source of this discrepancy between the two is unclear and may be due to some of the patients' not showing blindsight. Furthermore, the slight nasal versus temporal hemifield asymmetry that was measured in normal subjects by Walker et al. could have been due to asymmetric projections through the retinogeniculostriate pathway (Williams et al., 1995).

To further investigate unconscious visual processing in blindsight, and in particular whether there is retinotectal involvement in this form of unconscious vision, we used single-pulse TMS to induce transient and reversible scotomas in otherwise neurologically normal individuals (Ro et al., 2004). By placing the stimulating coil over the posterior occipital regions of the scalp and skull, as in our studies examining feedback processing for conscious vision (see figures 19.2 and 19.4), and time locking the TMS to the presentation of transient, centrally presented visual distractors, we assessed whether unconscious distractors might differentially influence performance on different types of tasks. In particular, we produced visual suppression of central distractors while subjects made either saccadic eye movements or manual button press responses to peripherally presented targets. Of most interest were the response latencies to peripheral targets when subjects were completely unaware, due to the TMS-induced scotoma, of the centrally presented distractor as assessed by subjective report after each trial.

Figure 19.5 (top panel) illustrates the mean latencies from the saccade task, whereas figure 19.5 (bottom panel) shows the mean response latencies from the manual button-press task. The main and most important result obtained in this study is that even though subjects were unaware of the distractors due to the TMS, and thus the distractor-present trials were phenomenally identical to the distractor-absent trials when TMS was delivered, subjects were nonetheless delayed in making saccades to peripheral targets when an unconscious distractor was presented. In contrast to these results obtained with the saccadic eye movement task, the manual RTs showed a very different pattern of results (see figure 19.5, bottom panel). Notably, when subjects were unaware of the foveal distractors due to the TMS-induced scotoma under these conditions, there was no influence of these unconscious distractors on the manual button-press responses made to the peripheral targets. This difference between the saccade and manual tasks was apparent in the paired comparisons, as well as the significant two-way interaction for the manual, but not the saccade task, and the three-way Task (saccade vs. manual) × Awareness (aware/no TMS vs. unaware/TMS) × Distractor (present vs. absent) interaction. This result suggests that the effects of the TMS on visual cortex are effective in producing a complete and transient lesion of it and, as a result, allow for an examination of extrageniculate visual function without any awareness. Furthermore, they suggest in contrast to visual suppression by metacontrast masking, which produces priming time courses that are almost identical for saccadic latencies as for two-choice manual and vocal responses (Schwarzbach & Vorberg, this volume; Vorberg et al., 2004), inducing visual suppression with TMS is not the same as inducing visual suppression with masks, as we have argued elsewhere (Breitmeyer et al., 2004b).

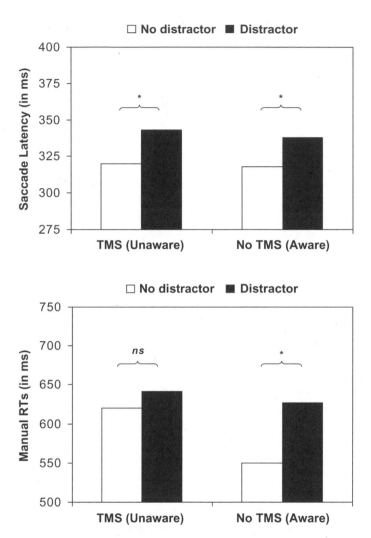

Figure 19.5
Data from a transcranial magnetic stimulation (TMS) experiment inducing blindsight in normal observers. Subjects were significantly slower to make saccades when a visual distractor was presented, regardless of whether or not subjects were aware of the distractor (top). However, when responses were indirect manual responses, the unconscious distractor had no influences on target responses (bottom). *p < .02; *ns*, not significant.

Thus, the preponderance of evidence, apart from a few exceptions (also see Fendrich et al., 1992) suggests that the more primitive retinotectal visual pathway, along with its projections to the dorsal visual stream (Goodale et al., this volume; Goodale & Milner, 1992; Milner & Goodale, 1995), may be heavily involved with unconscious vision. Contrary to frequent assumptions that it is a vestigial system, the pathway from the retina to the superior colliculus may therefore be important in guiding many of our automatic behaviors without awareness. The existence of this pathway, with its deprived access to color and complex form information, may also explain why the types of visual information that are processed unconsciously are raw, primitive, and physically based, subject to little influence from higher forms of perception. Furthermore, as described above, this pathway may process information much faster than the visual pathways, structures, and processes involved with conscious vision. Based on these and similar types of results, figure 19.6 (top panel) illustrates the projection pathways from the retina to the superior colliculus and the dorsal stream that are likely to be directly involved with unconscious vision.

By process of elimination and also via studies in visual agnosics, conscious vision, therefore, likely involves projections from the retina through the primary visual cortex to the ventral stream (Farah, 1990; Goodale et al., this volume; Goodale & Milner, 1992; Milner & Goodale, 1995). Further evidence for the neural basis of conscious perception may be gleaned from patients with hemispatial neglect. The areas typically damaged in neglect are the superior temporal gyrus (Karnath et al., 2001) and/or inferior parietal lobule (Mort et al., 2003; Vallar, 1993). Demonstrations of object-based neglect suggest that these brain regions may be involved with the final output stages of the ventral visual stream into consciousness. Based on our work, as well as that of others (Lamme & Roelfsema, 2000), which suggests that conscious visual processes involve feedback loops and longer processing times, figure 19.6 (bottom panel) depicts the likely processing mechanisms involved with conscious vision. As no studies have demonstrated loss of visual awareness after damage beyond the superior temporal gyrus and inferior parietal lobule, this may be one of the final stages of conscious visual processing.

19.4 Why Is There Unconscious Visual Information Processing?

In terms of the magnitude and extent of the visual information that we are typically confronted with at any given instance, it makes sense that the visual system, through top-down, feedback control, economizes and selectively chooses which limited information enters our awareness. If such were not the case, it is easy to see how we would instantaneously run into a situation of information overload. However, the repeated demonstrations of unconscious vision suggest that our capacity to

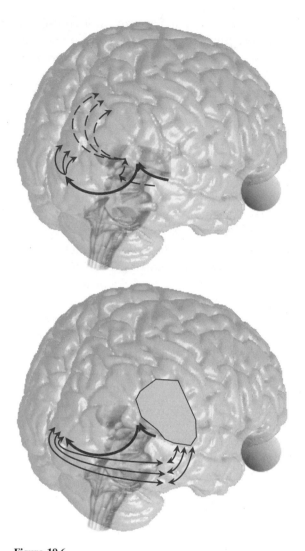

Figure 19.6
The neural pathways mediating unconscious (top panel) and conscious (bottom panel) vision in humans.
Note the extrageniculate/retinotectal projections from the retina that contribute to unconscious vision
in the top panel. The shaded, outlined region in the bottom panel depicts the areas (i.e., STG/IPL) that,
when damaged, typically produce hemispatial neglect (Karnath et al., 2001; Mort et al., 2003; Vallar, 1993).
Also note the feedback projections for conscious, but not unconscious vision. Solid lines represent
primary visual pathway projections; dashed lines represent secondary, extrageniculate projections.

"see" may be much larger than typically conceived and has yet to be estimated or quantified. It therefore seems that conscious vision may serve very different purposes than might be expected based on typical accounts of information overload and limited capacity for the processing of visual information.

If it is true that conscious vision takes longer than unconscious vision, as our TMS study demonstrating feedback processing has suggested, it may be that conscious vision may be more veridical than unconscious vision due to the extra processing time involved with conscious vision. This, of course, assumes that the amount of information processed per unit of time is equal between these two forms of vision and that the amount of information extracted is greater with longer processing times. However, plenty of studies have demonstrated that unconscious vision may be more accurate, being subject to lesser influence from top-down processes under some circumstances. For example, experiments using visual illusions have shown little to no processing of the illusions in vision for action, which is suggested to be unconscious under Milner and Goodale's framework (Aglioti et al., 1995; Gentilucci et al., 1996; Haffenden & Goodale, 2000b; but see Franz, 2001; Franz et al., 2000; Pavani et al., 1999). In contrast, vision for (conscious) perception does show the effects of these visual illusions, suggesting that conscious vision may frequently be less veridical than unconscious vision (but see studies on neglect briefly reviewed above, which show preserved illusory processing without awareness). Thus, veridicality also does not seem to provide a sufficient or at least a very straightforward answer to the question of why these different types of vision exist.

The temporal dynamics of unconscious and conscious vision suggest that faster (unconscious) vision may be utilized for information and behaviors that are coded extremely efficiently and more or less automatically (e.g., reflexively as in the case of dodging oncoming objects or efficiently triggered saccadic eye movements via the superior colliculus in response to abrupt visual onsets). In contrast, conscious vision may be used for slower, purposive interactions, such as when we want to pay attention to something, or when learning new forms of behavior, such as when driving for the first time. Future work along similar lines as reviewed here may be informative regarding the reasons why we have two very different forms of vision.

19.5   Conclusions: How Is Unconscious and Conscious Visual Information Processed?

To summarize and conclude, unconscious versus conscious vision appears to be processed in different ways and under different temporal dynamics. Unconscious vision may reflect fast and direct, bottom-up neuronal processing streams that may nonetheless guide (primarily motor) behavior (cf. Goodale et al., this volume;

Goodale & Milner, 1992; Milner & Goodale, 1995). Consistent with the notion of direct, bottom-up processing in unconscious vision, several studies have shown that unconscious visual information is only primitively and coarsely represented. Conversely, conscious vision may reflect slower and indirect, top-down influences via feedback–reiterative projections that give rise to our visual perceptions. These slower, more contemplative forms of visual processing are likely to be limited, at least in comparison to unconscious vision, with respect to the amount of information that can be processed (i.e., we can only be aware of one object or visual event at a given time). However, conscious vision is often incorrect, as in cases of the perception of visual illusions or similarities in perceived colors despite changes in physical wavelength, which is typically not the case with unconscious vision. Thus, conscious vision, being slower and frequently clumsier, may have limited utility for most intents and purposes; we may be visually aware simply because we have the capacity for it and because it supports our ability to learn and engage in purposive behavior.

20 Epilogue

As highlighted in the introductory chapter, vision is, by definition, a highly dynamic process. The objective of this book has been to probe in detail the dynamic aspects of conscious and unconscious visual processing. A survey of the chapters indicates convergence and maturity at the methodological level. Several well-developed and well-studied paradigms, such as masking, priming, and rapid serial visual presentation, form the core of experimental approaches. Although the exact mechanisms whereby these stimulus paradigms control the time course and conscious registration of stimuli are not known, existing theories and models that are applicable to these paradigms provide a framework for interpreting the experimental findings. Furthermore, comparative investigations that combine traditional methods with newer techniques, such as functional magnetic resonance imaging and transcranial magnetic stimulation, will provide—as some studies already have (e.g., Beck et al., 2001; Dehaene et al., 2001; Ro et al., 2004)—a more integrative view of the spatial and temporal dynamics of visual information processing.

An emergent theme of the book is that substantial processing of stimuli at unconscious levels takes place in the visual system. Furthermore, these unconscious processes can selectively modulate behavioral responses as well as conscious registration of stimuli. Such a convergence of opinion, however, does not extend to all levels of processing among investigators. For example, Dehaene et al. (2001) argued that high-level information of masked words, such as their case-independent representations, is processed unconsciously, whereas Kouider and Dupoux (2004) would challenge such conclusions, arguing instead that in many cases "unconscious" effects of masked words can be explained by partial visibility of their individual letters or their fragments.

While converging on the general principle of unconscious processing in the visual system, the topics covered in the chapters also raise several interrelated questions and opposing views on the dynamical aspects and neural correlates of conscious versus unconscious processes. Among these questions that need to be investigated further are the following:

• Are there qualitative differences between neural processes correlated with conscious and unconscious vision, or is the difference merely a quantitative one? Similar to Moutoussis and Zeki (2002), Rolls (this volume) argues that the transition from unconscious to conscious vision is one of attaining neural-activation thresholds in stimulus-specific areas of the brain such as inferotemporal cortex rather than requiring activation of additional (different) cortical areas. In contrast, the view expressed by Crick and Koch (1998), supported by the results of several investigations (Beck et al., 2001; Dehaene et al., 2001; Grosbas & Paus, 2003; Lumer et al., 1998), indicate that in addition to stronger activation in stimulus-specific areas, activation of other areas such as frontal and parietal cortex is required.

• Is conscious perception related to distributed processing in the visual system, or does it emerge from specific modular substrates? Zeki (1997, 1998) has argued for a form of distributed processing in which, however, each attribute-specific perceptual processing system (module) can act autonomously as a "microconsciousness" module. On the other hand, Dehaene and Naccache (2001) have proposed the existence of a global neuronal work space in which consciousness results from the collective modular activities mobilized into this dynamically integrative work space.

• A closely related question is this one: Is there a unity in conscious perception? If yes, what are the neural mechanisms that provide such a unity? Do neuronal oscillations or their synchronization play a role in providing such a unity? And how do consciousness as state and consciousness as trait contribute to such unity? A possible answer is provided by a theory recently proposed by John (2003). Here consciousness results from momentarily stable, but dynamically changing, neural-field coherences resulting from the convergence of exogenous stimulus-specific and endogenous memory-specific cortical network activities producing fragmentary sensations that are bound by cortico-thalamic-cortical reverberations into a unified percept. Insofar as consciousness as state is tied especially to thalamic activity (see Breitmeyer & Stoerig, this volume) and consciousness as trait to attribute-specific cortical areas, John's (2003) theory provides a useful working model for the unity of consciousness and its dynamically changing flow.

• Is feedback (reentrant) processing necessary for conscious registration? Here Rolls (this volume) presents empirically grounded arguments against the presence of, and hence the need for, top-down reentrant activation of lower cortical areas. In contrast, the theory of object-substitution masking proposed by Enns et al. (this volume), as well as the work of others (Edelman, 1997; Edelman & Tononi, 2000; Pascual-Leone & Walsh, 2001; Zeki, 1993), indicates the need and special role of such activation for conscious perception.

• How can studies comparing normal to clinical subjects inform us about conscious and unconscious processing and their temporal dynamics? Vogeley et al. (1999) have suggested that the prefrontal cortical area is especially important for the development of the human self model (self-consciousness) and that deficits in this area contribute especially to the cognitive and ideational distortions of self characteristic of schizophrenics. These and related neural-network abnormalities in schizophrenics (Selemon et al., 1998; Thompson et al., 2001) may correlate with the deficits in early visual processing in schizophrenics reported by Wynn and Green (this volume). Clinical syndromes found in other psychiatric, neurological, or ophthalmological abnormalities also may shed light on the temporal dynamics of normal conscious and unconscious vision. For instance, the abnormally high intraocular pressures found in glaucoma patients may result in a decrease and slowdown of activity specific to the M pathway, thus upsetting the normal temporal interactions between P- and M-pathway activities.

• Do "early" and "late" cortical response levels correlate with unconscious stimulus-dependent and conscious percept-dependent processes? Is the emergence of perceptual consciousness a gradual or all-or-none process? Regarding the latter question, the microgenetic view outlined by Bachmann (this volume) is sympathetic to a gradual temporal evolution of conscious experience. In contrast, Dehaene et al. (2003) and Sergent and Dehaene (2004) have presented evidence favoring all-or-none transitions from unconscious processing to conscious perception. Such saltatory phase changes in neural activity may be accommodated by a microgenetic approach if here, as in phylogenesis, one accepts the existence of "punctuated equilibria."

• What is the relationship between neural response timing and the timing of conscious perception? The latter question has been of particular interest in a series of investigations conducted by Libet and coworkers (Libet, 1985, 2002, 2004). Although their claim that much of sensory, cognitive, and motor processing is done at unconscious levels is generally accepted, their interesting but controversial interpretations of findings regarding the relationship between neural timing and timing in consciousness, particularly with regard to subjective backward referral of conscious experiences to prior neural correlates, increasingly face criticism based on alternative accounts (Breitmeyer, 2002; Pockett, 2002, 2004; Pollen, 2004). For that reason, the relationship of neural timing to timing of conscious experiences remains an important but unsettled issue.

Besides these open issues, several others have to be addressed in future research. The chapters in this volume constitute a sampler of topics relevant to the understanding of temporal dynamics of conscious and unconscious vision. Some relevant topics may not have been covered adequately. For instance, under natural viewing conditions, our eyes move constantly, sampling different points of interest in the visual scene. The emphasis of this book has been "the first half second"—that is, the microgenesis of those "samples." A broader question of interest is to understand how these samples give rise to an integrated temporal stream that underlies our phenomenal experience during visual exploratory behavior. We believe that another workshop and book focusing on topics including free viewing, eye movements, scan patterns, attentional tracking, and natural scene perception can build upon the foundations laid by the present book and provide a more complete view of visual dynamics.

Finally, we hope that this volume and the above questions also raise some interesting issues and stimulate new avenues for thought among the interested philosophers of mind. Neurophilosophy is a burgeoning field, rife with problematic issues regarding, among other topics, the existence of unconscious processing, distinct types of consciousness (Block, 1995, 1996; Rosenthal, 2002), and temporal aspects of conscious experience (Libet, 1985, 2002, 2004; Dennett, 1990; Dennett & Kinsbourne, 1992).

Glossary

action potential   Sudden spike in electrical activity that travels down an axon and serves as the output of a neuron.

attentional blink   When two targets are presented in rapid temporal succession, the identification of the second target can be impaired when it follows the first target within an interval of about 500 ms. The term attentional blink refers to this temporary period of "attentional blindness."

backward masking   Masking in which a mask stimulus follows a target stimulus (see also *masking, forward masking, masking function, metacontrast, paracontrast*).

blindsight   A neurological deficit caused by destruction of early visual cortex (V1) in which patients deny seeing a visual object yet, under forced-choice response procedures, can detect its presence, location, motion direction, and rudimentary aspects of its wavelength composition and shape.

BOLD   Blood oxygen level dependent signal that is measured in fMRI experiments.

dissociation/double dissociation   Dissociation refers to a selective loss or impairment of a perceptual or cognitive function while other functions remain intact. Double dissociation between two functions occurs when two conditions exist where one condition leads to the impairment of one function but not the other and vice versa.

dorsal pathway (stream)   Pathway emerging from the primary visual cortex and projecting to the posterior parietal cortex. Alternative functional roles attributed to the dorsal pathway include visual localization of objects ("where") and "vision for action" (see also *ventral pathway*).

electroencephalogram/EEG   Overall pattern of electrical activity recorded on the surface of the cortex or the surface of the scalp.

event-related magnetic field/ERMF   Magnetic field fluctuations that accompany event-related potentials.

event-related potential/ERP   Electrical potential elicited by a stimulus, a response, or some other event, usually recorded from the surface of the scalp.

feedback   Injection of the output of a processing system back to its input.

fMRI   Functional magnetic resonance imaging, a technique for precisely localizing changes in brain activity based on differences in the magnetic properties of oxygenated and deoxygenated hemoglobin.

form/surface attributes   Perceptual aspects of an object that are determined by its boundaries or contours (e.g., orientation, curvature) and by the reflectance properties of areas enclosed by its boundaries (e.g., color, luminance, texture).

forward masking   Masking in which a mask stimulus precedes a target stimulus (see also *masking, backward masking, masking function, metacontrast, paracontrast*).

hemifield neglect   The reduction or failure of responding to or awareness of objects in the behavioral field contralateral to damage affecting the right or left parietal cortices. The more typical or severe form is left neglect produced by damage to the right parietal cortex.

inferotemporal (IT) cortex   The "endpoint" of the ventral pathway. It is believed to be involved in complex object recognition (see also *ventral pathway*).

koniocellular (K) pathway   A third retino-geniculo-cortical pathway in the primate visual system. Neurophysiological and functional properties of this pathway are not as well-known as those of M and P pathways (see also *magnocellular pathway, parvocellular pathway*).

lateralized readiness potential (LRP)   A difference between cortical EEG potentials recorded over the motor cortices of the left and right cerebral hemispheres shortly prior to execution of a motor response.

local field potential   Graded change in electrical potential recorded at a short distance from a neuron, caused by postsynaptic potentials.

magnetoencephalogram/MEG   Magnetic field fluctuations that accompany the EEG.

magnocellular (M) pathway   The pathway starting with parasol (alternatively termed as *magnocellularly projecting*, or *M*) ganglion cells in the primate retina going through layers 1–2 of the lateral geniculate nucleus (LGN) and terminating principally in layer 4Cα of the primary visual cortex V1. Cells in this pathway respond transiently to step stimuli and are sensitive to relatively low spatial and relatively high temporal frequencies (see also *koniocellular pathway, parvocellular pathway, V1*).

masking   Reduced visibility of a stimulus (called the target) due to the presence of another stimulus (called the mask) (see also *backward masking, forward masking, metacontrast, paracontrast, masking function*).

masking function   The change of visibility of a brief target stimulus produced by a brief mask stimulus as a function of the stimulus onset asynchrony (SOA) separating the two stimuli. Forward/backward masking functions can be (i) monotonic (also called type A) with maximum masking occurring at SOA = 0 or (ii) nonmonotonic with a U shape (U-shaped or Type B) or with an oscillatory shape (oscillatory or multimodal).

metacontrast   Backward masking using spatially contiguous target and mask stimuli (see also *masking, backward masking, forward masking, paracontrast, masking function*).

microgenesis   Short-term formation of a psychological process within a fraction of a second or few seconds.

paracontrast   Forward masking using spatially contiguous target and mask stimuli (see also *masking, backward masking, forward masking, metacontrast, masking function*).

parvocellular (P) pathway   The pathway starting with midget (alternatively termed as *parvocellularly projecting*, or *P*) ganglion cells in the primate retina going through layers 3–6 of the lateral geniculate nucleus (LGN) and terminating principally in layer 4Cβ of the primary visual cortex V1. Cells in this pathway respond with sustained discharges to step stimuli and are sensitive to relatively high spatial and relatively low temporal frequencies (see also *koniocellular pathway, magnocellular pathway*).

perceptual epoch   A brief (few hundred milliseconds) period during which a relatively spatiotemporally stabilized stimulus is processed. Perceptual epochs typically occur during fixation and smooth pursuit conditions.

pertention   A psychophysiological process that transforms preconscious perceptual data that are encoded within the specific cortical sensory systems into the explicitly experienced, directly reportable, conscious representation.

PET Positron emission tomography, a technique for precisely localizing changes in brain activity based on the decay of radioactive isotopes.

phenomenal microgenesis (PMG) Formational unfolding of an active mental representation of an object, scene, or event in the directly experienced, phenomenal format.

postsynaptic potential Graded change in the membrane electrical potential of a neuron that occurs when a neurotransmitter binds with a receptor, leading ion channels to open or close.

priming The "preparatory effect" of one stimulus on a subsequent stimulus.

reentrant process See *feedback*.

representational microgenesis (RMG) Formation of an active mental representation of an object, scene, or event irrespective of whether it is consciously experienced or not.

saccade An eye movement, whose speed correlates with its spatial extent, used to change fixation rapidly from one point in a visual scene to another.

schizophrenia A mental disease characterized by a positive symptomatology consisting of sensory hallucinations and cognitive delusions or a negative symptomatology consisting of lack of emotional facial expression, reduced thought and speech, and reduced desire for social and familial contact.

stimulus onset asynchrony (SOA) The time interval, in milliseconds, between the onsets of two stimuli, S1 and S2. At negative asynchronies, the onset of S2 occurs before that of the S1; at positvive asynchronies, the onset of S2 occurs after that of S1; and at a zero asynchrony, the onsets of the two stimuli occur simultaneously.

stimulus-dependent/percept-dependent processing Visual responses correlating with physical/perceptual properties of a stimulus (e.g., wavelengths/colors).

transcranial magnetic stimulation (TMS) The application of a brief magnetic pulse to a circumscribed area of the cranial surface that disrupts neural processing in the underlying and correspondingly circumscribed cerebral region.

V1 Also called the primary visual cortex, it is the first cortical recipient area for projections from the retina via the lateral geniculate nucleus (LGN). It is located in the occipital lobe and has a columnar organization.

ventral pathway (stream) Pathway emerging from the primary visual cortex and projecting to the inferotemporal (IT) cortex. Alternative functional roles attributed to the ventral pathway include visual identification of objects ("what") and "vision for perception" (identification, evaluation, planning) (see also *dorsal pathway, inferotemporal cortex*).

References

Abbott, L. F., Varela, K., Sen, K., & Nelson, S. B. (1997). Synaptic depression and cortical gain control. *Science, 275,* 220–223.

Addington, J., & Addington, D. (1998). Facial affect recognition and information processing in schizophrenia and bipolar disorder. *Schizophrenia Research, 32,* 171–181.

Aggelopoulos, N. C., Franco, L., & Rolls, E. T. (2005). Object perception in natural scenes: Encoding by inferior temporal cortex simultaneously recorded neurons. *Journal of Neurophysiology, 93,* 1342–1367.

Aglioti, S., DeSouza, J. F. X., & Goodale, M. A. (1995). Size-contrast illusions deceive the eye but not the hand. *Current Biology, 5,* 679–685.

Albert, M. L., Soffer, D., Silverberg, R., & Reches, A. (1979). The anatomic basis of visual agnosia. *Neurology, 29,* 876–879.

Alkire, M. T., Haier, R. J., & Fallon, J. H. (2000). Toward a unified theory of narcosis: Brain imaging evidence for a thalamocortical switch as the neurophysiologic basis of anesthetic-induced unconsciousness. *Consciousness and Cognition, 9,* 387–395.

Allison, T., Goff, W. R., Williamson, P. D., & Van Gilder, J. C. (1980). On the neural origin of early components of the human somatosensory evoked potential. In J. Desmedt (Ed.), *Clinical uses of cerebral, brainstem and spinal somatosensory evoked potentials* (pp. 51–68). Basel, Switzerland: Karger.

Allman, F., Miezin, F., & McGuiness, E. (1985). Stimulus specific responses from beyond the classical receptive field: Neuro-physiological mechanisms for local–global comparisons in visual neurons. *Annual Review of Neuroscience, 8,* 407–430.

Alpern, M. (1953). Metacontrast. *Journal of the Optical Society of America, 43,* 648–657.

Amassian, V. E., Cracco, R. Q., Maccabee, P. J., Cracco, J. B., Rudell, A., & Eberle, L. (1989). Suppression of visual perception by magnetic coil stimulation of human occipital cortex. *Electroencephalography and Clinical Neurophysiology, 74,* 458–462.

Amassian, V. E., Cracco, R. Q., Maccabee, P. J., Cracco, J. B., Rudell, A. P., & Eberle, L. (1993). Unmasking human visual perception with the magnetic coil and its relationship to hemispheric asymmetry. *Brain Research, 605,* 312–316.

Anbar, S., & Anbar, D. (1982). Visual masking: A unified approach. *Perception, 11,* 427–439.

Anders, S., Birbaumer, N., Sadowski, B., Erb, M., Mader, I., Grodd, W., & Lotze, M. (2004). Parietal somatosensory association cortex mediates affective blindsight. *Nature Neuroscience, 7,* 339–340.

Andersen, R. A., Snyder, L. H., Bradley, D. C., & Xing, J. (1997). Multimodal representation of space in the posterior parietal cortex and its use in planning movements. *Annual Review of Neuroscience, 20,* 303–330.

Andreasen, N. C., & Olsen, S. (1982). Negative vs. positive schizophrenia. *Archives of General Psychiatry, 39,* 789–794.

Anllo-Vento, L., Luck, S. J., & Hillyard, S. A. (1998). Spatio-temporal dynamics of attention to color: Evidence from human electrophysiology. *Human Brain Mapping, 6,* 216–238.

Ansorge, U., Klotz, W., & Neumann, O. (1998). Manual and verbal responses to completely masked (unreportable) stimuli: Exploring some conditions for the metacontrast dissociation. *Perception, 27,* 1177–1189.

Arnold, D. H., & Clifford, C. W. G. (2002). Determinants of asynchronous processing in vision. *Proceedings of the Royal Society of London, B, 269,* 579–583.

Arrington, K. F. (1994). The temporal dynamics of brightness filling-in. *Vision Research, 34,* 3371–3387.

Aschersleben, G., & Bachmann, T. (submitted). *Synchronisation and metacontrast stimulation: Evidence for the dual-process attentional theory.*

Azouz, R., & Gray, C. M. (1999). Cellular mechanisms contributing to response variability of cortical neurons in vivo. *Journal of Neuroscience, 19,* 2209–2223.

Azzopardi, P., & Cowey, A. (1997). Is blindsight like normal, near-threshold vision? *Proceedings of the National Academy of Sciences, USA, 94,* 14190–14194.

Azzopardi, P., Fallah, M., Gross, C. G., & Rodman, H. T. (1998). Responses of neurons in visual areas MT and MTS after lesions of striate cortex in macaque monkeys. *Society of Neuroscience Abstracts, 24,* 648.

Baars, B. J. (1988). *A cognitive theory of consciousness.* Cambridge, England: Cambridge University Press.

Baars, B. J. (1997). *In the theater of consciousness: The workspace of the mind.* Oxford, England: Oxford University Press.

Baars, B. J. (2002). The conscious access hypothesis: Origins and recent evidence. *Trends in Cognitive Sciences, 6,* 47–52.

Baars, B. J., Ramsoy, T. Z., & Laureys, S. (2003). Brain, conscious experience and the observing self. *Trends in Neurosciences, 26,* 671–675.

Bach, M., & Meigen, T. (1992). Electrophysiological correlates of texture segregation in the human visual evoked potential. *Vision Research, 32,* 417–424.

Bachmann, T. (1984). The process of perceptual retouch: Nonspecific afferent activation dynamics in explaining visual masking. *Perception and Psychophysics, 35,* 69–84.

Bachmann, T. (1987). Different trends in perceptual pattern microgenesis as a function of the spatial range of local brightness averaging. *Psychological Research, 49,* 107–111.

Bachmann, T. (1988). Time course of the subjective contrast enhancement for a second stimulus in successively paired above-threshold transient forms: Perceptual retouch instead of forward masking. *Vision Research, 28,* 1255–1261.

Bachmann, T. (1989). Microgenesis as traced by the transient paired-forms paradigm. *Acta Psychologica, 70,* 3–17.

Bachmann, T. (1994). *Psychophysiology of visual masking: The fine structure of conscious experience.* Commack, NY: Nova Science.

Bachmann, T. (1999). Twelve spatiotemporal phenomena, and one explanation. In G. Ascersleben, T. Bachmann, & J. Müsseler (Eds.), *Cognitive contributions to the perception of spatial and temporal events* (pp. 173–212). Amsterdam: Elsevier.

Bachmann, T. (2000). *Microgenetic approach to the conscious mind.* Amsterdam: John Benjamins.

Bachmann, T., & Allik, J. (1976). Integration and interruption in the masking of form by form. *Perception, 5,* 79–97.

Bachmann, T., Luiga, I., & Põder, E. (2004a). Forward masking of faces by spatially quantized random and structured masks. *Psychological Research, 69,* 11–29.

Bachmann, T., Luiga, I., Põder, E., & Kalev, K. (2003). Perceptual acceleration of objects in stream: Evidence from flash-lag displays. *Consciousness and Cognition, 12,* 279–297.

Bachmann, T., Luiga, I., & Põder, E. (2005a). Variations in backward masking with different masking stimuli: I. Local interaction versus attentional switch. *Perception, 34,* 131–137.

Bachmann, T., Luiga, I., & Põder, E. (2005b). Variations in backward masking with different masking stimuli: II. The effects of spatially quantised masks in the light of local contour interaction, interchannel inhibition, perceptual retouch, and substitution theories. *Perception, 34,* 139–154.

Bachmann, T., & Oja, A. (2003). Flash-lag without change in feature space is alive and well at late intervals after stream onset. *Perception*, *325*, 126–127.

Bachmann, T., & Põder, E. (2001). Change in feature space is not necessary for the flash-lag effect. *Vision Research*, *41*, 1103–1106.

Bachmann, T., Põder, E., & Luiga, I. (2004b). Illusory reversal of temporal order: The bias to report a dimmer stimulus as the first. *Vision Research*, *44*, 241–246.

Bair, W., Cavanaugh, J. R., & Movshon, J. A. (2003). Time course and time–distance relationships for surround suppression in macaque V1 neurons. *Journal of Neuroscience*, *23*, 7690–7701.

Baizer, J. S., Ungerleider, L. G., & Desimone, R. (1991). Organization of visual inputs to the inferior temporal and posterior parietal cortex in macaques. *Journal of Neuroscience*, *11*, 168–190.

Baldo, M. V. C., Kihara, A. H., Namba, J., & Klein, S. A. (2002). Evidence for an attentional component of the perceptual misalignment between moving and flashed stimuli. *Perception*, *31*, 17–30.

Barbur, J. L. (1995). A study of pupil response components in human vision. In J. G. Robbins, M. B. A. Djamgoz, & A. Taylor (Eds.), *Basic and clinical perspectives in vision research* (pp. 3–18). New York: Plenum.

Barnes, G. R., & Asselman, P. T. (1991). The mechanism of prediction in human smooth pursuit eye movements. *Journal of Physiology*, *439*, 439–461.

Bartels, A., & Zeki, S. (1999). The clinical and functional measurement of cortical (in)activity in the visual brain, with special reference to the two subdivisions (V4 and V4α) of the human colour centre. *Philosophical Transactions of the Royal Society of London, B*, *354*, 1371–1382.

Battaglia, F., & Treves, A. (1998). Stable and rapid recurrent processing in realistic autoassociative memories. *Neural Computation*, *10*, 431–450.

Baumann, R., van der Zwaan, R., & Peterhans, E. (1997). Figure-ground segregation at contours: A neural mechanisms in the visual cortex of the alert monkey. *European Journal of Neuroscience*, *9*, 1290–1303.

Beck, D. M., Rees, G., Frith, C. D., & Lavie, N. (2001). Neural correlates of change detection and change blindness. *Nature Neuroscience*, *4*, 645–650.

Bedell, H. E., Chung, S. T. L., Öğmen, H., & Patel, S. S. (2003). Color and motion: Which is the tortoise and which is the hare? *Vision Research*, *43*, 2403–2412.

Bedwell, J. S., Brown, J. M., & Miller, L. S. (2003). The magnocellular visual system and schizophrenia: What can the color red tell us? *Schizophrenia Research*, *63*, 273–284.

Behrendt, R. P. (2003). Hallucinations: Synchronisation of thalamocortical gamma oscillations underconstrained by sensory input. *Consciousness and Cognition*, *12*, 413–451.

Benardete, E. A., & Kaplan, E. (1997). The receptive field of the primate P retinal ganglion cell: I. Linear dynamics. *Visual Neuroscience*, *14*, 169–185.

Benson, D. F., & Greenberg, J. P. (1969). Visual form agnosia. *Archives of Neurology*, *20*, 82–89.

Berti, A., & Rizzolatti, G. (1992). Visual processing without awareness: Evidence from unilateral neglect. *Journal of Cognitive Neuroscience*, *4*, 345–351.

Biederman, I., & Gerhardstein, P. C. (1993). Recognizing depth-rotated objects: Evidence and conditions for three-dimensional viewpoint invariance. *Journal of Experimental Psychology: Human Perception and Performance*, *19*, 1162–1182.

Bisiach, E. (1993). Mental representation in unilateral neglect and related disorders: The twentieth Bartlett memorial lecture. *Quarterly Journal of Experimental Psychology*, *46A*, 435–461.

Blake, R. (1998). What can be "perceived" in the absence of visual awareness? *Current Directions in Psychological Science*, *6*, 157–162.

Blake, R., & Fox, R. (1974). Adaptation to "invisible" gratings and the site of binocular rivalry suppression. *Nature*, *249*, 488–490.

Blake, R., & Logothetis, N. K. (2002). Visual competition. *Nature Reviews Neuroscience*, *3*, 13–23.

Blakemore, C., & Tobin, E. A. (1972). Lateral inhibition between orientation detectors in the cat's visual cortex. *Experimental Brain Research*, *15*, 439–440.

Block, N. (1995). On a confusion of a function of consciousness. *Behavioral and Brain Sciences, 18,* 227–287.

Block, N. (1996). How can we find the neural correlate of consciousness? *Trends in Neuroscience, 19,* 456–459.

Blythe, I. M., Kennard, C., & Ruddock, K. H. (1987). Residual vision in patients with retrogeniculate lesions of the visual pathways. *Brain, 110* (Pt 4), 887–905.

Bogen, J. E. (1995). On the neurophysiology of consciousness: I. An overview. *Consciousness and Cognition, 4,* 52–62.

Bogen, J. E. (1997). Some neurophysiological aspects of consciousness. *Seminars in Neurology, 17,* 95–103.

Booth, M. C. A., & Rolls, E. T. (1998). View-invariant representations of familiar objects by neurons in the inferior temporal visual cortex. *Cerebral Cortex, 8,* 510–523.

Borges, J. L. (1979). *A universal history of infamy.* New York: Dutton.

Braddick, O. J. (1993). Segmentation versus integration in visual motion processing. *Trends in Neuroscience, 16,* 263–267.

Braff, D. L., & Saccuzzo, D. P. (1981). Information processing dysfunction in paranoid schizophrenia: A two-factor deficit. *American Journal of Psychiatry, 138,* 1051–1056.

Braff, D. L., & Saccuzzo, D. P. (1982). Effect of antipsychotic medication on speed of information processing in schizophrenic patients. *American Journal of Psychiatry, 139,* 1127–1130.

Braff, D. L., Saccuzzo, D. P., & Geyer, M. A. (1992). Information processing dysfunctions in schizophrenia: Studies of visual backward masking, sensorimotor gating, and habituation (J. R. Steinhauer, J. H. Gruzelier, & J. Zubin, Trans.). In J. R. Steinhauer & J. H. Gruzelier (Eds.), *Neuropsychology, psychophysiology, and information processing* (pp. 305–334). New York: Elsevier.

Breitmeyer, B. G. (1975). Simple reaction time as a measure of the temporal response properties of transient and sustained channels. *Vision Research, 15,* 1411–1412.

Breitmeyer, B. G. (1978). Disinhibition in metacontrast masking of vernier acuity targets: Sustained channels inhibit transient channels. *Vision Research, 18,* 1401–1405.

Breitmeyer, B. G. (1984). *Visual masking.* Oxford, England: Oxford University Press.

Breitmeyer, B. G. (2002). In support of Pockett's critique of Libet's studies of the time course of consciousness. *Consciousness and Cognition, 11,* 280–283.

Breitmeyer, B. G., Ehrenstein, A., Pritchard, K., Hiscock, M., & Crisan, J. (1999). The roles of location specificity and masking mechanisms in the attentional blink. *Perception & Psychophysics, 61,* 798–809.

Breitmeyer, B. G., & Ganz, L. (1976). Implications of sustained and transient channels for theories of visual pattern masking, saccadic suppression, and information processing. *Psychological Review, 83,* 1–36.

Breitmeyer, B. G., Levi, D. M., & Harwerth, R. S. (1981a). Flicker masking in spatial vision. *Vision Research, 21,* 1377–1385.

Breitmeyer, B. G., & Öğmen, H. (2000). Recent models and findings in visual backward masking: A comparison, review, and update. *Perception & Psychophysics, 62,* 1572–1595.

Breitmeyer, B. G., Öğmen, H., & Chen, J. (2004a). Unconscious priming by color and form: Different processes and levels. *Consciousness and Cognition, 13,* 138–157.

Breitmeyer, B. G., Öğmen, H., & Chen, J. (2005). Nonconscious priming by forms and their parts. *Visual Cognition, 12,* 720–736.

Breitmeyer, B. G., Öğmen, H., Mardon, L., & Todd, S. (in press). Para- and metacontrast reveal differences between the processing of form and contrast. *Vision Research.*

Breitmeyer, B. G., Ro, T., & Öğmen, H. (2004b). A comparison of masking by visual and transcranial magnetic stimulation: Implications for the study of conscious and unconscious visual processing. *Consciousness and Cognition, 13,* 829–843.

Breitmeyer, B. G., Ro, T., & Singhal, N. S. (2004c). Nonconscious color priming occurs at stimulus- not percept-dependent levels of visual processing. *Psychological Science, 15,* 198–202.

Breitmeyer, B. G., & Rudd, M. E. (1981). A single-transient masking paradigm. *Perception & Psychophysics, 30*, 604–606.

Breitmeyer, B. G., Rudd, M., & Dunn, K. (1981b). Flicker masking in spatial vision. *Journal of Experimental Psychology: Human Perception and Performance, 7*, 770–779.

Brenner, E., & Smeets, J. B. J. (2000). Motion extrapolation is not responsible for the flash-lag effect. *Vision Research, 40*, 1645–1648.

Brenner, E., Smeets, J. B. J., & van den Berg, A. V. (2001). Smooth eye movements and spatial localisation. *Vision Research, 41*, 2253–2259.

Bridgeman, B. (1971). Metacontrast and lateral inhibition. *Psychological Review, 78*, 528–539.

Bridgeman, B. (1978). Distributed sensory coding applied to simulations of iconic storage and metacontrast. *Bulletin of Mathematical Biology, 40*, 605–623.

Bridgeman, B. (1980). Temporal response characteristics of cells in monkey striate cortex measured with metacontrast masking and brightness discrimination. *Brain Research, 196*, 347–364.

Bridgeman, B., & Leff, S. (1979). Interaction of stimulus size and retinal eccentricity in metacontrast masking. *Journal of Experimental Psychology: Human Perception and Performance, 5*, 101–109.

Bridgeman, B., Lewis, S., Heit, G., & Nagle, M. (1979). Relation between cognitive and motor-oriented systems in visual position perception. *Journal of Experimental Psychology: Human Perception and Performance, 5*, 692–700.

Bringuier, V., Chavane, F., Glaeser, L., & Fregnac, Y. (1999). Horizontal propagation of visual activity in the synaptic integration field of area 17 neurons. *Science, 283*, 695–699.

Broadbent, D. (1958). *Perception and communication*. Oxford, England: Pergamon.

Broadbent, D. E., & Broadbent, M. H. P. (1987). From detection to identification: Response to multiple targets in rapid serial visual presentation. *Perception and Psychophysics, 42*, 105–113.

Brooks, B., & Jung, R. (1973). Neuronal physiology of the visual cortex. In R. Jung (Ed.), *Handbook of sensory physiology*: 325–440. *Vol. VII/3. Central processing of visual information. Part B*. New York: Springer-Verlag.

Brown, J. (1977). *Mind, brain, and consciousness*. New York: Academic Press.

Brown, J. W. (1988). *The life of the mind*. Hillsdale, NJ: Erlbaum.

Bruce, C. J., & Goldberg, M. E. (1985). Primate frontal eye fields: I. Single neurons discharging before saccades. *Journal of Neurophysiology, 53*, 603–635.

Bruce, V., & Green, P. (1989). *Visual perception: Physiology, psychology and ecology*. London: Erlbaum.

Bullier, J. (2001). Integrated model of visual processing. *Brain Research Reviews, 36*, 96–107.

Bullier, J., McCourt, M. E., & Henry, G. H. (1988). Physiological studies on the feedback connection to the striate cortex from cortical areas 18 and 19 of the cat. *Experimental Brain Research, 70*, 90–98.

Burt, P., & Sperling, G. (1981). Time, distance, and feature trade-offs in visual apparent motion. *Psychological Review, 88*, 171–195.

Butler, P. D., DeSanti, L. A., Maddox, J., Harkavy-Friedman, J. M., Amador, X. F., Goetz, R. R., Javitt, D. C., & Gorman, J. M. (2002). Visual backward-masking deficits in schizophrenia: Relationship to visual pathway function and symptomatology. *Schizophrenia Research, 59*, 199–209.

Butler, P. D., Harkavy-Friedman, J. M., Amador, X. F., & Gorman, J. M. (1996). Backward masking in schizophrenia: Relationship to medication status, neuropsychological functioning, and dopamine metabolism. *Biological Psychiatry, 40*, 295–298.

Butler, P. D., Schechter, I., Zemon, V., Schwartz, S. G., Greenstein, V. C., Gordon, J., Schroeder, C. E., & Javitt, D. C. (2001). Dysfunction of early-stage visual processing in schizophrenia. *American Journal of Psychiatry, 158*, 1126–1133.

Cadenhead, K. S., Geyer, M. A., Butler, R. W., Perry, W., Sprock, J., & Braff, D. L. (1997). Information processing deficits of schizophrenia patients: Relationship to clinical ratings, gender and medication status. *Schizophrenia Research, 28*, 51–62.

Cadenhead, K. S., Kumar, C., & Braff, D. L. (1996). Clinical and experimental characteristics of "hypothetically psychosis prone" college students. *Journal of Psychiatry Research, 30,* 331–340.

Cadenhead, K. S., Serper Y., & Braff, D. L. (1998). Transient versus sustained visual channels in the visual backward masking deficits of schizophrenia patients. *Biological Psychiatry, 43,* 132–138.

Cai, R. H., Jacobson, K., Baloh, R., Schlag-Rey, M., & Schlag, J. (2000). Vestibular signals can distort the perceived spatial relationship of retinal stimuli. *Experimental Brain Research, 135,* 275–278.

Calis, G., Sterenborg, J., & Maarse, F. (1984). Initial microgenetic steps in single-glance face recognition. *Acta Psychologica, 55,* 215–230.

Cant, J. S., Westwood, D. A., Valyear, K. F., & Goodale, M. A. (2005). No evidence for visuomotor priming in a visually guided action task. *Neuropsychologia, 43,* 216–226.

Caputo, G. (1998). Texture brightness filling-in. *Vision Research, 38,* 841–851.

Caputo, G., & Casco, C. (1999). A visual evoked potential correlate of global figure–ground segmentation. *Vision Research, 39,* 1597–1610.

Carpenter, G. A., & Grossberg, S. (1981). Adaptation and transmitter gating in vertebrate photoreceptors. *Journal of Theoretical Neurobiology, 1,* 1–42.

Carpenter, G., & Grossberg, S. (1987). A massively parallel architecture for a self-organizing neural pattern recognition machine. *Computer Vision, Graphics, and Image Processing, 37,* 54–115.

Carrasco, M., Evert, D. L., Change, I., & Katz, S. M. (1995). The eccentricity effect: Target eccentricity affects performance on conjunction searches. *Perception & Psychophysics, 57,* 1241–1261.

Carrasco, M., Ling, S., & Read, S. (2004). Attention alters appearance. *Nature Neuroscience, 7,* 208–209.

Cave, C. B., Blake, R., & McNamara, T. P. (1998). Binocular rivalry disrupts visual priming. *Psychological Science, 9,* 299–302.

Cavonius, C. R., & Reeves, A. J. (1983). The interpretation of metacontrast and contrast-flash spectral sensitivity functions. In J. D. Mollon & L. T. Sharpe (Eds.), *Color vision: Physiology and psychophysics* (pp. 471–478). London: Academic Press.

Chance, F. S., Nelson, S. B., & Abbott, L. F. (1998). Synaptic depression and the temporal response characteristics of V1 cells. *Journal of Neuroscience, 18,* 4785–4799.

Cheesman, J., & Merikle, P. M. (1986). Distinguishing conscious from unconscious perceptual processes. *Canadian Journal of Psychology, 40,* 343–367.

Chelazzi, L. (1999). Serial attention mechanisms in visual search: A critical look at the evidence. *Psychological Research, 62,* 195–219.

Chelazzi, L., Duncan, J., Miller, E. K., & Desimone, R. (1998). Responses of neurons in inferior temporal cortex during memory-guided visual search. *Journal of Neurophysiology, 80,* 2918–2940.

Chelazzi, L., Miller, E. K., Duncan, J., & Desimone, R. (2001). Responses of neurons in macaque area V4 during memory-guided visual search. *Cerebral Cortex, 11,* 761–772.

Cho, Y. S., & Francis, G. (2003). Backward masking with sparse masks: Models and experiments [Abstract]. *Journal of Vision, 3,* 742a, http://journalofvision.org/3/9/742/, DOI:10.1167/3.9.742.

Chun, M. M., & Jiang, Y. (1998). Contextual cueing: Implicit learning and memory of visual context guides spatial attention. *Cognitive Psychology, 36,* 28–71.

Chun, M. M., & Potter, M. C. (1995). A two-stage model for multiple target detection in rapid serial visual presentation. *Journal of Experimental Psychology: Human Perception and Performance, 21,* 109–127.

Churchland, P. S. (1981). On the alleged backwards referral of experiences and its relevance to the mind–body problem. *Philosophy of Science, 48,* 165–181.

Churchland, P. S. (2002). *Brain-wise: Studies in neurophilosophy.* London: MIT Press/Bradford.

Clark, V. P., & Hillyard, S. A. (1996). Spatial selective attention affects early extrastriate but not striate components of the visual evoked potential. *Journal of Cognitive Neuroscience, 8,* 387–402.

Clifford, C. W. G., Arnold, D., & Pearson, J. (2003). A paradox of temporal perception revealed by a stimulus oscillating in colour and orientation. *Vision Research, 43,* 2245–2253.

Cohen, A., & Ivry, R. B. (1991). Density effects in conjunction search: Evidence for a coarse location mechanism of feature integration. *Journal of Experimental Psychology: Human Perception and Performance, 17*, 891–901.

Cohen, M. A., & Grossberg, S. (1984). Neural dynamics of brightness perception: Features, boundaries, diffusion, and resonance. *Perception & Psychophysics, 36*, 428–456.

Coles, M. G. H. (1989) Modern mind–brain reading: Psychophysiology, physiology, and cognition. *Psychophysiology, 26*, 251–269.

Coletta, N. J., & Williams, D. R. (1987). Psychophysical estimate of extrafoveal cone spacing. *Journal of the Optical Society of America, A, 4*, 1503–1513.

Coltheart, M. (1983). Iconic memory. *Philosophical Transactions of the Royal Society of London, B, 302*, 283–294.

Coltheart, V. (Ed.). (1999). *Fleeting memories: Cognition of brief visual stimuli.* Cambridge, MA: MIT Press.

Corrigan, P. W., Green, M. F., & Toomey, R. (1994). Cognitive correlates to social cue perception in schizophrenia. *Psychiatry Research, 53*, 141–151.

Corthout, E., Uttl, B., Walsh, V., Hallett, M., & Cowey, A. (1999a). Timing of activity in early visual cortex as revealed by transcranial magnetic stimulation. *NeuroReport, 10*, 2631–2634.

Corthout, E., Uttl, B., Ziemann, U., Cowey, A., & Hallett, M. (1999b). Two periods of processing in the (circum)striate visual cortex as revealed by transcranial magnetic stimulation. *Neuropsychologia, 37*, 137–145.

Cowey, A., & Stoerig, P. (1991). Reflections on blindsight. In D. Milner & M. Rugg (Eds.), *The neuropsychology of consciousness* (pp. 11–37). Oxford, England: Academic Press.

Cowey, A., & Stoerig, P. (2001). Detection and discrimination of chromatic targets in hemianopic macaque monkeys and humans. *European Journal of Neuroscience, 14*, 1320–1330.

Cowey, A., & Stoerig, P. (2004). Stimulus cueing in blindsight. *Progress in Brain Research, 144*, 261–277.

Cowey, A., Stoerig, P., & Hodinott-Hill, I. (2003). Chromatic priming in hemianopic visual fields. *Experimental Brain Research, 152*, 95–105.

Craighero, L., Fadiga, L., Umiltà, C. A., & Rizzolatti, G. (1996). Evidence for visuomotor priming effect. *Neuroreport, 8*, 347–349.

Craik, F. I. M., Moroz, T. M., Moscovitch, M., Stuss, D. T., Winocur, G., Tulving, E., & Kapur, S. (1999). In search of the self: A positron emission tomography study. *Psychological Science, 10*, 26–34.

Creem, S. H., & Proffitt, D. R. (2001). Grasping objects by their handles: A necessary interaction between cognition and action. *Journal of Experimental Psychology: Human Perception and Performance, 27*, 218–228.

Crick, F. (1984). Function of the thalamic reticular complex: The searchlight hypothesis. *Proceedings of the National Academy of Sciences, USA, 81*, 4586–4590.

Crick, F. (1994). *The astonishing hypothesis.* New York: Scribner.

Crick, F., & Koch, C. (1990). Towards a neurobiological theory of consciousness. *Seminar in the Neurosciences, 2*, 263–275.

Crick, F., & Koch, C. (1995). Are we aware of neural activity in primary visual cortex? *Nature, 375*, 121–123.

Crick, F., & Koch, C. (1998). Consciousness and neuroscience. *Cerebral Cortex, 8*, 97–107.

Crick, F., & Koch, C. (2003). A framework for consciousness. *Nature Neuroscience, 6*, 119–126.

Croner, L. J., & Kaplan, E. (1995). Receptive fields of P and M ganglion cells across the primate retina. *Vision Research, 35*, 7–24.

Culham, J. C., & Kanwisher, N. G. (2001). Neuroimaging of cognitive functions in human parietal cortex. *Current Opinion in Neurobiology, 11*, 157–163.

Cutting, J. E., & Millard, R. T. (1984). Three gradients and the perception of flat and curved surfaces. *Journal of Experimental Psychology: General, 113*, 198–216.

Czeisler, C. A., Shanahan, D. L., Klerman, E. B., Martens, H., Brotman, D. J., Emens, J. S., Klein, T., & Rizzo, J. F. (1995). Suppression of melatonin secretion in some blind patients by exposure to bright light. *New England Journal of Medicine, 322,* 6–11.

Czisch, M., Wetter, T. C., Kaufmann, C., Pollmächer, T., Holsboer, F., & Auer, D. P. (2002). Altered processing of acoustic stimuli during sleep: Reduced auditory activation and visual deactivation detected by a combined fMRI/EEG study. *Neuroimage, 16,* 251–258.

Dacey, D. M. (1993). The mosaic of midget ganglion cells in the human retina. *Journal of Neuroscience, 13,* 5334–5355.

Dacey, D. M., & Lee, B. B. (1994). The "blue-on" opponent pathway in primate retina originates from a distinct bistratified ganglion cell type. *Nature, 367,* 731–735.

Daini, R., Angelelli, P., Antonucci, G., Cappa, S. F., & Valler, G. (2001). Illusions of length in spatial unilateral neglect. *Cortex, 37,* 710–714.

Damasio, A. R. (1994). *Descartes' error.* New York: Putnam.

Damasio, A. R., Damasio, H., & van Hoesen, G. W. (1982). Prosopagnosia: Anatomic basis and behavioral mechanisms. *Neurology, 32,* 331–341.

D'Aquili, E. G., & Newberg, A. B. (1999). *The mystical mind.* Minneapolis, MN: Fortress Press.

Das, A., & Gilbert, C. D. (1999). Topography of contextual modulations mediated by short-range interactions in primary visual cortex. *Nature, 399,* 655–661.

Davenport, J. L., & Potter, M. C. (2005). The locus of semantic priming in RSVP target search. *Memory & Cognition, 33,* 241–248.

DeAngelis, G. C., Freeman, R. D., & Ohzawa, I. (1994). Length and width tuning of neurons in the cat's primary visual cortex. *Journal of Neurophysiology, 71,* 347–374.

de Gelder, B., de Haan, E., & Heywood, C. (Eds.). (2001a). *Out of mind: Varieties of unconscious processes.* Oxford, England: Oxford University Press.

de Gelder, B., Vroomen, J., & Pourtois, G. (2001b). Covert affective cognition and affective blindsight. In B. de Gelder, E. de Haan, & C. Heywood (Eds.), *Out of mind* (pp. 205–221). Oxford, England: Oxford University Press.

de Gelder, B., Vroomen, J., Pourtois, G., & Weiskrantz, L. (1999). Non-conscious recognition of affect in the absence of striate cortex. *Neuroreport, 10,* 3759–3763.

Dehaene, S., & Naccache, L. (2001). Towards a cognitive neuroscience of consciousness: Basic evidence and a workspace framework. *Cognition, 79,* 1–37.

Dehaene, S., Naccache, N., Cohen, L., Le Bihan, D., Mangin, J.-F., Poline, J.-B., & Riviere, D. (2001). Cerebral mechanisms of word masking and unconscious repetition priming. *Nature Neuroscience, 4,* 752–758.

Dehaene, S., Naccache, L., Le Clec'H, G., Koechlin, E., Mueller, M., Dehaene-Lambertz, G., van de Moortele, P.-F., & Le Bihan, D. (1998). Imaging unconscious semantic priming. *Nature, 395,* 597–600.

Dehaene, S., Sergent, C., & Changeaux, J.-P. (2003). A neuronal network model linking subjective reports and objective physiological data during conscious perception. *Proceedings of the National Academy of Sciences, USA, 100,* 8520–8525.

Dember, W. N., & Purcell, D. G. (1967). Recovery of masked visual targets by inhibition of the masking stimulus. *Science, 157,* 335–336.

De Monasterio, F. M. (1978). Properties of concentrically organized X and Y ganglion cells of macaque retina. *Journal of Neurophysiology, 41,* 1394–1417.

Dennett, D. C. (1991). *Consciousness explained.* Boston: Little, Brown.

Dennett, D. C., & Kinsbourne, M. (1992). Time and the observer: The where and when of consciousness in the brain. *Behavioral and Brain Sciences, 15,* 183–247.

Deouell, L. Y., Bentin, S., & Soroker, N. (2000a). Electrophysiological evidence for an early (preattentive) information processing deficit in patients with right hemisphere damage and unilateral neglect. *Brain, 123,* 353–365.

Deouell, L. Y., Hämäläinen, H., & Bentin, S. (2000b). Unilateral neglect after right hemisphere damage: Contributions from event-related potentials. *Audiology & Neuro-Otology, 5,* 225–234.

Desimone, R., & Schein, S. J. (1987). Visual properties of neurons in area V4 of the macaque: Sensitivity to stimulus form. *Journal of Neurophysiology, 57,* 835–868.

Desimone, R., & Ungerleider, L. (1989). Neural mechanisms of visual processing in monkeys. In F. Boller & J. Grafman (Eds.), *Handbook of neuropsychology* (Vol. 2, pp. 267–299). Amsterdam: Elsevier.

De Weerd, P., Desimone, R., & Ungerleider, L. G. (2003). Generalized deficits in visual selective attention after V4 and TEO lesions in macaques. *European Journal of Neuroscience, 18,* 1671–1691.

DeYoe, E. A., & Van Essen, D. C. (1988). Concurrent processing streams in monkey visual cortex. *Trends in Neuroscience, 11,* 219–226.

Dijkerman, H. C., Lê, S., Démonet, J.-F., & Milner, A. D. (2004). Visuomotor performance in a case of visual form agnosia due to early brain damage. *Cognitive Brain Research, 20,* 12–25.

Di Lollo, V. (1980). Temporal integration in visual memory. *Journal of Experimental Psychology: General, 109,* 75–97.

Di Lollo, V., Enns, J. T., & Rensink, R. (2000). Competition for consciousness among visual events: The psychophysics of reentrant visual processes. *Journal of Experimental Psychology: General, 129,* 481–507.

Di Lollo, V., Kawahara, J.-I., Ghorashi, S. M., & Enns, J. T. (2005). The attentional blink: Resource depletion or temporary loss of control? *Psychological Research, 69,* 191–200.

Di Lollo, V., Von Mühlenen, A., Enns, J. T., & Bridgeman, B. (2004). Decoupling stimulus duration from brightness in metacontrast masking: Data and models. *Journal of Experimental Psychology: Human Perception and Performance, 30,* 733–745.

Dimberg, U., Thunberg, M., & Elmehed, K. (2000). Unconscious facial reactions to emotional facial expressions. *Psychological Science, 11,* 86–89.

Dinse, H. R., & Kruger, K. (1994). The timing of processing along the visual pathway in the cat. *Neuroreport, 5,* 893–897.

Di Russo, F., Martinez, A., & Hillyard, S. A. (2003). Source analysis of event-related cortical activity during visuo-spatial attention. *Cerebral Cortex, 13,* 486–499.

Dixon, N. F. (1981). *Preconscious processing.* Chichester, England: Wiley.

Dodds, C., Machado, L., Rafal, R., & Ro, T. (2002). A temporal/nasal asymmetry for blindsight in a localisation task: Evidence for extrageniculate mediation. *Neuroreport, 13,* 655–658.

Dolan, R. J. (2002). Emotion, cognition, and behavior. *Science, 298,* 1191–1194.

Doniger, G. M., Foxe, J. J., Murray, M. M., Higgins, B. A., & Javitt, D. C. (2002). Impaired visual object recognition and dorsal/ventral stream interaction in schizophrenia. *Archives of General Psychiatry, 59,* 1011–1020.

Dow, B. M., Snyder, A. Z., Vautin, R. G., & Bauer, R. (1981). Magnification factor and receptive field size in foveal striate cortex of the monkey. *Experimental Brain Research, 44,* 213–228.

Driver, J., Baylis, G., & Rafal, R. (1992). Preserved figure–ground segmentation and symmetry perception in a patient with neglect. *Nature, 360,* 73–75.

Driver, J., & Mattingley, J. B. (1998). Parietal neglect and visual awareness. *Nature Neuroscience, 1,* 17–22.

Driver, J., & Vuilleumier, P. (2001). Perceptual awareness and its loss in unilateral neglect and extinction. *Cognition, 79,* 39–88.

Duncan, J. (1985). Two techniques for investigating perception without awareness. *Perception & Psychophysics, 38,* 296–298.

Eagleman, D. M. (2001). Visual illusions and neurobiology. *Nature Reviews Neuroscience, 2,* 920–926.

Eagleman, D. M., & Sejnowski, T. J. (2000a). Motion integration and postdiction in visual awareness. *Science, 287,* 2036–2038.

Eagleman, D. M., & Sejnowski, T. J. (2000b). The position of moving objects. *Science, 289,* 1107a.

Eason, R., Harter, M., & White, C. (1969). Effects of attention and arousal on visually evoked cortical potentials and reaction time in man. *Physiology and Behavior, 4,* 283–289.

Eckstein, M. P. (1998). The lower visual search efficiency for conjunctions is due to noise and not serial attentional processing. *Psychological Science, 9,* 111–118.

Edelman, G. M. (1987). *Neural Darwinism*. New York: Basic Books.

Edelman, G. M. (2003). Naturalizing consciousness: A theoretical framework. *Proceedings of the National Academy of Sciences, USA, 100*, 5520–5524.

Edelman, G. M., & Tononi, G. (2000). *A universe of consciousness: How matter becomes imagination*. New York: Basic Books.

Efron, R. (1967). The duration of the present. *Annals of the New York Academy of Sciences, 138*, 713–729.

Efron, R. (1970). The minimum duration of a perception. *Neurophysiologist, 8*, 57–63.

Efron, R. (1973). Conservation of temporal information by perceptual systems. *Perception and Psychophysics, 14*, 518–530.

Egelhaaf, M., Borst, A., & Reichardt, W. (1989). Computational structure of a biological motion-detection system as revealed by local detector analysis in the fly's nervous system. *Journal of the Optical Society of America, A, 6*, 1070–1087.

Eggermont, J. J. (1990). *The correlative brain*. Berlin, Germany: Springer-Verlag.

Eimer, M. (1996). The N2pc component as an indicator of attentional selectivity. *Electroencephalography and Clinical Neurophysiology, 99*, 225–234.

Eimer, M., & Schlaghecken, F. (1998). Effects of masked stimuli on motor activation: Behavioral and electrophysiological evidence. *Journal of Experimental Psychology: Human Perception and Performance, 24*, 1737–1747.

Eimer, M., & Schlaghecken, F. (2001). Response facilitation and inhibition in manual, vocal, and oculomotor performance: Evidence for a modality-unspecific mechanism. *Journal of Motor Behavior, 33*, 16–26.

Eimer, M., & Schlaghecken, F. (2002). Link between conscious awareness and response inhibition: Evidence from masked priming. *Psychonomic Bulletin & Review, 9*, 514–520.

Eimer, M., Schuboe, A., & Schlaghecken, F. (2002). Locus of inhibition in the masked priming of response alternatives. *Journal of Motor Behavior, 34*, 3–10.

Elder, J. H., & Zucker, S. W. (1998). Evidence for boundary-specific grouping. *Vision Research, 38*, 143–152.

Elliffe, M. C. M., Rolls, E. T., & Stringer, S. M. (2002). Invariant recognition of feature combinations in the visual system. *Biological Cybernetics, 86*, 59–71.

Engel, A. K., Koenig, P., Kreiter, A. K., Schillen, T. B., & Singer, W. (1992). Temporal coding in the visual cortex: New vistas on integration in the nervous system. *Trends in Neuroscience, 15*, 218–226.

Enns, J. T. (2002). Visual binding in the standing wave illusion. *Psychonomic Bulletin & Review, 9*, 489–496.

Enns, J. T. (2004). Object substitution and its relation to other forms of visual masking. *Vision Research, 44*, 1321–1331.

Enns, J. T., & Di Lollo, V. (1997). Object substitution: A new form of masking in unattended visual locations. *Psychological Science, 8*, 135–139.

Enns, J. T., & Di Lollo, V. (2000). What's new in visual masking? *Trends in Cognitive Sciences, 4*, 345–352.

Enns, J. T., & Rensink, R. A. (1990). Influence of scene-based properties on visual search. *Science, 9*, 721–723.

Erdelyi, M. H. (2004). Subliminal perception and its cognates: Theory, indeterminacy, and time. *Consciousness and Cognition 13*, 73–91.

Eriksen, C. W. (1966). Temporal luminance summation effects in backward and forward masking. *Perception & Psychophysics, 1*, 87–92.

Ernst, M. O., & Banks, M. S. (2002). Humans integrate visual and haptic information in a statistically optimal fashion. *Nature, 415*, 429–433.

Farah, M. J. (1990). *Visual agnosias*. Cambridge, MA: MIT Press.

Farah, M. J. (2004). *Visual agnosia* (2nd ed.). Cambridge, MA: MIT Press.

Farah, M. J., Levinson, K. L., & Klein, K. L. (1995a). Face perception and within-category discrimination in prosopagnosia. *Neuropsychologia, 33*, 661–674.

Farah, M. J., Wilson, K. D., Drain, H. M., & Tanaka, J. R. (1995b). The inverted face inversion effect in prosopagnosia: Evidence for mandatory, face-specific perceptual mechanisms. *Vision Research*, *35*, 2089–2093.

Fehrer, E., & Raab, D. (1962). Reaction time to stimuli masked by metacontrast. *Journal of Experimental Psychology*, *63*, 143–147.

Felleman, D. J., & Van Essen, D. C. (1991). Distributed hierarchical processing in the primate cerebral cortex. *Cerebral Cortex*, *1*, 1–47.

Fendrich, R., Wessinger, C. M., & Gazzaniga, M. S. (1992). Residual vision in a scotoma: Implications for blindsight. *Science*, *258*, 1489–1491.

Findlay, J. M., & Gilchrist, I. D. (2003). *Active vision: The psychology of looking and seeing.* Oxford, England: Oxford University Press.

Fischer, B., & Ramsperger, E. (1984). Human express saccades: Extremely short reaction times of goal directed eye movements. *Experimental Brain Research*, *57*, 191–195.

Flanagan, J. R., & Beltzner, M. A. (2000). Independence of perceptual and sensorimotor predictions in the size–weight illusion. *Nature Neuroscience*, *3*, 737–741.

Flavell, J. H., & Draguns, J. G. (1957). A microgenetic approach to perception and thought. *Psychological Bulletin*, *54*, 197–217.

Forster, K. I. (1970). Visual perception of rapidly presented word sequences of varying complexity. *Perception & Psychophysics*, *8*, 215–221.

Foxe, J. J., & Simpson, G. V. (2002). Flow of activation from V1 to frontal cortex in humans: A framework for defining "early" visual processing. *Experimental Brain Research*, *142*, 139–150.

Francis, G. (1997). Cortical dynamics of lateral inhibition: Metacontrast masking. *Psychological Review*, *104*, 572–594.

Francis, G. (2000). Quantitative theories of metacontrast masking. *Psychological Review*, *104*, 768–785.

Francis, G. (2003a). Developing a new quantitative account of backward masking. *Cognitive Psychology*, *46*, 198–226.

Francis, G. (2003b). Online simulations of models for backward masking. *Behavior Research Methods, Instruments, & Computers*, *35*, 512–519.

Francis, G., Grossberg, S., & Mingolla, E. (1994). Cortical dynamics of feature binding and reset: Control of visual persistence. *Vision Research*, *34*, 1089–1104.

Francis, G., & Herzog, M. (2004). Testing quantitative models of backward masking. *Psychonomic Bulletin & Review*, *11*, 104–112.

Francis, G., & Kim, H. (1999). Motion parallel to line orientation: Disambiguation of motion percepts. *Perception*, *28*, 1243–1255.

Francis, G., & Kim, H. (2001). Perceived motion in orientational afterimages: Direction and speed. *Vision Research*, *41*, 161–172.

Francis, G., & Rothmayer, M. (2003). Interactions of afterimages for orientation and color: Experimental data and model simulations. *Perception & Psychophysics*, *65*, 508–522.

Franco, L., Rolls, E. T., Aggelopoulos, N. C., & Treves, A. (2004). The use of decoding to analyze the contribution to the information of the correlations between the firing of simultaneously recorded neurons. *Experimental Brain Research*, *155*, 370–384.

Franz, V. H. (2001). Action does not resist visual illusions. *Trends in Cognitive Sciences*, *5*, 457–459.

Franz, V. H., Gegenfurtner, K. R., Bulthoff, H. H., & Fahle, M. (2000). Grasping visual illusions: No evidence for a dissociation between perception and action. *Psychological Science*, *11*, 20–25.

Freedman, D. J., Riesenhuber, M., Poggio, T., & Miller, E. K. (2002). Visual categorization and the primate prefrontal cortex: Neurophysiology and behavior. *Journal of Neurophysiology*, *88*, 929–941.

Friedrich, F. J., Egly, R., Rafal, R. D., & Beck, D. (1998). Spatial attention deficits in humans: A comparison of superior parietal and temporo-parietal junction lesions. *Neuropsychology*, *12*, 193–207.

Frith, C., Perry, R., & Lumer, E. (1999). The neural correlates of conscious experience: An experimental framework. *Trends in Cognitive Science*, *3*, 105–114.

Froehlich, W. D. (1984). Microgenesis as a functional approach to information processing through search. In W. D. Froehlich, G. Smith, J. G. Draguns, & U. Hentchel (Eds.), *Psychological processes in cognition and personality* (pp. 19–52). Washington, DC: Hemisphere.

Fry, G. A. (1934). Depression of the activity aroused by a flash of light by applying a second flash immediately afterwards to adjacent areas of the retina. *American Journal of Physiology, 108,* 701–707.

Gabbiani, F., Krapp, H. G., Koch, C., & Laurent, G. (2002). Multiplicative computation in a visual neuron sensitive to looming. *Nature, 420,* 320–324.

Gail, A., Brinksmeyer, H. J., & Eckhorn, R. (2004). Perception-related modulations of local field potential power and coherence in primary visual cortex of awake monkey during binocular rivalry. *Cerebral Cortex, 14,* 300–313.

Gallant, J. L., Conner, C. E., Rahshit, S., Lewis, J. W., & VanEssen, D. C. (1996). Neural responses to polar, hyperbolic and Cartesian gratings in area V4 of the macaque monkey. *Journal of Neurophysiology, 76,* 2718–2739.

Gandhi, S. P., Heeger, D. J., & Boynton, G. M. (1999). Spatial attention affects brain activity in human primary visual cortex. *Proceedings of the National Academy of Sciences, USA, 96,* 3314–3319.

Ganel, T., & Goodale, M. A. (2003). Visual control of action but not perception requires analytical processing of object shape. *Nature, 426,* 664–667.

Garofeanu, C., Króliczak, G., Goodale, M. A., & Humphrey, G. K. (2004). Naming and grasping common objects: A priming study. *Experimental Brain Research, 159,* 55–64.

Gaudiano, P. (1992). A unified neural network of spatio-temporal processing in X and Y retinal ganglion cells: II. Temporal adaptation and simulation of experimental data. *Biological Cybernetics, 67,* 23–34.

Gawne, T. J., & Richmond, B. J. (1993). How independent are the messages carried by adjacent inferior temporal cortical neurons? *Journal of Neuroscience, 13,* 2758–2771.

Gegenfurter, K. R. (2003). Cortical mechanisms of color vision. *Nature Reviews, 4,* 563–572.

Gelb, A., & Goldstein, K. (1922). Psychologische Analysen hirnpathologischer Stoerungen der Raumwahrnehmung. *Bericht ueber den IX. Kongress for Experimentelle Psychologie* (pp. 23–80). Jena, Germany: Fischer Verlag.

Genova, B., Mateeff, S., Bonnet, C., & Hohnsbein, J. (2000). Mechanisms of simple and choice reaction to changes in direction of visual motion. *Vision Research, 40,* 3049–3058.

Gentilucci, M., Chieffi, S., Deprati, E., Saetti, M. C., & Toni, I. (1996). Visual illusion and action. *Neuropsychologia, 34,* 369–376.

Georgopoulos, A. P., Kalaska, J. F., Caminiti, R., & Massey, J. T. (1982). On the relations between the direction of two-dimensional arm movements and cell discharge in primate motor cortex. *Journal of Neuroscience, 2,* 1527–1537.

Georgopoulos, A. P., Schwartz, A. B., & Kettner, R. E. (1986). Neuronal population coding of movement direction. *Science, 233,* 1416–1419.

Gibbon, J., Malapani, C., Dale, C. L., & Gallistel, C. R. (1997). Toward a neurobiology of temporal cognition: Advances and challenges. *Current Opinion in Neurobiology, 7,* 170–184.

Giesbrecht, B. L., Bischof, W. F., & Kingstone, A. (2003). Visual masking during the attentional blink: Tests of the object substitution hypothesis. *Journal of Experimental Psychology: Human Perception and Performance, 29,* 238–255.

Girard, P., Hupe, J. M., & Bullier, J. (2001). Feedforward and feedback connections between areas V1 and V2 of the monkey have similar rapid conduction velocities. *Journal of Neurophysiology, 85,* 1328–1331.

Gold, J. I., & Shadlen, M. N. (2001). Neural computations that underlie decisions about sensory stimuli. *Trends in Cognitive Sciences, 5,* 10–16.

Gomez Gonzales, C. M., Clark, V. P., Fan, S., Luck, S. J., & Hillyard, S. A. (1994). Sources of attention-sensitive visual event-related potentials. *Brain Topography, 7,* 41–51.

Goodale, M. A., & Haffenden, A. M. (1998). Frames of reference for perception and action in the human visual system. *Neuroscience & Biobehavioral Reviews, 22,* 161–172.

Goodale, M. A., & Haffenden, A. M. (2003). Interactions between dorsal and ventral streams of visual processing. In A. Siegel, R. Andersen, H.-J. Freund, & D. Spencer (Eds.), *Advances in neurology: Vol. 93. The parietal lobe* (pp. 249–267). Philadelphia: Lippincott-Raven.

Goodale, M. A., Jakobson, L. S., & Keillor, J. M. (1994). Differences in the visual control of pantomimed and natural grasping movements. *Neuropsychologia, 32,* 1159–1178.

Goodale, M. A., & Milner, A. D. (1992). Separate visual pathways for perception and action. *Trends in Neuroscience, 15,* 20–25.

Goodale, M. A., & Milner, A. D. (2004). *Sight unseen: An exploration of conscious and unconscious vision.* Oxford, England: Oxford University Press.

Goodale, M. A., Milner, A. D., Jakobson, L. S., & Carey, D. P. (1991). A neurological dissociation between perceiving objects and grasping them. *Nature, 349,* 154–156.

Goodale, M. A., Pelisson, D., & Prablanc, C. (1986). Large adjustments in visually guided reaching do not depend on vision of the hand or perception of target displacement. *Nature, 320,* 748–750.

Goodale, M. A., Westwood, D. A., & Milner, A. D. (2003). Two distinct modes of control for object-directed action. In C. A. Heywood, A. D. Milner, & C. Blakemore (Eds.), *The roots of visual awareness: Progress in brain research* (pp. 131–144).

Gordon, A. M., Forssberg, H., Johansson, R. S., & Westling, G. (1991). Visual size cues in the programming of manipulative forces during precision grip. *Experimental Brain Research, 83,* 477–482.

Gordon, A. M., Westling, G., Cole, K. J., & Johansson, R. S. (1993). Memory representations underlying motor commands used during manipulation of common and novel objects. *Journal of Neurophysiology, 69,* 1789–1796.

Gouras, P. (1969). Antidromic responses of orthodromically identified ganglion cells in monkey retina. *Journal of Physiology, London, 204,* 407–419.

Green, M. F. (1996). What are the functional consequences of neurocognitive deficits in schizophrenia? *American Journal of Psychiatry, 153,* 321–330.

Green, M. F., Glahn, D., Engel, S. A., Nuechterlein, K. H., Sabb, F., Strojwas, M., & Cohen, M. S. (2005). Regional brain activity associated with visual backward masking. *Journal of Cognitive Neuroscience, 17,* 13–23.

Green, M. F., Mintz, J., Salveson, D., Nuechterlein, K. H., Breitmeyer, B. G., Light, G. A., & Braff, D. L. (2003). Visual masking as a probe for abnormal gamma range activity in schizophrenia. *Biological Psychiatry, 53,* 1113–1119.

Green, M. F., & Nuechterlein, K. H. (1999). Should schizophrenia be treated as a neurocognitive disorder? *Schizophrenia Bulletin, 25,* 309–319.

Green, M. F., Nuechterlein, K. H., & Breitmeyer, B. G. (1997). Backward masking performance in unaffected siblings of schizophrenic patients. *Archives of General Psychiatry, 54,* 465–472.

Green, M. F., Nuechterlein, K. H., Breitmeyer, B. G., & Mintz, J. (1999). Backward masking in unmedicated schizophrenic patients in psychotic remission: Possible reflection of aberrant cortical oscillation. *American Journal of Psychiatry, 156,* 1367–1373.

Green, M. F., Nuechterlein, K. H., & Mintz, J. (1994a). Backward masking in schizophrenia and mania: I. Specifying a mechanism. *Archives of General Psychiatry, 51,* 939–944.

Green, M. F., Nuechterlein, K. H., & Mintz, J. (1994b). Backward masking in schizophrenia and mania: II. Specifying the visual channels. *Archives of General Psychiatry, 51,* 945–951.

Green, M., & Walker, E. (1984). Susceptibility to backward masking in schizophrenic patients with positive or negative symptoms. *American Journal of Psychiatry, 141,* 1273–1275.

Green, M., & Walker, E. (1986). Symptom correlates of vulnerability to backward masking in schizophrenia. *American Journal of Psychiatry, 143,* 181–186.

Gregory, R. (1998). Flagging the present with qualia. In S. Rose (Ed.), *From brains to consciousness? Essays on the new sciences of the mind* (pp. 200–209). London: Allen Lane/Penguin Press.

Grill-Spector, K., & Malach, R. (2004). The human visual cortex. *Annual Review of Neuroscience, 27,* 649–677.

Grinvald, A., Lieke, E. E., Frostig, R. D., & Hildescheim, R. (1994). Cortical point-spread function and long-range lateral interactions revealed by real-time optical imaging of macaque primary visual cortex. *Journal of Neuroscience, 14*, 2545–2568.

Grosbas, M.-H., & Paus, T. (2003). Transcranial magnetic stimulation of the human frontal eye field facilitates visual awareness. *European Journal of Neuroscience, 18*, 3121–3126.

Grossberg, S. (1972). A neural theory of punishment and avoidance: II. Quantitative theory. *Mathematical Biosciences, 15*, 253–285.

Grossberg, S. (1976a). Adaptive pattern classification and universal recoding: I. Parallel development and coding of neural feature detectors. *Biological Cybernetics, 23*, 121–134.

Grossberg, S. (1976b). Adaptive pattern classification and universal recoding: II. Feedback, expectation, olfaction, and illusions. *Biological Cybernetics, 23*, 187–202.

Grossberg, S. (1988). Nonlinear neural networks: Principles, mechanisms, and architectures. *Neural Networks, 1*, 17–61.

Grossberg, S. (1994). 3-D vision and figure–ground separation by visual cortex. *Perception & Psychophysics, 55*, 48–120.

Grossberg, S. (1999). The link between brain learning, attention, and consciousness. *Consciousness and Cognition, 8*, 1–44.

Grossberg, S., & Mingolla, E. (1985). Neural dynamics of form perception: Boundary completion, illusory figures, and neon color spreading. *Psychological Review, 92*, 173–211.

Growney, R., Weisstein, N., & Cox, S. I. (1977). Metacontrast as a function of spatial separation with narrow line targets and masks. *Vision Research, 17*, 1205–1210.

Grüsser, O. J., & Landis, T. (1991). *Visual agnosias and other disturbances of visual perception and cognition.* London: MacMillan.

Grunze, H. C., Rainnie, D. G., Hasselmo, M. E., Barkai, E., Hearn, E. F., & McCarley, R. W. (1996). NMDA-dependent modulation of CA1 local circuit inhibition. *Journal of Neuroscience, 16*, 2034–2043.

Gusel'nikov, V. I. (1976). [*Electrophysiology of the Brain*] (in Russian). Moscow: Vysshaya Shkola.

Haber, R. N. (Ed.). (1969). *Information processing approaches to visual perception.* New York: Holt, Rinehart & Winston.

Hadjikhani, N., Liu, A. K., Dale, A. M., Cavanagh, P., & Tootell, R. B. H. (1998). Retinotopy and color sensitivity in human visual cortical area V8. *Nature Neuroscience, 1*, 235–241.

Haffenden, A. M., & Goodale, M. A. (2000a). The effect of learned perceptual associations on visuomotor control varies with kinematic demands. *Journal of Cognitive Neuroscience, 12*, 950–964.

Haffenden, A. M., & Goodale, M. A. (2000b). Independent effects of pictorial displays on perception and action. *Vision Research, 40*, 1597–1607.

Haffenden, A. M., & Goodale, M. A. (2002a). Learned perceptual associations influence visuomotor programming under limited conditions: Cues as surface patterns. *Experimental Brain Research, 147*, 473–484.

Haffenden, A. M., & Goodale, M. A. (2002b). Learned perceptual associations influence visuomotor programming under limited conditions: Kinematic consistency. *Experimental Brain Research, 147*, 485–493.

Haffenden, A. M., Schiff, K. C., & Goodale, M. A. (2001). The dissociation between perception and action in the Ebbinghaus illusion: Nonillusory effects of pictorial cues on grasp. *Current Biology, 11*, 177–181.

Haig, A. R., Gordon, E., De Pascalis, V., Meares, R. A., Bahramali, H., & Harris, A. (2000). Gamma activity in schizophrenia: Evidence of impaired network binding? *Clinical Neurophysiology, 111*, 1461–1468.

Hallett, M. (2000). Transcranial magnetic stimulation and the human brain. *Nature, 406*, 147–150.

Hamker, F. H. (2004). A dynamic model of how feature cues guide spatial attention. *Vision Research, 44*, 501–521.

Hanlon, R. E. (Ed.). (1991). *Cognitive microgenesis: A neuropsychological perspective.* New York: Springer-Verlag.

Hansen, J. C., & Hillyard, S. A. (1980). Endogenous brain potentials associated with selective auditory attention. *Electroencephalography and Clinical Neurophysiology, 49*, 277–290.

Harter, M. R., & Guido, W. (1980). Attention to pattern orientation: Negative cortical potentials, reaction time, and the selection process. *Electroencephalography and Clinical Neurophysiology, 49*, 461–475.

Harter, M. R., & Previc, F. H. (1978). Size-specific information channels and selective attention: Visual evoked potential and behavioral measures. *Electroencephalography and Clinical Neurophysiology, 45*, 628–640.

Hartmann, J. A., Wolz, W. A., Roeltgen, D. P., & Loverso, F. L. (1991). Denial of visual perception. *Brain and Cognition, 16*, 29–40.

Harwerth, R. S., Boltz, R. L., & Smith, E. L. (1980). Psychophysical evidence for sustained and transient channels in the monkey visual system. *Vision Research, 20*, 15–22.

He, Z. J., & Nakayama, K. (1994). Perceived surface shape, not features, determines correspondence strength in apparent motion. *Vision Research, 34*, 2125–2135.

Hebb, D. O. (1949). *The organization of behavior*. New York: Wiley.

Heinze, H. J., Luck, S. J., Mangun, G. R., & Hillyard, S. A. (1990). Visual event-related potentials index focused attention within bilateral stimulus arrays: I. Evidence for early selection. *Electroencephalography and Clinical Neurophysiology, 75*, 511–527.

Heinze, H. J., Mangun, G. R., Burchert, W., Hinrichs, H., Scholz, M., Münte, T. F., Gös, A., Scherg, M., Johannes, S., & Hundeshagen, H. (1994). Combined spatial and temporal imaging of brain activity during visual selective attention in humans. *Nature, 372*, 543–546.

Heller, J., Hertz, J. A., Kjaer, T. W., & Richmond, B. J. (1995). Information flow and temporal coding in primate pattern vision. *Journal of Computational Neuroscience, 2*, 175–193.

Hellige, J. B., Walsh, D. A., Lawrence, V. W., & Prasse, M. (1979). Figural relationship effects and mechanisms of visual masking. *Journal of Experimental Psychology: Human Perception and Performance, 5*, 88–100.

Helmholtz, H. V. (1866). *Handbuch der physiologischen Optik* (1st ed.). Leipzig: Voss. (Trans. J. P. C. Southall, 1962. *Handbook of physiological optics*, 3rd ed. New York: Dover.)

Hendry, S. H., & Reid, R. C. (2000). The koniocellular pathway in primate vision. *Annual Review of Neuroscience, 23*, 127–153.

Henik, A., Rafal, R., & Rhodes, D. (1994). Endogenously generated and visually guided saccades after lesions of the human frontal eye fields. *Journal of Cognitive Neuroscience, 6*, 400–411.

Herzog, M. H., Dependahl, S., Schmonsees, U., & Fahle, M. (2004a). Valences in contextual vision. *Vision Research, 44*, 3131–3143.

Herzog, M. H., Ernst, U., Etzold, A., & Eurich, C. (2003a). Local interactions in neural networks explain global effects in gestalt processing and masking. *Neural Computation, 15*, 2091–2113.

Herzog, M. H., & Fahle, M. (2002). Effects of grouping on contextual modulation. *Nature, 415*, 433–436.

Herzog, M. H., Fahle, M., & Koch, C. (2001a). Spatial aspects of object formation revealed by a new illusion, shine-through. *Vision Research, 41*, 2325–2335. [Please read Erratum: *Vision Research, 42*, 271.]

Herzog, M. H., Harms, M., Ernst, U., Eurich, C., Mahmud, S., & Fahle, M. (2003b). Extending the shine-through effect to classical masking paradigms. *Vision Research, 43*, 2659–2667.

Herzog, M. H., & Koch, C. (2001). Seeing properties of an invisible element: Feature inheritance and shine-through. *Proceedings of the National Academy of Sciences, USA, 98*, 4271–4275.

Herzog, M. H., Koch, C., & Fahle, M. (2001b). Shine-through: Temporal aspects. *Vision Research, 41*, 2337–2346.

Herzog, M. H., Kopmann, S., & Brand, A. (2004b). Intact figure–ground-segmentation in schizophrenic patients. *Psychiatry Research, 129*, 55–63.

Herzog, M. H., Parish, L., Koch, C., & Fahle, M. (2003c). Fusion of competing features is not serial. *Vision Research, 43*, 1951–1960.

Herzog, M. H., Schmonsees, U., & Fahle, M. (2003d). Collinear contextual suppression. *Vision Research, 43*, 2915–2925.

Heywood, C. A., Kentridge, R. W., & Cowey, A. (2001). Colour and the cortex: Wavelength processing in cortical achromatopsia. In B. de Gelder, E. de Haan, & C. Heywood (Eds.), *Out of mind* (pp. 52–68). Oxford, England: Oxford University Press.

Hikosaka, O., Miyauchi, S., & Shimojo, S. (1993). Voluntary and stimulus-induced attention detected as motion sensation. *Perception, 22*, 517–526.

Hillyard, S. A., Hink, R. F., Schwent, V. L., & Picton, T. W. (1973). Electrical signs of selective attention in the human brain. *Science, 182*, 177–179.

Hillyard, S. A., & Münte, T. F. (1984). Selective attention to color and location: An analysis with event-related brain potentials. *Perception and Psychophysics, 36*, 185–198.

Hillyard, S. A., Vogel, E. K., & Luck, S. J. (1998). Sensory gain control (amplification) as a mechanism of selective attention: Electrophysiological and neuroimaging evidence. *Philosophical Transactions of the Royal Society of London, B, 353*, 1257–1270.

Hobson, J. A., & Steriade, M. (1986). The neuronal basis of behavioral state control: Internal regulatory systems of the brain. In F. Bloom & V. Mountcastle (Eds.), *Handbook of physiology* (Vol. 4, pp. 701–823). Baltimore: American Physiological Society.

Hochberg, J. (1968). In the mind's eye. In R. N. Haber (Ed.), *Contemporary theory and research in visual perception* (pp. 309–331). New York: Holt, Rhinehart & Winston.

Hochstein, S., & Ahissar, M. (2002). View from the top: Hierarchies and reverse hierarchies in the visual system. *Neuron, 36*, 791–804.

Hoeger, R. (1997). Speed of processing and stimulus complexity in low-frequency and high-frequency channels. *Perception, 26*, 1039–1045.

Hopf, J.-M., Boelmans, K., Schoenfeld, A. M., Luck, S. J., & Heinze, H.-J. (2004). Attention to features precedes attention to locations in visual search: Evidence from electromagnetic brain responses in humans. *Journal of Neuroscience, 24*, 1822–1832.

Hopf, J.-M., Luck, S. J., Girelli, M., Hagner, T., Mangun, G. R., Scheich, H., & Heinze, H.-J. (2000). Neural sources of focused attention in visual search. *Cerebral Cortex, 10*, 1233–1241.

Hopf, J.-M., Vogel, E. K., Woodman, G. F., Heinze, H.-J., & Luck, S. J. (2002). Localizing visual discrimination processes in time and space. *Journal of Neurophysiology, 88*, 2088–2095.

Hu, Y., & Goodale, M. A. (2000). Grasping after a delay shifts size-scaling from absolute to relative metrics. *Journal of Cognitive Neuroscience, 12*, 856–868.

Hubel, D. H. (1988). *Eye, brain, and vision*. New York: Scientific American Library.

Hubel, D. H., & Wiesel, T. N. (1968). Receptive fields and functional architecture of monkey striate cortex. *Journal of Physiology, London, 195*, 215–243.

Hughes, H. C., Nozawa, G., & Kitterle, F. (1996). Global precedence, spatial frequency channels, and the statistics of natural images. *Journal of Cognitive Neuroscience, 8*, 197–230.

Humphreys, G. W., & Bruce, V. (1989). *Visual cognition*. Hove, England: Erlbaum.

Humphreys, G. W., Romani, C., Olson, A., Riddoch, M. J., & Duncan, J. (1994). Non-spatial extinction following lesions of the parietal lobe in humans. *Nature, 372*, 357–359.

Hupe, J. M., James, A. C., Girard, P., Payne, B., & Bullier, J. (2001). Feedback connections act on the early part of the responses in monkey visual cortex. *Journal of Neurophysiology, 85*, 134–145.

Hupe, J. M., James, A. C., Payne, B., Lomber, S. G., Girard, P., & Bullier, J. (1998). Cortical feedback improves discrimination between figure and background by V1, V2 and V3 neurons. *Nature, 394*, 784–787.

Husain, M., & Rorden, C. (2003). Non-spatially lateralized mechanisms in hemispatial neglect. *Nature Reviews, 4*, 26–36.

Huxter, J., Burgess, N., & O'Keefe, J. (2003). Independent rate and temporal coding in hippocampal pyramidal cells. *Nature, 425*, 828–832.

Hyun, J.-S., & Luck, S. J. (submitted). *Allocation of attention during feature detection and feature localization*.

Intrilligator, J., & Cavanagh, P. (2001). The spatial resolution of visual attention. *Cognitive Psychology, 43*, 171–216.

Ishai, A., Ungerleider, L. G., Martin, A., Schouten, J. L., & Haxby, J. V. (1999). Distributed representation of objects in the human ventral visual pathway. *Proceedings of the National Academy of Sciences, USA, 96*, 9379–9384.

Ito, M., & Komatsu, H. (2004). Representation of angles embedded within contour stimuli in area V2 of macaque monkeys. *Journal of Neuroscience, 24*, 3313–3324.

Jahanshahi, M., & Rothwell, J. (2000). Transcranial magnetic stimulation studies of cognition: An emerging field. *Experimental Brain Research, 131*, 1–9.

James, T. W., Culham, J., Humphrey, G. K., Milner, D. A., & Goodale, M. A. (2003). Ventral occipital lesions impair object recognition but not object-directed grasping: An fMRI study. *Brain, 126*, 2463–2475.

James, T. W., Humphrey, G. K., Gati, J. S., Menon, R. S., & Goodale, M. A. (2002). Differential effects of viewpoint on object-driven activation in dorsal and ventral streams. *Neuron, 35*, 793–801.

Jaśkowski, P. (1996). Simple reaction time and perception of temporal order: Dissociations and hypotheses. *Perceptual and Motor Skills, 82*, 707–730.

Jaśkowski, P., Skalska, B., & Verleger, R. (2003). How the self controls its "automatic pilot" when processing subliminal information. *Journal of Cognitive Neuroscience, 15*, 911–920.

Jaśkowski, P., van der Lubbe, R., Schlotterbeck, E., & Verleger, R. (2002). Traces left on visual selective attention by stimuli that are not consciously identified. *Psychological Science, 13*, 48–54.

Jasper, H. H. (1949). Diffuse projection systems: The integrative action of the thalamic reticular system. *Electroencephalography and Clinical Neurophysiology, 1*, 405–420.

Jeannerod, M., Decety, D., & Michel, F. (1994). Impairment of grasping movement following a bilateral posterior parietal lesion. *Neuropsychologia, 32*, 369–380.

Jennett, B. (2002). The vegetative state. *Journal of Neurology, Neurosurgery and Psychiatry, 73*, 355–356.

Jiang, Y., & Chun, M. M. (2001a). The spatial gradient of visual masking by object substitution. *Vision Research, 41*, 3121–3131.

Jiang, Y., & Chun, M. M. (2001b). Asymmetric object substitution masking. *Journal of Experimental Psychology: Human Perception and Performance, 27*, 895–918.

John, E. R. (2003). A theory of consciousness. *Current Directions in Psychological Science, 12*, 244–250.

Johnson, J. S., & Olshausen, B. A. (2003). Timecourse of neural signatures of object recognition. *Journal of Vision, 3*, 499–512.

Jolicoeur, P., & Dell'Acqua, R. (1998). The demonstration of short-term consolidation. *Cognitive Psychology, 36*, 138–202.

Jones, E. G. (1998). A new view of specific and nonspecific thalamocortical connections. In H. H. Jasper, L. Descarries, V. F. Castellucci, & S. Rossignol (Eds.), *Consciousness at the frontiers of neuroscience: Advances in neurology* (Vol. 77, pp. 49–71). Philadelphia: Lipincott-Ravell.

Jones, E. G., & Burton, H. (1976). A projection from the medial pulvinar to the amygdala in primates. *Brain Research, 104*, 142–147.

Julesz, B. (1972). *Foundations of Cyclopean perception*. Chicago: University of Chicago Press.

Julesz, B. (1981). Textons, the elements of texture perception, and their interactions. *Nature, 290*, 91–97.

Julesz, B., & White, B. (1969). Short term visual memory and the Pulfrich phenomenon. *Nature, 222*, 639–641.

Jung, R. (1973). Visual perception and neurophysiology. In R. Jung (Ed.), *Handbook of sensory physiology: Vol. VII/3a. Central processing of visual information: Part A* (pp. 1–152). New York: Springer-Verlag.

Kaas, J. H. (2000). Why does the brain have so many visual areas? In M. S. Gazzaniga (Ed.), *Cognitive neuroscience* (pp. 448–472). Malden, MA: Blackwell.

Kaas, J. H., & Huerta, M. F. (1988). The subcortical visual system of primates. In H. D. Steklis & J. Erwin (Eds.), *Comparative primate biology: Vol. 4. Neurosciences* (pp. 327–391). New York: Wiley-Liss.

Kahneman, D. (1968). Method, findings, and theory in studies of visual masking. *Psychological Bulletin, 70*, 404–425.

Kamitani, Y., & Shimojo, S. (1999). Manifestation of scotomas created by transcranial magnetic stimulation of human visual cortex. *Nature Neuroscience, 2*, 767–771

Kammer, T. (1999). Phosphenes and transient scotomas induced by magnetic stimulation of the occipital lobe: Their topographic relationship. *Neuropsychologia, 37*, 191–198.

Kammer, T., Scharnowski, F., & Herzog, M. H. (2003). Combining backward masking and transcranial magnetic stimulation in human observers. *Neuroscience Letters, 343*, 171–174.

Kang, K., Shelley, M., & Sompolinsky, H. (2003). Mexican hats and pinwheels in visual cortex. *Proceedings of the National Academy of Sciences, USA, 100*, 2848–2853.

Kanwisher, N. G. (1987). Repetition blindness: Type recognition without token individuation. *Cognition, 27*, 117–143.

Kanwisher, N., McDermott, J., & Chun, M. M. (1997). The fusiform face area: A module in human extrastriate cortex specialized for face perception. *Journal of Neuroscience, 17*, 4302–4311.

Kapadia, M. K., Ito, M., Gilbert, C. D., & Westheimer, G. (1995). Improvement in visual sensitivity by changes in local context: Parallel studies in human observers and in V1 of alert monkeys. *Neuron, 15*, 843–856.

Kaplan, E., & Shapley, R. M. (1986). The primate retina contains two types of retinal ganglion cells, with high and low contrast sensitivity. *Proceedings of the National Academy of Sciences USA, 83*, 2755–2757.

Karnath, H. O., Ferber, S., & Himmelbach, M. (2001). Spatial awareness is a function of the temporal not the posterior parietal lobe. [Comment in: *Nature*. 2001, June 21; 411(6840): 903–4 UI: 21312029]. *Nature, 411*, 950–953.

Karnath, H. O., Fruhmann Berger, M., Küker, W., & Rorden, C. (2004). The anatomy of spatial neglect based on voxelwise statistical analysis: A study of 140 patients. *Cerebral Cortex, 14*, 1164–1172.

Kastner, S., Demmer, I., & Ziemann, U. (1998). Transient visual field defects induced by transcranial magnetic stimulation over human occipital pole. *Experimental Brain Research, 118*, 19–26.

Kastner, S., De Weerd, P., & Ungerleider, L. G. (2000). Texture segregation in the human visual cortex: A functional MRI study. *Journal of Neurophysiology, 83*, 2453–2457.

Kastner, S., Pinsk, M. A., De Weerd, P., Desimone, R., & Ungerleider, L. G. (1999). Increased activity in human visual cortex during directed attention in the absence of visual stimulation. *Neuron, 22*, 751–761.

Keane, J. R. (1979). Blinking to sudden illumination: A brain stem reflex present in neocortical death. *Archives of Neurology, 36*, 52–53.

Kee, K. S., Kern, R. S., & Green, M. F. (1998). Perception of emotion and neurocognitive functioning in schizophrenia: What's the link? *Psychiatry Research, 81*(1), 57–65.

Kentridge, R. W., & Heywood, C. A. (2001). Attention and alerting: Cognitive processes spared in blindsight. In B. de Gelder, E. de Haan, & C. Heywood (Eds.), *Out of mind* (pp. 163–181). Oxford, England: Oxford University Press.

Kentridge, R. W., Heywood, C. A., & Weiskrantz, L. (2004). Spatial attention speeds discrimination without awareness in blindsight. *Neuropsychologia, 42*, 831–835.

Keri, S., Antal, A., Benedek, G., & Janka, Z. (2000). Visual information processing in patients with schizophrenia: Evidence for the impairment of central mechanism. *Neuroscience Letters, 293*(1), 69–71.

Keri, S., Kelemen, O., Benedek, G., & Janka, Z. (2001). Different trait markers for schizophrenia and bipolar disorder: A neurocognitive approach. *Psychological Medicine, 31*, 915–922.

Kerkhoff, G. (2001). Spatial neglect in humans. *Progress in Neurobiology, 63*, 1–27.

Kerzel, D., & Gegenfurtner, K. R. (2003). Neuronal processing delays are compensated in the sensorimotor branch of the visual system. *Current Biology, 13*, 1975–1978.

Khurana, B., & Nijhawan, R. (1995). Extrapolation or attentional shift?—Reply. *Nature, 378*, 566.

Khurana, B., Watanabe, K., & Nijhawan, R. (2000). The role of attention in motion extrapolation: Are moving objects 'corrected' or flashed objects attentionally delayed? *Perception, 29*, 675–692.

Kiefer, M. (2002). The N400 is modulated by unconsciously perceived masked words: Further evidence for an automatic spreading activation account of N400 priming effects. *Brain Research. Cognitive Brain Research, 13*, 27–39.

Kihlstrom, J. F. (1996). Perception without awareness of what is perceived, learning without awareness of what is learned. In V. Velman (Ed.), *The science of consciousness* (pp. 23–46). London: Routledge.

Kim, H., & Francis, G. (1998). A computational and perceptual account of motion lines. *Perception, 27,* 785–797.

Kinoshita, S., & Lupker, S. (2003). *Masked priming.* New York: Psychology Press.

Klapp, S. T., & Hinkley, L. B. (2002). The negative compatibility effect: Unconscious inhibition influences reaction time and response selection. *Journal of Experimental Psychology: General, 131,* 255–269.

Klotz, W., & Neumann, O. (1999). Motor activation without conscious discrimination in metacontrast masking. *Journal of Experimental Psychology: Human Perception and Performance, 25,* 976–992.

Klotz, W., & Wolff, P. (1995). The effect of a masked stimulus on the response to the masking stimulus. *Psychological Research, 58,* 92–101.

Knierim, J. J., & VanEssen, D. C. (1992). Neuronal responses to static texture patterns in area-V1 of the alert macaque monkey. *Journal of Neurophysiology, 67,* 961–980.

Knill, D. C., & Richards, W. (Eds.). (1996). *Perception as Bayesian inference.* Cambridge, England: Cambridge University Press.

Koch, C. (2004). *The quest for consciousness: A neurobiological approach.* Englewood, CO: Roberts.

Koch, C., & Crick, F. (2001a). The zombie within. *Nature, 411,* 893.

Koch, C., & Crick, F. (2001b). Neural basis of consciousness. In *International encyclopedia of the social and behavioral sciences* (pp. 2600–2604). Amsterdam: Elsevier.

Koch, C., & Segev, I. (1989). *Methods in neuronal modeling.* Cambridge, MA: MIT Press.

Koechlin, E., Anton, J. L., & Burnod, Y. (1999). Bayesian inference in populations of cortical neurons: A model of motion integration and segregation in area MT.

Koffka, K. (1935). *Principles of Gestalt psychology.* New York: Harcourt Brace.

Kolers, P. A. (1962). Intensity and contour effects in visual masking. *Vision Research, 2,* 277–294.

Kolers, P. A. (1972). *Aspects of motion perception.* New York: Pergamon Press.

Kolers, P. A., & Rosner, B. S. (1960). On visual masking (metacontrast): Dichoptic observation. *American Journal of Psychology, 73,* 2–21.

Kouider, S., & Dupoux, E. (2004). Partial awareness creates the "illusion" of subliminal semantic priming. *Psychological Science, 15,* 75–81.

Kóvacs, G., Vogels, R., & Orban, G. A. (1995). Cortical correlates of pattern backward-masking. *Proceedings of the National Academy of Sciences, USA, 92,* 5587–5591.

Kovács, I., Papathomas, T. V., Yang, M., & Fehér, Á. (1996). When the brain chages its mind: Interocular grouping during binocular rivalry. *Proceedings of the National Academy of Sciences, USA, 93,* 15508–15511.

Kragh, U., & Smith, G. (1970). *Percept-genetic analysis.* Lund, Sweden: Gleerup.

Kreegipuu, K., & Allik, J. (2003). Perceived onset time and position of a moving stimulus. *Vision Research, 43,* 1625–1635.

Kreiman, G., Fried, I., & Koch, C. (2002). Single-neuron correlates of subjective vision in the human medial temporal lobe. *Proceedings of the National Academy of Sciences, USA, 99,* 8378–8383.

Krekelberg, B., & Lappe, M. (2000). A model of the perceived relative positions of moving objects based upon a slow averaging process. *Vision Research, 40,* 201–215.

Krekelberg, B., & Lappe, M. (2001). Neuronal latencies and the position of moving objects. *Trends in Neurosciences, 24,* 335–339.

Kremers, J. (1999). Spatial and temporal response properties of the major retino-geniculate pathways of Old and New World monkeys, *Documenta Ophthalmologica, 95,* 229–245.

Kulikowski, J. J., & Tolhurst, D. J. (1973). Psychophysical evidence for sustained and transient detectors in human vision. *Journal of Physiology, 232,* 149–162.

Kwon, J. S., O'Donnell, B. F., Wallenstein, G. V., Greene, R. W., Hirayasu, Y., Nestor, P. G., et al. (1999). Gamma frequency-range abnormalities to auditory stimulation in schizophrenia. *Archives of General Psychiatry, 56,* 1001–1005.

LaBerge, D. (1995). *Attentional processing*. Cambridge, MA: Harvard University Press.

Ladavas, E., Cimatti, D., Del Pesce, M., & Tuozzi, G. (1993a). Emotional evaluation with and without conscious stimulus identification: Evidence from a split-brain patient. *Cognition and Emotion, 7*, 95–114.

Ladavas, E., Paladini, R., & Cubelli, R. (1993b). Implicit associative priming in a patient with left visual neglect. *Neuropsychologia, 31*, 1307–1320.

Ladavas, E., Zeloni, G., Zaccara, G., & Gangemi, P. (1997). Eye movements and orienting of attention in patients with visual neglect. *Journal of Cognitive Neuroscience, 9*, 67–74.

Lamme, V. A. F. (1995). The neurophysiology of figure–ground segregation in primary visual cortex. *Journal of Neuroscience, 15*, 1605–1615.

Lamme, V. A. F. (2000). Neural mechanisms of visual awareness: A linking proposition. *Brain and Mind, 1*, 385–406.

Lamme, V. A. F. (2003). Why visual attention and awareness are different. *Trends in Cognitive Sciences, 7*, 12–18.

Lamme, V. A. F., Rodriquez-Rodriquez, V., & Spekreijse, H. (1999). Separate processing dynamics for texture elements, boundaries and surfaces in primary visual cortex of the macaque monkey. *Cerebral Cortex, 9*, 406–413.

Lamme, V. A. F., & Roelfsema, P. R. (2000). The distinct modes of vision offered by feedforward and recurrent processing. *Trends in Neuroscience, 23*, 571–579.

Lamme, V. A. F., & Spekreijse, H. (1998). Neuronal synchrony does not represent texture segregation. *Nature, 396*, 362–366.

Lamme, V. A., Super, H., Landman, R., Roelfsema, P. R., & Spekreijse, H. (2000). The role of primary visual cortex (V1) in visual awareness. *Vision Research, 40*, 1507–1521.

Lamme, V. A. F., Super, H., & Spekreijse, H. (1998a). Feedforward, horizontal, and feedback processing in the visual cortex. *Current Opinion in Neurobiology, 8*, 529–535.

Lamme, V. A. F., VanDijk, B. W., & Spekreijse, H. (1992). Texture segregation is processed by primary visual-cortex in man and monkey—Evidence from VEP experiments. *Vision Research, 32*, 797–807.

Lamme, V. A. F., Zipser, K., & Spekreijse, H. (1998b). Figure–ground activity in primary visual cortex is suppressed by anesthesia. *Proceedings of the National Academy of Sciences, USA, 95*, 3263–3268.

Lamme, V. A. F., Zipser, K., & Spekreijse, H. (2002). Masking interrupts figure–ground signals in V1. *Journal of Cognitive Neuroscience, 14*, 1044–1053.

Landahl, H. D. (1967). A neural net model for masking phenomena. *Bulletin of Mathematical Biophysics, 29*, 227–232.

Landy, M. S., & Bergen, J. R. (1991). Texture segregation and orientation gradient. *Vision Research, 31*, 679–691.

Lange, N. N. (1892a). The law of perception. I–II. (in Russian). *Voprosy Filosofii I Psikhologii, Spetsial'nyi Otdel, 13*, 18–37.

Lange, N. N. (1892b). The law of perception. III. (in Russian). *Voprosy Filosofii I Psikhologii, Spetsial'nyi Otdel, 14*, 44–54.

Lange, N. N. (1892c). The law of perception. IV–V. (in Russian). *Voprosy Filosofii I Psikhologii, Spetsial'nyi Otdel, 15*, 55–68.

Lange, N. N. (1892d). The law of perception. VI–VII. (in Russian). *Voprosy Filosofii I Psikhologii, Spetsial'nyi Otdel, 16*, 25–38.

Lappe, M., & Krekelberg, B. (1998). The position of moving objects. *Perception, 27*, 1437–1449.

Laureys, S., Antoine, S., Boly, M., Elincx, S., Faymonville, M.-E., Berré, J., Sadzot, B., Ferring, M., De Tiege, X., Van Bogaert, T., Hansen, I., Damas, P., Mavroudakis, N., Lambermont, B., del Fiore, G., Aerts, J., Delguedre, C., Phillips, C., Franck, G., Vincent, J.-L., Lamy, M., Luxen, A., Moonen, G., Goldman, S., & Maquet, P. (2002). Brain function in the vegetative state. *Acta Neurologica Belgica, 102*, 177–185.

Lawrence, D. H. (1971). Two studies of visual search for word targets with controlled rates of presentation. *Perception and Psychophysics, 10*, 85–89.

Lee, T. S., Mumford, D., Romero, R., & Lamme, V. A. F. (1998). The role of the primary visual cortex in higher level vision, *Vision Research*, *38*, 2429–2454.

Lee, B. B., Pokorny, J., Smith, V. C., Martin, P. R., & Valberg, A. (1990). Luminance and chromatic modulation sensitivity of macaque ganglion cells and human observers. *Journal of the Optical Society of America, A*, *7*, 2223–2236.

Lee, K.-H., Williams, L. M., Breakspear, M., & Gordon, E. (2003). Synchronous gamma activity: A review and contribution to an integrative neuroscience model of schizophrenia. *Brain Research Reviews*, *41*, 57–78.

Lee, S. H., & Blake, R. (2004). A fresh look at interocular grouping during binocular rivalry. *Vision Research*, *44*, 983–991.

Lee, T. S., & Mumford, D. (2003). Hierarchical Bayesian inference in the visual cortex. *Journal of the Optical Society of America, A*, *20*, 1434–1448.

Lee, T. S., Mumford, D., Romero, R., & Lamme, V. A. F. (1998). The role of the primary visual cortex in higher level vision. *Vision Research*, *38*, 2429–2454.

Lee, T., Mumford, D., & Schiller, P. (1995). Neuronal correlates of boundary and medial axis representations in primate visual cortex. *Journal of Investigative Ophthalmology and Visual Science*, *36*, 477.

Lee, T. S., Yang, C. F., Romero, R. D., & Mumford, D. (2002). Neural activity in early visual cortex reflects behavioral experience and higher-order perceptual saliency. *Nature Neuroscience*, *5*, 589–597.

Leeuwenberg, E., Mens, L., & Calis, G. (1985). Knowledge within perception: Masking caused by incompatible interpretation. *Acta Psychologica*, *55*, 91–102.

Legge, G. (1978). Sustained and transient mechanisms in human vision: Temporal and spatial properties. *Vision Research*, *18*, 341–376.

Lennie, P. (1981). The physiological basis of variations in visual latency. *Vision Research*, *21*, 815–824.

Lennie, P. (1998). Single units and visual cortical organization. *Perception*, *27*, 889–935.

Leopold, D. A., & Logothetis, N. K. (1996). Activity changes in early visual cortex reflect monkeys' percepts during binocular rivalry. *Nature*, *379*, 549–552.

Leopold, D. A., & Logothetis, N. K. (1999). Multistable phenomena: Changing views in perception. *Trends in Cognitive Sciences*, *3*, 254–264.

Leuthold, H., & Kopp, B. (1998). Mechanisms of priming by masked stimuli: Inferences from event-related brain potentials. *Psychological Science*, *9*, 263–269.

Leventhal, A. G., Thompson, K. G., Liu, D., Zhou, Y., & Ault, S. J. (1995). Concomitant sensitivity to orientation, direction, and color of cells in layers 2, 3, and 4 of monkey striate cortex. *Journal of Neuroscience*, *15*, 1808–1818.

Li, C. Y., & Li, W. (1994). Extensive integration field beyond the classical receptive field of cat's striate cortical neurons: Classification and tuning properties. *Vision Research*, *34*, 2337–2355.

Li, W., Thier, P., & Wehrhahn, C. (2000). Contextual influence on orientation discrimination of humans and responses of neurons in V1 of alert monkeys. *Journal of Neurophysiology*, *83*, 941–954.

Li, Z. P. (2000). Can V1 mechanisms account for figure–ground and medial-axis effects? In S. A. Solla, T. K. Leen, & K.-R. Muller (Eds.), *Advances in neural information processing systems* (Vol. 12, pp. 134–142). Cambridge, MA: MIT Press.

Li, Z. P. (2003). V1 mechanisms and some figure–ground and border effects. *Journal of Physiology*, *97*, 503–515.

Libet, B. (1966). Brain stimulation and the threshold of conscious experience. In J. C. Eccles (Ed.), *Brain and conscious experience* (pp. 165–181). Berlin, Germany: Springer-Verlag.

Libet, B. (1973). Electrical stimulation of cortex in human subjects and conscious sensory aspects. In A. Iggo (Ed.), *Handbook of sensory physiology: Vol. 2. Somatosensory systems* (pp. 743–790). Berlin, Germany: Springer-Verlag.

Libet, B. (1985). Unconscious cerebral initiative and the role of conscious will in voluntary action. *Behavioral and Brain Sciences*, *8*, 529–566.

Libet, B. (1993). *Neurophysiology of consciousness: Selected papers and new essays by Benjamin Libet*. Boston: Birkhäuser.

Libet, B. (2002). The timing of mental events: Libet's experimental findings and their implications. *Consciousness and Cognition*, *11*, 291–299.

Libet, B. (2004). *Mind time*. Cambridge, MA: Harvard University Press.

Lissauer, H. (1890). Ein Fall von Seelenblindheit nebst einem Baeitrage zur Theorie derselben. *Archiv der Psychiatrie und Nervenkrankheiten*, *21*, 222–270.

Lit, A. (1960). The magnitude of the Pulfrich stereophenomenon as a function of target velocity. *Journal of Experimental Psychology*, *59*, 165–175.

Liu, J., Harris, A., & Kanwisher, N. (2002). Stages of processing in face perception: An MEG study. *Nature Neuroscience*, *5*, 910–916.

Liu, T., & Cooper, L. A. (2001). The influence of task requirements on priming in object decision and matching. *Memory & Cognition*, *29*, 874–882.

Livingstone, M., & Hubel, D. (1988). Segregation of form, color, movement, and depth: Anatomy, physiology, and perception. *Science*, *240*, 740–749.

Lleras, A., & Enns, J. T. (2004). Negative compatibility or object updating? A cautionary tale of mask-dependent priming. *Journal of Experimental Psychology: General*, *133*, 475–493.

Lleras, A., & Moore, C. M. (2003). When the target becomes the mask: Using apparent motion to isolate the object-level component of object substitution masking. *Journal of Experimental Psychology: Human Perception and Performance*, *29*, 106–120.

Lleras, A., Rensink, R. A., & Enns, J. T. (in press). Rapid resumption of interrupted search reveals new role for memory in human vision, *Psychological Science*.

Llinás, R. R. (2001). *I of the vortex: From neurons to self*. Cambridge, MA: MIT Press.

Llinás, R., & Pare, D. (1996). The brain as a closed system modulated by the senses. In R. Llinas & P. S. Churchland (Eds.), *The mind–brain continuum* (pp. 1–8). Cambridge, MA: MIT Press.

Loftus, G. R., & Masson, M. E. (1994). Using confidence intervals in within-subject designs. *Psychonomic Bulletin & Review*, *1*, 476–490.

Logan, G. D. (1996). The CODE theory of visual attention: An integration of space-based and object-based attention. *Psychological Review*, *103*, 603–649.

Luck, S. J. (1995). Multiple mechanisms of visual-spatial attention: Recent evidence from human electrophysiology. *Behavioural Brain Research*, *71*, 113–123.

Luck, S. J., Chelazzi, L., Hillyard, S. A., & Desimone, R. (1997a). Neural mechanisms of spatial selective attention in areas V1, V2, and V4 of macaque visual cortex. *Journal of Neurophysiology*, *77*, 24–42.

Luck, S. J., Fan, S., & Hillyard, S. A. (1993). Attention-related modulation of sensory-evoked brain activity in a visual search task. *Journal of Cognitive Neuroscience*, *5*, 188–195.

Luck, S. J., & Ford, M. A. (1998). On the role of selective attention in visual perception. *Proceedings of the National Academy of Sciences, USA*, *95*, 825–830.

Luck, S. J., Girelli, M., McDermott, M. T., & Ford, M. A. (1997b). Bridging the gap between monkey neurophysiology and human perception: An ambiguity resolution theory of visual selective attention. *Cognitive Psychology*, *33*, 64–87.

Luck, S. J., Heinze, H. J., Mangun, G. R., & Hillyard, S. A. (1990). Visual event-related potentials index focused attention within bilateral stimulus arrays: II. Functional dissociation of P1 and N1 components. *Electroencephalography and Clinical Neurophysiology*, *75*, 528–542.

Luck, S. J., & Hillyard, S. A. (1990). Electrophysiological evidence for parallel and serial processing during visual search. *Perception & Psychophysics*, *48*, 603–617.

Luck, S. J., & Hillyard, S. A. (1994a). Electrophysiological correlates of feature analysis during visual search. *Psychophysiology*, *31*, 291–308.

Luck, S. J., & Hillyard, S. A. (1994b). Spatial filtering during visual search: Evidence from human electrophysiology. *Journal of Experimental Psychology: Human Perception and Performance*, *20*, 1000–1014.

Luck, S. J., & Hillyard, S. A. (1995). The role of attention in feature detection and conjunction discrimination: An electrophysiological analysis. *International Journal of Neuroscience, 80*, 281–297.

Luck, S. J., Hillyard, S. A., Mouloua, M., Woldorff, M. G., Clark, V. P., & Hawkins, H. L. (1994). Effects of spatial cuing on luminance detectability: Psychophysical and electrophysiological evidence for early selection. *Journal of Experimental Psychology: Human Perception and Performance, 20*, 887–904.

Luck, S. J., Vogel, E. K., & Shapiro, K. L. (1996). Word meanings can be accessed but not reported during the attentional blink. *Nature, 383*, 616–618.

Lumer, E. D., Friston, K. J., & Rees, G. (1998). Neural correlates of perceptual rivalry in the human brain. *Science, 280*, 1930–1934.

Luria, A. R. (1969). *The mind of a mnemonist*. London: Jonathan Cape.

MacDonald, A. W., III, Cohen, J. D., Stenger, V. A., & Carter, C. S. (2000). Dissociating the role of the dorsolateral prefrontal and anterior cingulate cortex in cognitive control. *Science, 288*, 1835–1838.

Mack, A., & Rock, I. (1998). *Inattentional blindness*. Cambridge, MA: MIT Press.

MacKay, D. M. (1958). Perceptual stability of a stroboscopically lit visual field containing self-luminous objects. *Nature, 181*, 507–508.

MacKay, D. M. (1973). Lateral interaction between neural channels sensitive to texture density. *Nature, 245*, 159–161.

Macknik, S. L., & Livingstone, M. S. (1998). Neuronal correlates of visibility and invisibility in the primate visual system. *Nature Neuroscience, 1*, 144–149.

Macknik, S. L., Martinez-Conde, S., & Haglund, M. M. (2000). The role of spatiotemporal edges in visibility and visual masking. *Proceedings of the National Academy of Sciences, USA, 97*, 7556–7560.

Maffei, L., & Fiorentini, A. (1976). The unresponsive regions of visual cortical receptive fields. *Vision Research, 16*, 1131–1139.

Magoun, H. W. (1958). *The waking brain*. Springfield, IL: C. C. Thomas.

Maki, W. S., Frigen, K., & Paulson, K. (1997). Associative priming by targets and distractors during rapid serial visual presentation: Does word meaning survive the attentional blink? *Journal of Experimental Psychology: Human Perception and Performance, 23*, 1014–1034.

Malach, R., Amir, Y., Harel, M., & Grinvald, A. (1993). Relationship between intrinsic connections and functional architecture revealed by optical imaging and in vivo targeted biocytin injections. *Proceedings of the National Academy of Sciences, USA, 90*, 10469–10473.

Mangun, G. R., & Hillyard, S. A. (1991). Modulations of sensory-evoked brain potentials indicate changes in perceptual processing during visual-spatial priming. *Journal of Experimental Psychology: Human Perception and Performance, 17*, 1057–1074.

Manly, T., Woldt, K., Watson, P., & Warburton, E. (2002). Is motor perseveration in unilateral neglect "driven" by the presence of neglected leftsided stimuli? *Neuropsychologia, 40*, 1794–1803.

Marcel, A. J. (1983a). Conscious and unconscious perception: Experiments on visual masking and word recognition. *Cognitive Psychology, 15*, 197–237.

Marcel, A. J. (1983b). Conscious and unconscious perception: An approach to the relations between phenomenal experience and perceptual processes. *Cognitive Psychology, 15*, 238–300.

Marcus, D. S., & Van Essen, D. C. (2002). Scene segmentation and attention in primate cortical areas V1 and V2. *Journal of Neurophysiology, 88*, 2648–2658.

Marr, D. (1982). *Vision: A computational investigation into the human representation and processing of visual information*. San Francisco: Freeman.

Martin, E., Thiel, T., Joeri, P., Loenneker, T., Ekatodramis, E., Huisman, T., Hennig, J., & Marcar, V. L. (2000). Effect of pentobarbital on visual processing in man. *Human Brain Mapping, 10*, 132–139.

Martin, K. A. C. (1992). Parallel pathways converge. *Current Biology, 2*, 555–557.

Martinez, A., Di Russo, F., Anllo-Vento, L., Sereno, M. I., Buxton, R. B., & Hillyard, S. A. (2001). Putting spatial attention on the map: Timing and localization of stimulus selection processes in striate and extrastriate visual areas. *Vision Research, 41*, 1437–1457.

Marzi, C. A., Tassinari, G., Lutzemberger, L., & Aglioti, A. (1986). Spatial summation across vertical meridian in henianopics. *Neuropsychologia, 24*, 749–758.

Mateeff, S., Genova, B., & Hohnsbein, J. (1999). The simple reaction time to changes in direction of visual motion. *Experimental Brain Research, 124*, 391–394.

Mateeff, S., & Hohnsbein, J. (1988). Perceptual latencies are shorter for motion towards the fovea than for motion away. *Vision Research, 28*, 711–719.

Matell, M. S., & Meck, W. H. (2000). Neuropsychological mechanisms of interval timing behavior. *Bioessays, 22*, 94–103.

Matin, E. (1975). The two-transient (masking) paradigm. *Psychological Review, 82*, 451–461.

Mattingley, J. B., Bradshaw, J. L., & Bradshaw, J. A. (1995). The effects of unilateral visuospatial neglect on perception of Müller–Lyer illusory figures. *Perception, 24*, 415–433.

Mattler, U. (2003). Priming of mental operations by masked stimuli. *Perception & Psychophysics, 65*, 167–187.

Maunsell, J. H. R., Ghose, G. G., Assas, J. A., McAdams, C. J., Boudreau, C. E., & Noerager, B. D. (1999). Visual response latencies of magnocellular and parvocellular LGN neurons in macaque monkeys. *Visual Neuroscience, 16*, 1–14.

Maunsell, J. H. R., & Gibson, J. R. (1992). Visual response latencies in striate cortex of the macaque monkey. *Journal of Neurophysiology, 68*, 1332–1344.

Maunsell, J. H., & Van Essen, D. C. (1983). Functional properties of neurons in middle temporal visual area of the macaque monkey: I. Selectivity for stimulus direction, speed, and orientation. *Journal of Neurophysiology, 49*, 1127–1147.

McCarley, R. W., Hsiao, J., Freedman, R., Pfefferbaum, A., & Donchin, E. (1996). Neuroimaging and the cognitive neuroscience of schizophrenia. *Schizophrenia Bulletin, 22*, 703–726.

McCarter, A., & Roehrs, T. (1976). A spatial frequency analogue to Mach bands. *Vision Research, 16*, 1317–1321.

McElree, B., & Carrasco, M. (1999). The temporal dynamics of visual search: Evidence for parallel processing in feature and conjunction searches. *Journal of Experimental Psychology: Human Perception and Performance, 25*, 1517–1539.

McGlinchey-Berroth, R., Milberg, W. P., Verfaellie, M., Alexander, M., & Kilduff, P. T. (1993). Semantic processing in the neglected visual field: Evidence from a lexical decision task. *Cognitive Neuropsychology, 10*, 79–108.

McIntosh, R. (2000). Seeing size and weight. *Trends in Cognitive Sciences, 4*, 442–444.

Meadows, J. C. (1974). Disturbed perception of colours associated with localized cerebral lesions. *Brain, 97*, 615–632.

Merikle, P. M., & Daneman, M. (1998). Psychological investigations of nonconscious perception. *Journal of Consciousness Studies, 5*, 5–18.

Merikle, P. M., & Joordens, S. (1997). Parallels between perception without attention and perception without awareness. *Consciousness and Cognition, 6*, 219–236.

Merikle, P. M., Joordens, S., & Stolz, J. A. (1995). Measuring the relative magnitude of unconscious influences. *Consciousness and Cognition, 4*, 422–439.

Metzger, W. (1932). Versuch einer gemeinsamen Theorie der Phänomene Fröhlich's und Hazelhoff's und Kritik ihrer Verfahren zur Messung der Empfindungszeit. *Psychological Research/Psychologische Forschung, 16*, 176–200.

Metzinger, T. (Ed.). (1995). *Conscious experience*. Paderborn, Germany: Schöningh/Imprint Academic.

Metzinger, T. (2000). *Neural correlates of consciousness*. Cambridge, MA: MIT Press.

Michaels, C. F., & Turvey, M. T. (1979). Central sources of visual masking: Indexing structures supporting seeing at a single, brief glance. *Psychological Research, 41*, 1–61.

Mignard, M., & Malpeli, J. G. (1991). Paths of information flow through visual cortex. *Science, 251*, 1249–1251.

Milner, A. D., Dijkerman, H. C., Pisella, L., McIntosh, R. D., Tilikete, C., Vighetto, A., & Rossetti, Y. (2001). Grasping the past: Delay can improve visuomotor performance. *Current Biology, 11*, 1–20.

Milner, A. D., & Goodale, M. A. (1995). *The visual brain in action*. Oxford, England: Oxford University Press.

Milner, A. D., Paulignan, Y., Dijkerman, H. C., Michel, F., & Jeannerod, M. (1999). A paradoxical improvement of misreaching in optic ataxia: New evidence for two separate neural systems for visual localization. *Proceedings of the Royal Society of London, B, 266*, 2225–2229.

Milner, A. D., Perrett, D. I., Johnston, R. S., Benson, P. J., Jordan, T. R., Heeley, D. W., Bettucci, D., Mortara, F., Mutani, R., & Terazzi, E., Davidson, D. L. W. (1991). Perception and action in "visual form agnosia." *Brain, 114*, 405–428.

Milner, B., & Teuber, H.-L. (1968). Alteration of perception and memory in man. In L. Weiskrantz (Ed.), *Analysis of behavioral change* (pp. 268–376). New York: Harper & Row.

Mithen, S. (1996). *The prehistory of the mind*. London: Thames & Hudson.

Moran, J., & Desimone, R. (1985). Selective attention gates visual processing in the extrastriate cortex. *Science, 229*, 782–784.

Mordkoff, J. T., Yantis, S., & Egeth, H. E. (1990). Detecting conjunctions of color and form in parallel. *Perception & Psychophysics, 48*, 157–568.

Morris, J. S., Öhman, A., & Dolan, R. J. (1998). Conscious and unconscious emotional learning in the human amygdala. *Nature, 393*, 467–470.

Mort, D. J., Malhotra, P., Mannan, S. K., Rorden, C., Pambakian, A., Kennard, C., & Husain, M. (2003). The anatomy of visual neglect. *Brain, 126*, 1986–1997.

Moruzzi, G., & Magoun, W. (1949). Brainstem reticular formation and activation of the EEG. *Electroencephalography and Clinical Neurophysiology, 1*, 455–473.

Motter, B. C. (1994). Neural correlates of attentive selection for color or luminance in extrastriate area V4. *Journal of Neuroscience, 14*, 2178–2189.

Moutoussis, K., & Zeki, S. (1997a). A direct demonstration of perceptual asynchrony in vision. *Proceedings of the Royal Society of London, B, 264*, 393–399.

Moutoussis, K., & Zeki, S. (1997b). Functional segregation and temporal hierarchy of the visual perceptive systems. *Proceedings of the Royal Society of London, B, 264*, 1407–1414.

Moutoussis, K., & Zeki, S. (2002). The relationship between cortical activation and perception investigated with invisible stimuli. *Proceedings of the National Academy of Sciences, USA, 99*, 9527–9532.

Mumford, D. (1992). On the computational architecture of the neocortex: II. The role of cortico-cortical loops. *Biological Cybernetics, 66*, 241–251.

Munk, M. H., Nowak, L. G., Girard, P., Chounlamountri, N., & Bullier, J. (1995). Visual latencies in cytochrome oxidase bands of macaque area V2. *Proceedings of the National Academy of Sciences, USA, 92*, 988–992.

Munk, M. H. J., Roelfsema, P. R., König, P., Engel, A. K., & Singer, W. (1996). Role of reticular activation in the modulation of intracortical synchronization. *Science, 272*, 271–274.

Müsseler, J., Stork, S., & Kerzel, D. (2002). Comparing mislocalizations with moving stimuli: The Fröhlich effect, the flash-lag, and representational momentum. *Visual Cognition, 9*, 120–138.

Naatanen, R. (1975). Selective attention and evoked potentials in humans—A critical review. *Biological Psychology, 2*, 237–307.

Naccache, L., Blandin, E., & Dehaene, S. (2002). Unconscious masked priming depends on temporal attention. *Psychological Science, 13*, 416–424.

Naccache, L., & Dehaene, S. (2001). The priming method: Imaging unconscious repetition priming reveals an abstract representation of number in parietal lobes. *Cerebral Cortex, 11*, 966–974.

Nakayama, K., & Shimojo, S. (1992). Experiencing and perceiving visual surfaces. *Science, 257*, 1357–1363.

Nakayama, K., Shimojo, S., & Silverman, G. H. (1989). Stereoscopic depth—Its relation to image segmentation, grouping, and the recognition of occluded objects. *Perception, 18*, 55–68.

Namba, J., & Baldo, M. V. C. (2004). The modulation of the flash-lag effect by voluntary attention. *Perception, 33*, 621–631.

Navon, D. (1977). Forest before trees: The precedence of global features in visual perception. *Cognitive Psychology, 9*, 353–383.

Navon, D., & Purcell, D. G. (1981). Does integration produce masking or protect from it? *Perception, 10*, 71–84.

Neill, W. T., Hutchison, K. A., & Graves, D. F. (2002). Masking by object substitution: Dissociation of masking and cuing effects. *Journal of Experimental Psychology: Human Perception and Performance, 28*, 682–694.

Neisser, U. (1967). *Cognitive psychology*. New York: Appleton-Century-Crofts.

Nelkin, N. (1996). *Consciousness and the origins of thought*. Cambridge, England: Cambridge University Press.

Neumann, O. (1990). Direct parameter specification and the concept of perception. *Psychological Research, 52*, 207–215.

Neumann, O., & Klotz, W. (1994). Motor responses to nonreportable, masked stimuli: Where is the limit of direct parameter specification? In C. Umilta & M. Moscovitch (Eds.), *Attention and performance* (Vol. 15, pp. 123–150). Cambridge, MA: MIT Press.

Newman, J. (1995). Thalamic contributions to attention and consciousness. *Consciousness and Cognition, 4*, 172–193.

Niedeggen, M., Wichmann, P., & Stoerig, P. (2001). Change detection and time to consciousness. *European Journal of Neuroscience, 14*, 1–10.

Nijhawan, R. (1994). Motion extrapolation in catching. *Nature, 370*, 256–257.

Nijhawan, R. (2001). The flash-lag phenomenon: Object and eye movements. *Perception, 30*, 263–282.

Nijhawan, R. (2002). Neural delays, visual motion and the flash-lag effect. *Trends in Cognitive Sciences, 6*, 387–393.

Nishida, S., & Johnston, A. (2002). Marker correspondence, not processing latency, determines temporal binding of visual attributes. *Current Biology, 12*, 359–368.

Nissen, M. J. (1985). Accessing features and objects: Is location special? In M. I. Posner & O. S. M. Marin (Eds.), *Attention and performance* (Vol. 11, pp. 205–219). Hillsdale, NJ: Erlbaum.

Noesselt, T., Hillyard, S. A., Woldorff, M. G., Schoenfeld, A., Hagner, T., Jäncke, L., Tempelmann, C., Hinrichs, H., Heinze, H. J. (2002). Delayed striate cortical activation during spatial attention. *Neuron, 35*, 575–587.

Nothdurft, H. C. (1985). Orientation sensitivity and texture segmentation in patterns with different line orientation. *Vision Research, 25*, 551–560.

Nothdurft, H. C. (1991). Texture segmentation and pop-out from orientation contrast. *Vision Research, 31*, 1073–1078.

Nothdurft, H. C. (1992). Feature analysis and the role of similarity in pre-attentive vision. *Perception & Psychophysics, 52*, 355–375.

Nowak, L. G., & Bullier, J. (1997). The timing of information transfer in the visual system. In J. Kaas, K. Rockland, & A. Peters (Eds.), *Cerebral cortex: Extrastriate cortex in primates* (pp. 205–241). New York: Plenum Press.

Nowak, L. G., Munk, M. H. J., Girard, P., & Bullier, J. (1985). Visual latencies in areas V1 and V2 of the macaque monkey. *Visual Neuroscience, 12*, 371–384.

Nunez, P. L. (1981). *Electric fields of the brain*. New York: Oxford University Press.

Öğmen, H. (1993). A neural theory of retino–cortical dynamics. *Neural Networks, 6*, 245–273.

Öğmen, H., Breitmeyer, B. G., & Melvin, R. (2003). What and where in visual masking. *Vision Research, 43*, 1337–1350.

Öğmen, H., Breitmeyer, B. G., Todd, S., & Mardon, L. (2004a). Double dissociation in target recovery: effect of contrast. *Journal of Vision, 4*, 74a.

Öğmen, H., & Gagné, S. (1990). Neural models for sustained and on–off units of insect lamina. *Biological Cybernetics, 63*, 51–60.

Öğmen, H., Patel, S. S., Bedell, H. E., & Camuz, K. (2004b). Differential latencies and the dynamics of the position-computation process for moving targets, assessed with the flash-lag effect. *Vision Research, 44*, 2109–2128.

Olk, B., Harvey, M., Dow, L., & Murphy, P. J. S. (2001). Illusion processing in hemispatial neglect. *Neuropsychologia, 39*, 611–625.

Olson, I. R., Chun, M. M., & Allison, T. (2001). Contextual guidance of attention: Human intracranial event-related potential evidence for feedback modulation in anatomically early, temporally late stages of visual processing. *Brain, 124*, 1417–1425.

Oostenveld, R., Praamstra, P., Stegeman, D. F., & van Oosterom, A. (2001). Overlap of attention and movement-related activity in lateralized event related brain potentials. *Clinical Neurophysiology, 112*, 477–484.

Optican, L. M., & Richmond, B. J. (1987). Temporal encoding of two-dimensional patterns by single units in primate inferior temporal cortex: III. Information theoretic analysis. *Journal of Neurophysiology, 57*, 162–178.

Oram, M. W., & Perrett, D. I. (1992). Time course of neural responses discriminating different views of the face and head. *Journal of Neurophysiology, 68*, 70–84.

O'Regan, J. K., & Noë, A. (2001). A sensorimotor account of vision and visual consciousness. *Behavioral and Brain Sciences, 24*, 939–1031.

O'Regan, J. K., Rensink, R. A., & Clark, J. J. (1999). Change-blindness as a result of "mudsplashes." *Nature, 398*, 34.

O'Shea, R. P., & Crassini, B. (1984). Binocular rivalry occurs without simultaneous presentation of rival stimuli. *Perception & Psychophysics, 36*, 266–276.

Ortells, J. J., Daza, M. T., & Fox, E. (2003). Semantic activation in the absence of perceptual awareness. *Perception & Psychophysics, 65*, 1307–1317.

Overgaard, M., Nielsen, J. F., & Fuglsang-Frederiksen, A. (2004). A TMS study of the ventral projections from V1 with implications for the finding of neural correlates of consciousness. *Brain and Cognition, 54*, 58–64.

Pandya, D. N., & Barnes, C. L. (1987). Architecture and connections of the frontal lobe. In E. Perecman (Ed.), *The frontal lobes revisited* (pp. 41–72). New York: Institute for Research in Behavioral Neuroscience.

Panzeri, S., Schultz, S. R., Treves, A., & Rolls, E. T. (1999). Correlations and the encoding of information in the nervous system. *Proceedings of the Royal Society B, 266*, 1001–1012.

Panzeri, S., & Treves, A. (1996). Analytical estimates of limited sampling biases in different information measures. *Network, 7*, 87–107.

Paradiso, M. A., & Hahn, S. (1996). Filling-in percepts produced by luminance modulation. *Vision Research, 36*, 2657–2663.

Paradiso, M. A., & Nakayama, K. (1991). Brightness perception and filling-in. *Vision Research, 31*, 1221–1236.

Pascual-Leone, A., & Walsh, V. (2001). Fast backprojections from the motion to the primary visual area necessary for visual awareness. *Science, 292*, 510–512.

Pascual-Leone, A., Walsh, V., & Rothwell, J. (2000). Transcranial magnetic stimulation in cognitive neuroscience—Virtual lesion, chronometry, and functional connectivity. *Current Opinion in Neurobiology, 10*, 232–237.

Pasley, B. N., Mayes, L. C., & Schultz, R. T. (2004). Subcortical discrimination of unperceived objects during binocular rivalry. *Neuron, 42*, 163–172.

Pasupathy, A., & Connor, C. E. (2002a). Population coding of shape in area V4. *Nature Neuroscience, 5*, 1332–1338.

Pasupathy, A., & Connor, C. E. (2002b). Responses to contour features in macaque area V4. *Journal of Neurophysiology, 82*, 2490–2502.

Patel, S. S., Öğmen, H., Bedell, H. E., & Sampath, V. (2000). Flash-lag effect: Differential latency, not post-diction. *Science*, *290*, 1051a.

Pavani, F., Boscagli, I., Benvenuti, F., Rabuffetti, M., & Farne, A. (1999). Are perception and action affected differently by the Titchener circles illusion? *Experimental Brain Research*, *127*, 95–101.

Pena, J. L., & Konishi, M. (2001). Auditory spatial receptive fields created by multiplication. *Science*, *292*, 249–252. Comment by L. Helmuth. *Science*, *292*, 185.

Penn, D. L., Corrigan, P. W., Bentall, R. P., Racenstein, J. M., & Newman, L. (1997). Social cognition in schizophrenia. *Psychological Bulletin*, *121*, 114–132.

Perenin, M.-T. (1978). Discrimination of motion direction in perimetrically blind fields. *Neuroreport*, *2*, 397–400.

Perenin, M. T., & Rossetti, Y. (1996). Grasping without form discrimination in a hemianopic field. *Neuroreport*, *7*, 793–797.

Pessoa, L., & De Weerd, P. (2003). *Filling-in*. Oxford, England: Oxford University Press.

Pessoa, L., & Ungerleider, L. G. (2004). Neural correlates of change detection and change blindness in a working memory task. *Cerebral Cortex*, *14*, 511–520.

Petersen, S. E., Miezin, F. M., & Allman, J. M. (1988). Transient and sustained responses in four extrastriate visual areas of the owl monkey. *Experimental Brain Research*, *70*, 55–60.

Petry, S. (1978). Perceptual changes during metacontrast. *Vision Research*, *18*, 1337–1341.

Pins, D., & Ffytche, D. (2003). The neural correlates of conscious vision. *Cerebral Cortex*, *13*, 461–474.

Place, E. J., & Gilmore, G. C. (1980). Perceptual organization in schizophrenia. *Journal of Abnormal Psychology*, *89*, 409–418.

Plum, F., & Posner, J. B. (1982). *The diagnosis of stupor and coma*. Oxford: Oxford University Press.

Pockett, S. (2002). On subjective back-referral and how long it takes to become conscious of a stimulus: A reinterpretation of Libet's data. *Consciousness and Cognition*, *11*, 144–161.

Pockett, S. (2004). Hypnosis and the death of "subjective backwards referral." *Consciousness and Cognition*, *13*, 621–625.

Poeppel, E. (1986). Long-range colour-generating interaction across the retina. *Nature*, *320*, 523–525.

Poeppel, E., Held, R., & Frost, D. (1973). Residual visual function after brain wounds involving the central visual pathways in man. *Nature*, *243*, 295–296.

Pollen, D. A. (1999). On the neural correlates of visual perception. *Cerebral Cortex*, *9*, 4–13.

Pollen, D. A. (2004). Brain stimulation and conscious experience. *Consciousness and Cognition*, *13*, 626–645.

Posner, M. I. (1994). Attention: The mechanism of consciousness. *Proceedings of the National Academy of Sciences, USA*, *91*, 7398–7403.

Posner, M. I., & Petersen, S. E. (1990). The attention system of the human brain. *Annual Review of Neuroscience*, *13*, 25–42.

Posner, M. I., Walker, J. A., Friedrich, F. J., & Rafal, R. D. (1984). Effects of parietal injury on covert orienting of attention. *Journal of Neuroscience*, *4*, 1863–1874.

Potter, M. C. (1975). Meaning in visual search. *Science*, *187*, 965–966.

Potter, M. C. (1976). Short-term conceptual memory for pictures. *Journal of Experimental Psychology: Human Learning and Memory*, *2*, 509–522.

Potter, M. C. (1982). *Very short-term memory: In one eye and out the other*. Paper presented at the 23rd annual meeting of the Psychonomic Society, Minneapolis, MN.

Potter, M. C. (1984). Rapid serial visual presentation (RSVP): A method for studying language processing. In D. Kieras & M. Just (Eds.), *New methods in reading comprehension research* (pp. 91–118). Hillsdale, NJ: Erlbaum.

Potter, M. C. (1993). Very short-term conceptual memory. *Memory & Cognition*, *21*, 156–161.

Potter, M. C. (1999). Understanding sentences and scenes: The role of conceptual short term memory. In V. Coltheart (Ed.), *Fleeting memories* (pp. 13–46). Cambridge, MA: MIT Press.

Potter, M. C., Chun, M. M., Banks, B. S., & Muckenhoupt, M. (1998). Two attentional deficits in serial target search: The visual attentional blink and an amodal task-switch deficit. *Journal of Experimental Psychology: Learning, Memory, and Cognition, 24*, 979–992.

Potter, M. C., Dell'Acqua, R., Pesciarelli, F., Job, R., Peressotti, F., & O'Connor, D. H. (2005). Bidirectional semantic priming in the attentional blink. *Psychonomic Bulletin & Review, 12*, 460–465.

Potter, M. C., Fox, L. F., & Meyer, C. T. (in preparation a). *Sentence priming and the attentional blink.*

Potter, M. C., Kroll, J. F., & Harris, C. (1980). Comprehension and memory in rapid sequential reading. In R. Nickerson (Ed.), *Attention and performance* (Vol. 8, pp. 395–418). Hillsdale, NJ: Erlbaum.

Potter, M. C., Kroll, J. F., Yachzel, B., Carpenter, E., & Sherman, J. (1986). Pictures in sentences: Understanding without words. *Journal of Experimental Psychology: General, 115*, 281–294.

Potter, M. C., & Levy, E. I. (1969). Recognition memory for a rapid sequence of pictures. *Journal of Experimental Psychology, 81*, 10–15.

Potter, M. C., Meyer, C. T., & Fox, L. F. (in preparation b). *Unmasking effects in a high-speed attentional blink procedure.*

Potter, M. C., & O'Connor, D. H. (2000). *Location uncertainty in a two-stream attentional blink.* Unpublished manuscript.

Potter, M. C., Staub, A., & O'Connor, D. H. (2002). The time course of competition for attention: Attention is initially labile. *Journal of Experimental Psychology: Human Perception and Performance, 28*, 1149–1162.

Pouget, A., Dayan, P., & Zemel, R. S. (2003). Inference and computation with population codes. *Annual Reviews in Neuroscience, 26*, 381–410.

Pouget, A., Deneve, S., & Duhamel, J. R. (2002). A computational perspective on the neural basis of multisensory spatial representations. *Nature Reviews Neuroscience, 3*, 741–747.

Pribram, K. H. (1999). The self as me and I. *Consciousness and Cognition, 8*, 385–386.

Proverbio, A. M., Burco, F., del Zotto, M., & Zani, A. (2004). Blue piglets? Electrophysiological evidence for the primacy of shape over color in object recognition. *Cognitive Brain Research, 18*, 288–300.

Pugh, M. C., Ringach, D. L., Shapley, R., & Shelley, M. J. (2000). Computational modeling of orientation tuning dynamics in monkey primary visual cortex. *Journal of Computational Neuroscience, 8*(2), 143–159.

Purpura, K. P., & Schiff, N. D. (1997). The thalamic intralaminar nuclei: A role in visual awareness. *The Neuroscientist, 3*, 8–15.

Purushothaman, G., Öğmen, H., & Bedell, H. E. (2000). Gamma-range oscillations in backward-masking function and their putative neural correlates. *Psychological Review, 107*, 556–577.

Purushothaman, G., Patel, S. S., Bedell, H. E., & Öğmen, H. (1998). Moving ahead through differential latency. *Nature, 396*, 424.

Pylyshyn, Z. W. (2003). *Seeing and visualizing: It's not what you think.* Cambridge, MA: MIT Press.

Rafal, R. D. (1994). Neglect. *Current Opinion in Neurobiology, 4*, 2312–2316.

Rafal, R. D. (2000). Neglect II: Cognitive neuropsychological issues. In M. J. Farah & T. E. Feinberg (Eds.), *Patient-based approaches to cognitive neuroscience* (pp. 125–141). Cambridge, MA: MIT Press.

Rafal, R., Smith, J., Krantz, J., Cohen, A., & Brennan, C. (1990). Extrageniculate vision in hemianopic humans: Saccade inhibition by signals in the blind field. *Science, 250*, 118–121.

Raiguel, S. E., Lagae, L., Gulyas, B., & Orban, G. A. (1989). Response latencies of visual cells in macaque areas V1, V2 and V5. *Brain Research, 493*, 155–159.

Ramachandran, V. S. (1988). Perceiving shape from shading. *Scientific American, 259*, 76–83.

Ramachandran, V. S., & Cobb, S. (1995). Visual attention modulates metacontrast masking. *Nature, 373*, 66–68.

Rao, R. P. N. (2004). Bayesian computation in recurrent neural networks. *Neural Computation, 16*, 1–38.

Rao, R. P. N., Olshausen, B. A., & Lewicki, M. S. (Eds.). (2002). *Probabilistic models of the brain: perception and neural function.* Cambridge, MA: MIT Press.

Rao, S. C., Rainer, G., & Miller, E. K. (1997). Integration of what and where in the primate prefrontal cortex. *Science, 276*, 821–824.

Raymond, J. E., Shapiro, K. L., & Arnell, K. M. (1992). Temporary suppression of visual processing in an RSVP task: An attentional blink? *Journal of Experimental Psychology: Human Perception and Performance, 18*, 849–860.

Rees, G., Kreiman, G., & Koch, C. (2001). Neural correlates of consciousness in humans. *Nature Reviews Neuroscience, 3*, 261–270.

Reeves, A. (1982). Metacontrast U-shaped functions derive from two monotonic functions. *Perception, 11*, 415–426.

Reeves, A., & Sperling, G. (1986). Attention gating in short-term visual memory. *Psychological Review, 9*, 180–206.

Rensink, R. A. (2000). Seeing, sensing, and scrutinizing. *Vision Research, 40*, 1469–1487.

Rensink, R. A. (2002). Change detection. *Annual Review of Psychology, 53*, 245–277.

Rensink, R. A., O'Regan, J. K., & Clark, J. J. (1997). To see or not to see: The need for attention to perceive changes in scenes. *Psychological Science, 8*, 368–373.

Reppas, J. B., Niyogi, S., Dale, A. M., Sereno, M. I., & Tootell, B. H. (1997). Representation of motion boundaries in retinotopic human visual cortical areas. *Nature, 388*, 175–179.

Revonsuo, A., & Kamppinen, M. (Eds.). (1994). *Consciousness in philosophy and cognitive neuroscience.* Hillsdale, NJ: Erlbaum.

Ricci, R., Pia, L., & Gindri, P. (2004). Effects of illusory spatial anisometry in unilateral neglect. *Experimental Brain Research, 154*, 226–237.

Richards, W. (1973). Visual processing in scotomata. *Experimental Brain Research, 17*, 333–347.

Ringach, D. L. (1998). Tuning of orientation detectors in human vision. *Vision Research, 38*, 963–972.

Ringach, D. L., Hawken, M. J., & Shapley, R. (2003). Dynamics of orientation tuning in macaque V1: The role of global and tuned suppression. *Journal of Neurophysiology, 90*, 342–352.

Ritter, W., Simson, R., Vaughan, H. G., & Friedman, D. (1979). A brain event related to the making of a sensory discrimination. *Science, 203*, 1358–1361.

Ro, T., Breitmeyer, B., Burton, P., Singhal, N. S., & Lane, D. (2003). Feedback contributions to visual awareness in human occipital cortex. *Current Biology, 11*, 1038–1041.

Ro, T., Henik, A., Machado, L., & Rafal, R. (1997). Transcranial magnetic stimulation of the prefrontal cortex delays contralateral endogenous saccades. *Journal of Cognitive Neuroscience, 9*, 433–440.

Ro, T., & Rafal, R. D. (1996). Perception of geometric illusions in hemispatial neglect. *Neuropsychologia, 34*, 973–978.

Ro, T., Shelton, D., Lee, O. L., & Chang, E. (2004). Extrageniculate mediation of unconscious vision in transcranial magnetic stimulation-induced blindsight. *Proceedings of the National Academy of Sciences, USA, 101*, 9933–9935.

Ro, T., Singhal, N., Breitmeyer, B., & Garcia, J. (in preparation). *Unconscious processing of color and form.*

Robertson, E. M., Théoret, H., & Pascual-Leone, A. (2003). Studies in cognition: The problems solved and created by transcranial magnetic stimulation. *Journal of Cognitive Neuroscience, 15*, 948–960.

Robinson, D. L., & McClurkin, J. W. (1989). The visual superior colliculus and pulvinar. *Review of Oculomotor Research, 3*, 337–360.

Rock, I., & Palmer, S. (1990). The legacy of Gestalt psychology. *Scientific American, 263*, 48–61.

Roelfsema, P. R., Lamme, V. A. F., & Spekreijse, H. (1998). Object-based attention in the primary visual cortex of the macaque monkey. *Nature, 395*, 376–381.

Roelfsema, P. R., Lamme, V. A. F., Spekreijse, H., & Bosch, H. (2002). Figure–ground segregation in a recurrent network architecture. *Journal of Cognitive Neuroscience, 14*, 525–537.

Rogowitz, B. (1983). Spatial/temporal interactions: Backward and forward metacontrast masking with sine-wave gratings. *Vision Research*, *23*, 1057–1073.

Rolls, E. T. (1992). Neurophysiological mechanisms underlying face processing within and beyond the temporal cortical visual areas. *Philosophical Transactions of the Royal Society of London*, B, *335*, 11–21.

Rolls, E. T. (1997). Consciousness in neural networks? *Neural Networks*, *10*, 1227–1240.

Rolls, E. T. (1999). *The brain and emotion.* Oxford, England: Oxford University Press.

Rolls, E. T. (2000a). Functions of the primate temporal lobe cortical visual areas in invariant visual object and face recognition. *Neuron*, *27*, 205–218.

Rolls, E. T. (2000b). Précis of *the brain and emotion.* *Behavioral and Brain Sciences*, *23*, 177–233.

Rolls, E. T. (2004). A higher order syntactic thought (HOST) theory of consciousness. In R. J. Gennaro (Ed.), *Higher order theories of consciousness* (pp. 137–172). Amsterdam: John Benjamins.

Rolls, E. T., Aggelopoulos, N. C., Franco, L., & Treves, A. (2004). Information encoding in the inferior temporal cortex: Contributions of the firing rates and correlations between the firing of neurons. *Biological Cybernetics*, *90*, 19–32.

Rolls, E. T., & Deco, G. (2002). *Computational neuroscience of vision.* Oxford, England: Oxford University Press.

Rolls, E. T., Franco, L., Aggelopoulos, N. C., & Reece, S. (2003). An information theoretic approach to the contributions of the firing rates and correlations between the firing of neurons. *Journal of Neurophysiology*, *89*, 2810–2822.

Rolls, E. T., & Tovée, M. J. (1994). Processing speed in the cerebral cortex, and the neurophysiology of visual masking. *Proceedings of the Royal Society of London*, B, *257*, 9–15.

Rolls, E. T., & Tovée, M. J. (1995). The sparseness of the neuronal representation of stimuli in the primate temporal visual cortex. *Journal of Neurophysiology*, *73*, 713–726.

Rolls, E. T., Tovée, M. J., & Panzeri, S. (1999). The neurophysiology of backward visual masking: Information analysis. *Journal of Cognitive Neuroscience*, *11*, 335–346.

Rolls, E. T., Tovée, M. J., Purcell, D. G., Stewart, A. L., & Azzopardi, P. (1994). The responses of neurons in the temporal cortex of primates and face identification and detection. *Experimental Brain Research*, *101*, 473–484.

Rolls, E. T., & Treves, A. (1998). *Neural networks and brain function.* Oxford, England: Oxford University Press.

Rolls, E. T., Treves, A., Tovée, M., & Panzeri, S. (1997). Information in the neuronal representation of individual stimuli in the primate temporal visual cortex. *Journal of Computational Neuroscience*, *4*, 309–333.

Rosenthal, D. (1990). A theory of consciousness. *ZIF Report No. 40*, Zentrum für Interdisziplinäre Forschung, Bielefeld, Germany.

Rosenthal, D. M. (1993). Thinking that one thinks. In: M. Davies, & G. W. Humphreys (Eds.), *Consciousness*, 197–223. Oxford: Blackwell.

Rosenthal, D. M. (2002). How many kinds of consciousness? *Consciousness and Cognition*, *11*, 653–665.

Rosenthal, V. (2004). Microgenesis, immediate experience and visual processes in reading. In A. Carsetti (Ed.), *Seeing and thinking* (pp. 221–243) Amsterdam: Kluwer.

Roskies, A. L. (1999). The binding problem. *Neuron*, *24*, 7–9, and associated articles.

Rossi, A. F., Desimone, R., & Ungerleider, L. G. (2001). Contextual modulation in primary visual cortex of macaques. *Journal of Neuroscience*, *21*, 1698–1709.

Rossi, A. F., & Paradiso, M. A. (1996). Temporal limits of brightness induction and mechanisms of brightness perception. *Vision Research*, *36*, 1391–1398.

Rossi, A. F., & Paradiso, M. A. (1999). Neural correlates of perceived brightness in the retina, lateral geniculate nucleus, and striate cortex. *Journal of Neuroscience*, *19*, 6145–6156.

Rushton, D. (1975). Use of the Pulfrich pendulum for detecting abnormal delay in the visual pathway in multiple sclerosis. *Brain*, *98*, 283–296.

Ruz, M., Madrid, E., Lupiáñez, J., & Tudela, P. (2003). High density ERP indices of conscious and unconscious semantic priming. *Cognitive Brain Research, 17*, 719–731.

Ryle, G. (1949). *The concept of mind.* London: Hutchison Publishing Group.

Saarinen, J., Levi, D. M., & Shen, B. (1997). Integration of local pattern elements into a global shape in human vision. *Proceedings of the National Academy of Sciences, USA, 94*, 8267–8271.

Saccuzzo, D. S., Cadenhead, M. D., & Braff, D. L. (1996). Backward versus forward visual masking deficits in schizophrenic patients: Centrally, not peripherally, mediated? *American Journal of Psychiatry, 153*, 1564–1570.

Sagi, D., & Hochstein, S. (1985). Lateral inhibition between spatially adjacent spatial-frequency channels? *Perception & Psychophysics, 37*, 315–322.

Sagiv, N., & Bentin, S. (2001). Structural encoding of human and schematic faces: Holistic and part-based processes. *Journal of Cognitive Neuroscience, 13*, 937–951.

Sahani, M., & Dayan, P. (2003). doubly distributional population codes: Simutaneous representation of uncertainty and multiplicity. *Neural Computation, 15*, 2255–2279.

Salin, P., & Bullier, J. (1995). Corticocortical connections in the visual system: Structure and function, *Physiological Reviews, 75*, 107–154.

Salinas, E., & Abbott, L. F. (1996). A model of multiplicative neural responses in parietal cortex. *Proceedings of the National Academy of Sciences USA, 93*, 11956–11961.

Sander, F. (1962). Experimentelle Ergebnisse der Gestaltpsychologie. In F. Sander & H. Volkelt (Eds.), *Ganzgeitspsychologie.* Munich, Germany: Beck. (Reprinted from E. Becher, Ed., *10 Kongress bericht experimentelle Psychologie*, 1928, 23–87. Jena, Germany: Fischer.)

Sanocki, T. (1993). Time course of object identification: Evidence for a global-to-local contingency. *Journal of Experimental Psychology: Human Perception and Performance, 19*, 878–898.

Sarikaya, M., Wang, W., & Öğmen, H. (1998). Neural network model of on–off units in the fly visual system: Simulations of dynamic behavior. *Biological Cybernetics, 78*, 399–412.

Saunders, J. A., & Knill, D. C. (2003). Humans use continuous visual feedback from the hand to control fast reaching movements. *Experimental Brain Research, 152*, 341–352.

Schacter, D. L. (1987). Implicit memory: History and current status. *Journal of Experimental Psychology: Learning, Memory, and Cognition, 13*, 501–518.

Schacter, D. L., & Buckner, R. L. (1998). Priming and the brain. *Neuron, 20*, 185–195.

Schall, J. D., Hanes, D. P., Thompson, K. G., & King, D. J. (1995). Saccade target selection in frontal eye field of macaque: I. Visual and premovement activation. *Journal of Neuroscience, 15*, 6905–6918.

Scharf, B., & Lefton, L. A. (1970). Backward and forward masking as a function of stimulus and task parameters. *Journal of Experimental Psychology, 84*, 331–338.

Scharlau, I. (2004). Evidence against response bias in temporal order tasks with attention manipulation by masked primes. *Psychological Research, 68*, 224–236.

Scharlau, I., & Ansorge, U. (2003). Direct parameter specification of an attention shift: Evidence from perceptual latency priming. *Vision Research, 43*, 1351–1363.

Scharlau, I., & Neumann, O. (2003). Temporal parameters and time course of perceptual latency priming. *Acta Psychologica, 113*, 185–203.

Schechter, I., Butler, P. D., Silipo, G., Zemon, V., & Javitt, D. C. (2002). Magnocellular and parvocellular contributions to backward masking dysfunction in schizophrenia. *Schizophrenia Research, 64*, 91–101.

Scheibel, A. B. (1981). The problem of selective attention: A possible structural substrate. In O. Pompeiano and C. Ajmone (Eds.), *Brain mechanisms and perceptual awareness* (pp. 319–326). New York: Raven.

Schiff, N. D., & Purpura, K. P. (2002). Towards a neurophysiological foundation for cognitive neuromodulation through deep brain stimulation. *Thalamus & Related Systems, 2*, 55–69.

Schiller, P. H. (1965). Metacontrast interference as determined by a method of comparison. *Perceptual & Motor Skills, 20*, 279–285.

Schiller, P. H., Finlay, B. L., & Volman, S. F. (1976). Quantative studies of single cell properties in monkey striate cortex. I–V. *Journal of Neurophysiology, 39*, 1288–1374.

Schiller, P. H., & Smith, M. C. (1966). Detection in metacontrast. *Journal of Experimental Psychology, 71*, 32–39.

Schlag, J., & Schlag Rey, M. (2002). Delays and localization errors in the visual system. *Nature Reviews Neuroscience, 3*, 191–200.

Schlaghecken, F., & Eimer, M. (2001). Partial response activation to masked primes is not dependent on response readiness. *Perceptual Motor Skills, 92*, 208–222.

Schlaghecken, F., & Eimer, M. (2002). Motor activation with and without inhibition: Evidence for a threshold mechanism in motor control. *Perception & Psychophysics, 64*, 148–162.

Schmidt, K. E., Goebel, R., Lowel, S., & Singer, W. (1997). The perceptual grouping criterion of colinearity is reflected by anisotropies of connections in the primary visual cortex. *European Journal of Neuroscience, 9*, 1083–1089.

Schmidt, T. (2002). The finger in flight: Real-time motor control by visually masked color stimuli. *Psychological Science, 13*, 112–118.

Schmolesky, M. T., Wang, Y., Hanes, D. G., Thompson, K. G., Leutgeb, S., Schall, J. D., & Leventhal, A. G. (1998). Signal timing across the macaque visual system. *Journal of Neurophysiology, 79*, 3272–3278.

Schuck, J. R., & Lee, R. G. (1989). Backward masking, information-processing, and schizophrenia. *Schizophrenia Bulletin, 15*, 491–500.

Schürmann, M., Grumbt, M., Heide, W., & Verleger, R. (2003). Effects of same- and different-modality cues in a Posner task: Extinction-type, spatial, and non-spatial deficits after right-hemispheric stroke. *Cognitive Brain Research, 16*, 348–358.

Schwartz, B. D., McGinn, T., & Winstead, D. K. (1987). Disordered spatiotemporal processing in schizophrenics. *Biological Psychiatry, 22*, 688–698.

Schwartz, B. D., & Winstead, D. K. (1982). Visual processing deficits in acute and chronic schizophrenics. *Biological Psychiatry, 17*, 1377–1387.

Schweinberger, S. R., & Stief, V. (2001). Implicit perception in patients with visual neglect: Lexical specificity in repetition priming. *Neuropsychologia, 39*, 420–429.

Schyns, P. G., & Oliva, A. (1994). From blobs to boundary edges: Evidence for time- and spatial-scale-dependent scene recognition. *Psychological Science, 5*, 195–200.

Schyns, P. G., & Oliva, A. (1999). Dr. Angry & Mr. Smile: When categorization flexibly modifies the perception of faces in rapid visual presentations. *Cognition, 69*, 243–265.

Searle, J. (1992). *The rediscovery of mind*. Cambridge, MA: MIT Press.

Searle, J. (2000). Consciousness. *Annual Review of Neuroscience, 23*, 557–578.

Seiffert, A. E., & Di Lollo, V. (1997). Low-level masking in the attentional blink. *Journal of Experimental Psychology: Human Perception and Performance, 23*, 1061–1073.

Selemon, L. D., Rajkowska, G., & Goldman-Rakic, P. S. (1998). Elevated neuronal density in prefrontal area 46 in brains from schizophrenic patients: Application of three-dimensional, stereologic counting method. *Journal of Comparative Neurology, 392*, 402–412.

Sengpiel, F., Sen, A., & Blakemore, C. (1997). Characteristics of surround inhibition in cat area 17. *Experimental Brain Research, 116*, 216–238.

Sergent, C., & Dehaene, S. (2004). Is consciousness a gradual phenomenon? Evidence for an all-or-none bifurcation during the attentional blink. *Psychological Science, 15*, 720–728.

Sergi, M. J., & Green, M. F. (2003). Social perception and early visual processing in schizophrenia. *Schizophrenia Research, 59*, 233–241.

Shannon, C. E. (1948). A mathematical theory of communication. *AT&T Bell Laboratories Technical Journal, 27*, 379–423.

Shapiro, K. (2001). *The limits of attention: Temporal constraints on human information processing*. Oxford, England: Oxford University Press.

Shapiro, K., Driver, J., Ward, R., & Sorensen, R. E. (1997). Priming from the attentional blink: A failure to extract visual tokens but not visual types. *Psychological Science, 8*, 95–100.

Sheinberg, D. L., & Logothetis, N. K. (1997). The role of temporal cortical areas in perceptual organization. *Proceedings of the National Academy of Sciences, USA, 94*, 3408–3413.

Sherman, S. M., & Guillery, R. W. (1996). Functional organization of thalamocortical relays. *Journal of Neurophysiology, 76*, 1367–1395.

Shih, S. (2000). Recall of two visual targets embedded in RSVP streams of distractors depends on their temporal and spatial relationship. *Perception & Psychophysics, 62*, 1348–1355.

Silverstein, S. M., Knight, R. A., Schwarzkopf, S. B., West, L. L., Osborn, L. M., & Kamin, D. (1996). Stimulus configuration and context effects in perceptual organization in schizophrenia. *Journal of Abnormal Psychology, 105*, 410–420.

Sincich, L. C., & Horton, J. C. (2002). Divided by cytochrome oxidase: A map of the projections from V1 to V2 in macaques. *Science, 295*, 1734–1737.

Singer, W. (1994). Putative functions of temporal correlations in neocortical processing. In C. Koch & J. L. Davis (Eds.), *Large-scale neuronal theories of the brain* (pp. 201–237). Cambridge, MA: MIT Press.

Singer, W. (1999). Neuronal synchrony: A versatile code for the definition of relations? *Neuron, 24*, 49–65.

Singer, W. (2000). Response synchronization: A universal coding strategy for the definition of relations. In M. Ganzzaniga (Ed.), *The new cognitive neurosciences* (2nd ed., pp. 325–338). Cambridge, MA: MIT Press.

Slaghuis, W. L., & Bakker, V. J. (1995). Forward and backward visual masking of contour by light in positive- and negative-symptom schizophrenia. *Journal of Abnormal Psychology, 104*, 41–54.

Slaghuis, W. L., & Bishop, A. M. (2001). Luminance flicker sensitivity in positive- and negative-symptom schizophrenia. *Experimental Brain Research, 138*, 88–99.

Slaghuis, W. L., & Curran, C. E. (1999). Spatial frequency masking in positive- and negative-symptom schizophrenia. *Journal of Abnormal Psychology, 108*, 42–50.

Solso, R. L. (2003). *The psychology of art and the evolution of the conscious brain.* Cambridge, MA: MIT Press.

Somers, D. C., Dale, A. M., Seiffert, A. E., & Tootell, R. B. H. (1999). Functional MRI reveals spatially specific attentional modulation in human primary visual cortex. *Proceedings of the National Academy of Sciences, USA, 96*, 1663–1668.

Spencer, K. M., Nestor, P. G., Niznikiewicz, M. A., Salisbury, D. F., Shenton, M. E., & McCarley, R. W. (2003). Abnormal neural synchrony in schizophrenia. *The Journal of Neuroscience, 23*, 7407–7411.

Spencer, T. J., & Shuntich, R. (1970). Evidence for an interruption theory of backward masking. *Journal of Experimental Psychology, 85*, 198–203.

Sperry, R. (1969). A modified concept of consciousness. *Psychological Review, 76*, 532–536.

Sperry, R. (1970). An objective approach to subjective experience. *Psychological Review, 77*, 585–590.

Spillmann, L. (1971). Foveal perceptive fields in the human visual system measured with simultaneous contrast in grids and bars. *Pfluegers Archiv der gesamten Physiologie, 326*, 281–299.

Seriade, M. (2000). Corticothalamic resonance, states of vigilance and mentation. *Neuroscience, 101*, 243–276.

Steriade, M., & McCarley, R. (1990). *Brainstem control of wakefulness and sleep.* New York: Plenum.

Sternberg, S. (1969). The discovery of processing stages: Extensions of Donders' method. In W. G. Koster (Ed.), *Attention and performance II* (pp. 276–315). Amsterdam: North-Holland.

Sternberg, S., & Knoll, R. L. (1973). The perception of temporal order: Fundamental issues and a general model. In S. Kornblum (Ed.), *Attention and performance* (Vol. 4, pp. 629–686). New York: Academic Press.

Stewart, A. L., & Purcell D. G. (1970). U-shaped masking functions in visual backward masking: Effects of target configuration and retinal position. *Perception & Psychophysics, 7*, 253–256.

Stewart, A. L., & Purcell, D. G. (1974). Visual backward masking by a flash of light: A study of U-shaped detection functions. *Journal of Experimental Psychology, 103*, 553–566.

Stigler, R. (1910). Chronophotische Studien über den Umgebungskontrast. *Pflügers Archiv der Gesamten Physiologie, 135,* 365–435.

Stigler, R. (1926). Die Untersuchung des zeitlichen Verlaufes des optischen Erregung mittels des Metakontrastes. In E. Aberhalden (Ed.), *Handbuch des Biologischen Arbeitsmethoden* (Pt. 6, Whole No. 6, pp. 949–968). Berlin, Germany: Urban & Schwarzenberg.

Stober, R. S., Brussel, E. M., & Komoda, M. K. (1978). Differential effects of metacontrast on target brightness and clarity. *Bulletin of the Psychonomic Society, 12,* 433–436.

Stoerig, P. (1996). Varieties of vision: From blind responses to conscious recognition. *Trends in Neurosciences, 19,* 401–406.

Stoerig, P. (1997). There is no single correlate of conscious vision. *Journal of NIH Research, 9,* 37–41.

Stoerig, P. (2002). Neural correlates of consciousness as state and trait. In L. Nadel (Ed.), *Encyclopedia of cognitive neuroscience* (pp. 233–240). London: Macmillan.

Stoerig, P., & Brandt, S. (1993). The visual system and levels of perception: Properties of neuromental organization. *Theoretical Medicine, 14,* 117–135.

Stoerig, P., & Cowey, A. (1989). Wavelength sensitivity in blindsight. *Nature, 342,* 916–918.

Stoerig, P., & Cowey, A. (1992). Wavelength discrimination in blindsight. *Brain, 115,* 425–444.

Stoerig, P., & Cowey, A. (1997). Blindsight in man and monkey. *Brain, 120,* 535–559.

Stoerig, P., Hubner, M., & Poeppel, E. (1985). Signal detection analysis of residual vision in a field defect due to post-geniculate lesion. *Neuropsychologia, 23,* 589–599.

Stoffer, T. H. (1993). The time course of attentional zooming: A comparison of voluntary and involuntary allocation of attention to the levels of compound stimuli. *Psychological Research/Psychologische Forschung, 56,* 14–25.

Stoper, A. E., & Mansfield, J. G. (1978). Metacontrast and paracontrast suppression of a contourless area. *Vision Research, 18,* 1669–1674.

Sugase, Y., Yamane, S., Ueno, S., & Kawano, K. (1999). Global and fine information coded by single neurons in the temporal visual cortex. *Nature, 400,* 869–873.

Super, H., Spekreijse, H., & Lamme, V. A. F. (2001). Two distinct modes of sensory processing observed in monkey primary visual cortex (V1). *Nature Neuroscience, 4,* 304–310.

Supèr, H., Spekreijse, H., & Lamme, V. A. F. (2003). Figure–ground activity in primary visual cortex (V1) of the monkey matches the speed of behavioral response. *Neuroscience Letters, 344,* 75–78.

Tallon-Baudry, C., & Bertrand, O. (1999). Oscillatory gamma activity in humans and its role in object representation. *Trends in Cognitive Sciences, 3,* 151–162.

Tallon-Baudry, C., Bertrand, O., Delpuech, C., & Pernier, J. (1996). Stimulus specificity of phase-locked and non-phase-locked 40 Hz visual responses in humans. *Journal of Neuroscience, 16,* 4240–4249.

Tallon-Baudry, C., Kreiter, A., & Bertrand, O. (1999). Sustained and transient oscillatory responses in the gamma and beta bands in a visual short-term memory task in humans. *Visual Neuroscience, 16,* 449–459.

Tata, M. S. (2002). Attend to it now or lose it forever: Selective attention, metacontrast masking and object substitution. *Perception & Psychophysics, 64,* 1028–1038.

Taylor, J. L., & McCloskey, D. I. (1990). Triggering of preprogrammed movements as reactions to masked stimuli. *Journal of Neurophysiology, 63,* 439–446.

Teller, D. Y. (1984). Linking propositions. *Vision Research, 24,* 1233–1246.

Theeuwes, J., Kramer, A. F., Hahn, S., & Irwin, D. E. (1998). Our eyes do not always go where we want them to go: Capture of the eyes by new objects. *Psychological Science, 9,* 379–385.

Thompson, K. G., & Schall, J. D. (2000). Antecedents and correlates of visual detection and awareness in macaque prefrontal cortex. *Vision Research, 40,* 1523–1538.

Thompson-Schill, S. L., & Gabrieli, J. D. E. (1999). Priming of visual and functional knowledge on a semantic classification task. *Journal of Experimental Psychology: Learning, Memory, and Cognition, 25,* 41–53.

Thorpe, S., Fize, D., & Mariot, C. (1996). Speed of processing in the human visual system. *Nature, 381*, 520–522.

Tolhurst, D. J., & Lewis, P. R. (1992). Effect of myelination on the conduction velocity of optic nerve fibres. *Ophthalmic and Physiological Optics, 12*, 241–243.

Tong, F. (2001). Competing theories of binocular rivalry: A possible resolution. *Brain and Mind, 2*, 55–83.

Tong, F. (2003). Primary visual cortex and visual awareness. *Nature Reviews Neuroscience, 4*, 219–229.

Tong, F., & Engel, S. A. (2001). Interocular rivalry revealed in the human blind-spot representation. *Nature, 411*, 195–199.

Tong, F., Nakayama, K., Moscovitch, M., Weinrib, O., & Kanwisher, N. (2000). Response properties of the human fusiform face area. *Cognitive Neuropsychology, 17*, 257–279.

Tootell, R. B., Dale, A. M., Sereno, M. I., & Malach, R. (1996). New images from human visual cortex. *Trends in Neuroscience, 19*, 481–489.

Tootell, R. B., Tsao, D., & Vanduffel, W. (2003). Neuroimaging weighs in: Humans meet macaques in "primate" visual cortex. *Journal of Neuroscience, 23*, 3981–3989.

Toth, J. P. (2000). Nonconscious forms of human memory. In E. Tulving & F. I. Craik (Eds.), *The Oxford handbook of memory* (pp. 245–265). Oxford, England: Oxford University Press.

Tovée, M. J., & Rolls, E. T. (1995). Information encoding in short firing rate epochs by single neurons in the primate temporal visual cortex. *Visual Cognition, 2*, 35–58.

Tovée, M. J., Rolls, E. T., Treves, A., & Bellis, R. P. (1993). Information encoding and the responses of single neurons in the primate temporal visual cortex. *Journal of Neurophysiology, 70*, 640–654.

Townsend, J. T. (1990). Serial vs. parallel processing: Sometimes they look like Tweedledum and Tweedledee but they can (and should) be distinguished. *Psychological Science, 1*, 46–54.

Traub, R. D., Whittington, M. A., Stanford, I. M., & Jeffreys, J. G. R. (1996). A mechanism for generation of long-range synchronous fast oscillations in the cortex. *Nature, 383*, 621–624.

Treisman, A. (1988). Features and objects: The Fourteenth Bartlett Memorial Lecture. *Quarterly Journal of Experimental Psychology, 40, A*, 201–237.

Treisman, A. M., & Gelade, G. (1980). A feature-integration theory of attention. *Cognitive Psychology, 12*, 97–136.

Treue, S., & Martinez Trujillo, J. C. (1999). Feature-based attention influences motion processing gain in macaque visual cortex. *Nature, 399*, 575–579.

Treves, A. (1993). Mean-field analysis of neuronal spike dynamics. *Network, 4*, 259–284.

Treves, A., Panzeri, S., Rolls, E. T., Booth, M., & Wakeman, E. A. (1999). Firing rate distributions and efficiency of information transmission of inferior temporal cortex neurons to natural visual stimuli. *Neural Computation, 11*, 611–641.

Trevethan, C. T., & Sahraie, A. (2003). Spatial and temporal processing in a subject with cortical blindness following occipital surgery. *Neuropsychologia, 41*, 1296–1306.

Tsunoda, K., Yamane, Y., Nishizaki, M., & Tanifuji, M. (2001). Complex objects are represented in macaque inferotemporal cortex by the combination of feature columns. *Nature Neuroscience, 4*, 832–838.

Tucker, M., & Ellis, R. (1998). On the relations between seen objects and components of potential actions. *Journal of Experimental Psychology: Human Perception and Performance, 24*, 830–846.

Tucker, M., & Ellis, R. (2004). Action priming by briefly presented objects. *Acta Psychologica, 116*, 185–203.

Tulving, E., & Schacter, D. L. (1990). Priming and human memory systems. *Science, 247*, 301–306.

Turvey, M. T. (1973). On peripheral and central processes in vision: Inferences from an information-processing analysis of masking with patterned stimuli. *Psychological Review, 80*, 1–52.

Ullman, S. (2000). *High-level vision: Object recognition and visual cognition.* Cambridge, MA: MIT Press.

Undeutsch, U. (1942). Die Aktualgenese in ihrer Allgemein-Philosophischen und ihrer characterologischen Bedeutung. *Scientia, 72*, 37–42, 95–98.

Ungerleider, L. G. (1985). The corticocortical pathways for object recognition and spatial perception. In C. Chagas, R. Gattas, & C. Gross (Eds.), *Pattern recognition mechanisms* (pp. 21–37). Vatican City: Pontifical Academy of Sciences.

Ungerleider, L. G., & Mishkin, M. (1982). Two cortical visual systems. In D. J. Ingle, M. A. Goodale, & R. J. W. Mansfield (Eds.), *Analysis of visual behavior* (pp. 549–586). Cambridge, MA: MIT Press.

Valdes-Sosa, M., Bobes, M. A., Rodriguez, V., & Pinilla, T. (1998). Switching attention without shifting the spotlight: Object-based attentional modulation of brain potentials. *Journal of Cognitive Neuroscience, 10*, 137–151.

Vallar, G. (1993). The anatomical basis of spatial neglect in humans. In I. H. Robertson & J. C. Marshall (Eds.), *Unilateral neglect: Clinical and experimental studies* (pp. 27–62). Hillsdale, NJ: Erlbaum.

Vallar, G. (1998). Spatial hemineglect in humans. *Trends in Cognitive Science, 2*, 87–97.

Vallar, G., Daini, R., & Antonucci, G. (2000). Processing of illusion of length in spatial hemineglect: A study of line bisection. *Neuropsychologia, 38*, 1087–1097.

van Beers, R. J., Wolpert, D. M., & Haggard, P. (2001). Sensorimotor integration compensates for visual localization errors during smooth pursuit eye movements. *Journal of Neurophysiology, 85*, 1914–1922.

Van Essen, D. C., Anderson, C. H., & Felleman, D. J. (1992). Information processing in the primate visual system: An integrated systems perspective. *Science, 255*, 419–423.

Van Essen, D. C., Lewis, J. W., Drury, H. A., Hadjikhani, N., Tootell, R. B., Bakircioglu, M., & Miller, M. I. (2001). Mapping visual cortex in monkeys and humans using surface-based atlases. *Vision Research, 41*, 1359–1378.

VanRullen, R., Guyonneau, R., & Thorpe, S. J. (2005). Spike times make sense. *Trends in Neuroscience, 28*, 1–4.

VanRullen, R., & Koch, C. (2003a). Visual selective behavior can be triggered by a feedforward process. *Journal of Cognitive Neuroscience, 15*, 209–217.

VanRullen, R., & Koch, C. (2003b). Is perception discrete or continuous? *Trends in Cognitive Sciences, 7*, 207–213.

VanRullen, R., & Koch, C. (2003c). Competition and selection during visual processing of natural scenes and objects. *Journal of Vision, 3*, 75–85.

Van Voorhis, S. T., & Hillyard, S. A. (1977). Visual evoked potentials and selective attention to points in space. *Perception & Psychophysics, 22*, 54–62.

Verleger, R. (1997). On the utility of P3 latency as an index of mental chronometry. *Psychophysiology, 34*, 131–156.

Verleger, R. (1998). Towards an integration of P3 research with cognitive neuroscience. [Author's response on continuing commentary.] *Behavioral and Brain Sciences, 21*, 150–154.

Verleger, R., Heide, W., Butt, C., Wascher, E., & Kömpf, D. (1996). Online brain potential correlates of right parietal patients' attentional deficit. *Electroencephalography and Clinical Neurophysiology, 99*, 444–457.

Verleger, R., Heide, W., & Kömpf, D. (2002). Effects of stimulus-induced saccades on manual response times in healthy elderly and in patients with right-parietal lesions. *Experimental Brain Research, 144*, 17–29.

Verleger, R., Jaskowski, P., Aydemir, A., van der Lubbe, R. H. J., & Groen, M. (2004). Qualitative differences between conscious and non-conscious processing? On inverse priming induced by masked arrows. *Journal of Experimental Psychology: General, 133*, 494–515.

Visser, T. A. W., Bischoff, W. F., & DiLollo, V. (1999). Attentional switching in spatial and non-spatial domains: Evidence from the attentional blink. *Psychological Bulletin, 125*, 458–469.

Viviani, P., & Aymoz, C. (2001). Colour, form and movement are not perceived simultaneously. *Vision Research, 41*, 2909–2918.

Vogel, E. K., & Luck, S. J. (2000). The visual N1 component as an index of a discrimination process. *Psychophysiology, 37*, 190–123.

Vogel, E. K., Luck, S. J., & Shapiro K. L. (1998). Electrophysiological evidence for a postperceptual locus of suppression during the attentional blink. *Journal of Experimental Psychology: Human Perception and Performance, 24,* 1656–1674.

Vogeley, K., Kurthen, M., Falkai, P., & Maier, W. (1999). Essential functions of the human self model are implemented in the prefrontal cortex. *Consciousness and Cognition, 8,* 343–363.

Vogels, R., & Orban, G. A. (1994). Activity of inferior temporal neurons during orientation discrimination with successively presented gratings. *Journal of Neurophysiology, 71,* 1428–1451.

von der Heydt, E. P., Peterhans, E., & Duersteler, M. R. (1992). Periodic-pattern-selective cells in monkey visual cortex. *Journal of Neuroscience, 12,* 1416–1434.

von Holst, E., & Mittelstädt, H. (1950). Das reafferenzprinzip: Wechselwirkungen zwischen Zentralnervensystem und Peripherie. *Naturwissenschaften, 37,* 464–476.

Vorberg, D., Mattler, U., Heinecke, A., Schmidt, T., & Schwarzbach, J. (2003). Different time courses for visual perception and action priming. *Proceedings of the National Academy of Sciences, USA, 100,* 6275–6280.

Vorberg, D., Mattler, U., Heinecke, A., Schmidt, T., & Schwarzbach, J. (2004). Invariant time-course of priming with and without awareness. In C. Kaernbach, E. Schröger, & H. Müller (Eds.), *Psychophysics beyond sensation: Laws and invariants of human cognition* (pp. 271–288). Mahwah, NJ: Erlbaum.

Vuilleumier, P. O., & Rafal, R. D. (2000). A systematic study of visual extinction: Between- and within-field deficits of attention in hemispatial neglect. *Brain, 123,* 1263–1279.

Vuilleumier, P., Schwartz, S., Clarke, K., Husain, M., & Driver, J. (2002b). Testing memory for unseen visual stimuli in patients with extinction and spatial neglect. *Journal of Cognitive Neuroscience, 14,* 875–886.

Wachtler, T., Sejnowski, T. J., & Albright, T. D. (2003). Representation of color stimuli in awake macaque primary visual cortex. *Neuron, 37,* 681–691.

Walker, G. A., Ohzawa, R. D., & Freeman, R. (1999). Asymmetric suppression outside the classical receptive field of the visual cortex. *Journal Neuroscience, 19,* 10536–10553.

Walker, R., Mannan, S., Maurer, D., Pambakian, A. L., & Kennard, C. (2000). The oculomotor distractor effect in normal and hemianopic vision. *Proceedings of the Royal Society of London, B, 267,* 431–438.

Wallis, G., & Rolls, E. T. (1997). Invariant face and object recognition in the visual system. *Progress in Neurobiology, 51,* 167–194.

Walsh, V., & Cowey, A. (2000). Transcranial magnetic stimulation and cognitive neuroscience. *Nature Reviews Neuroscience, 1,* 73–79.

Wapner, S., & Kaplan, B. (Eds.). (1983). *Toward a holistic developmental psychology.* Hillsdale, NJ: Erlbaum.

Ward, L. M. (2003). Synchronous neural oscillations and cognitive processes. *Trends in Cognitive Sciences, 7,* 553–559.

Wascher, E., Schatz, U., Kuder, T., & Verleger, R. (2001). Validity and boundary conditions of automatic response activation in the Simon task. *Journal of Experimental Psychology: Human Perception and Performance, 27,* 731–751.

Wauschkuhn, B., Verleger, R., Wascher, E., Klostermann, W., Burk, M., Heide, W., & Kömpf, D. (1998). Lateralised human cortical activity for shifting visuospatial attention and initiating saccades. *Journal of Neurophysiology, 80,* 2900–2910.

Wehrhahn, C., Li, W., & Westheimer, G. (1996). Patterns that impair discrimination of orientation in human vision. *Perception, 25,* 1053–1064.

Weichselgartner, E., & Sperling, G. (1987). Dynamics of automatic and controlled visual attention. *Science, 238,* 778–780.

Weiskrantz, L. (1996). Blindsight revisited. *Current Opinion in Neurobiology, 6,* 215–220.

Weiskrantz, L. (1997). *Consciousness lost and found.* Oxford, England: Oxford University Press.

Weiskrantz, L. (1998). *Blindsight: A case study and implications* (2nd ed.). Oxford, England: Oxford University Press.

Weiskrantz, L. (2001). Blindsight—Putting beta (β) on the back burner. In B. de Gelder, E. De Haan, & C. Heywood (Eds.), *Out of mind: Varieties of unconscious processes* (pp. 20–31). Oxford, England: Oxford University Press.

Weiskrantz, L., Rao, A., Hodinott-Hill, I., & Cowey, A. (2003). Brain potentials associated with conscious aftereffects induced by unseen stimuli in a blindsight subject. *Proceedings of the National Academy of Sciences, USA, 100*, 10500–10505.

Weiskrantz, L., Warrington, E. K., Sanders, M. D., & Marshall, J. (1974). Visual capacity in the hemianopic field following a restricted occipital ablation. *Brain, 97*, 709–728.

Weisstein, N. (1968). A Rashevsky–Landahl neural net: Simulation of metacontrast. *Psychological Review, 75*, 494–521.

Weisstein, N. (1972). Metacontrast. In D. Jameson & L. Hurvich (Eds.), *Handbook of sensory physiology: Vol. 7. Visual psychophysics* (pp. 233–272). Berlin, Germany: Springer-Verlag.

Weisstein, N., & Growney, R. L. (1969). Apparent movement and metacontrast: A note on Kahneman's formulation. *Perception & Psychophysics, 5*, 321–328.

Weisstein, N., Ozog, G., & Szoc, R. (1975). A comparison and elaboration of two models of metacontrast. *Psychological Review, 82*, 325–343.

Werner, H. (1935). Studies on contour: I. Qualitative analyses. *American Jorunal of Psychology, 47*, 40–64.

Werner, H. (1940). *Comparative psychology of mental development.* New York: Harper.

Werner, H. (1956). Microgenesis and aphasia. *Journal of Abnormal and Social Psychology, 52*, 347–353.

Westwood, D. A., & Goodale, M. A. (2003). Perceptual illusion and the real-time control of action. *Spatial Vision, 16*, 243–254.

Whalen, P. J., Rauch, S. L., Etcoff, N. L., McInerney, S. C., Lee, M. B., & Jenike, M. A. (1998). Masked presentations of emotional facial expressions modulate amygdala activity without explicit knowledge. *Journal of Neuroscience, 18*, 411–418.

Whitney, D. (2002). The influence of visual motion on spatial position. *Trends in Cognitive Sciences, 6*, 211–216.

Whitney, D., & Cavanagh, P. (2000). The position of moving objects. *Science, 289*, 1107.

Whitney, D., Murakami, I., & Cavanagh, P. (2000). Illusory spatial offset of a flash relative to a moving stimulus is caused by differential latencies for moving and flashed stimuli. *Vision Research, 40*, 137–149.

Whittington, M. A., Traub, R. D., & Jeffreys, J. (1995). Synchronized oscillations in interneuron networks driven by metabotropic glutamate receptor activation. *Nature, 373*, 612–615.

Wiesenfelder, H., & Blake, R. (1991). Apparent motion can survive binocular rivalry suppression. *Vision Research, 31*, 1589–1599.

Wiggs, C. L., & Martin, A. (1998). Properties and mechanisms of perceptual priming. *Current Opinion in Neurobiology, 8*, 227–233.

Wilbrand, H., & Saenger, A. (1900). *Die Neurologie des Auges* (Vol. 3). Wiesbaden, Germany: J. F. Bergmann.

Wilenius-Emet, M., Revonsuo, A., & Ojanen, V. (2004). An electrophysiological correlate of human visual awareness. *Neuroscience Letters, 354*, 38–41.

Wilke, M., Logothetis, N. K., & Leopold, D. A. (2003). Generalized flash suppression of salient visual targets. *Neuron, 39*, 1043–1052.

Williams, C., Azzopardi, P., & Cowey, A. (1995). Nasal and temporal retinal ganglion cells projecting to the midbrain: Implications for "blindsight." *Neuroscience, 65*, 577–586.

Williams, J. M., & Lit, A. (1983). Luminance-dependent visual latency for the Hess effect, the Pulfrich effect, and simple reaction time. *Vision Research, 23*, 171–179.

Williams, M. A., Morris, A. P., McGlone, F., Abbott, D. F., & Mattingley, J. B. (2004). Amygdala responses to fearful and happy facial expressions under conditions of binocular suppression. *Journal of Neuroscience, 24*, 2898–2904.

Williams, P., & Tarr, M. J. (1999). Orientation-specific possibility priming for novel three-dimensional objects. *Perception & Psychophysics*, *61*, 963–976.

Wilson, A. E., & Johnson R. M. (1985). Transposition in backward masking: The case of travelling gap. *Vision Research*, *25*, 283–288.

Wilson, H. R., Blake, R., & Lee, S.-H. (2001). Dynamics of travelling waves in visual perception. *Nature*, *412*, 907–910.

Wolbers, T., Schoell, E. D., Verleger, R., Kraft, S., McNamara, A., Jaskowski, P., & Büchel, C. (in press) Changes in connectivity profiles as a mechanism for strategic control over interfering subliminal information. *Cerebral Cortex*.

Woldorff, M. G., Gallen, C. C., Hampson, S. A., Hillyard, S. A., Pantev, C., Sobel, D., & Bloom, F. E. (1993). Modulation of early sensory processing in human auditory cortex during auditory selective attention. *Proceedings of the National Academy of Sciences, USA*, *90*, 8722–8726.

Woldorff, M. G., Liotti, M., Seabolt, M., Busse, L., Lancaster, J. L., & Fox, P. T. (2002). The temporal dynamics of the effects in occipital cortex of visual–spatial selective attention. *Cognitive Brain Research*, *15*, 1–15.

Wolfe, J. M., O'Neill, P., & Bennett, S. C. (1998). Why are there eccentricity effects in visual search? Visual and attentional hypotheses. *Perception & Psychophysics*, *60*, 140–156.

Wolff, P. (1997, December). *Einfluß der Alternativenzahl auf den Kongruenz-Inkongruenz-Effekt*. Paper presented at the Motorische Effekte nicht bewußt repräsentierter Reize, Bielefeld, Germany.

Wong, P. S., & Root, J. C. (2003). Dynamic variations in affective priming. *Consciousness and Cognition*, *12*, 147–168.

Woodman, G. F., & Luck, S. J. (1999). Electrophysiological measurement of rapid shifts of attention during visual search. *Nature*, *400*, 867–869.

Woodman, G. F., & Luck, S. J. (2003a). Dissociations among attention, perception, and awareness during object-substitution masking. *Psychological Science*, *14*, 605–611.

Woodman, G. F., & Luck, S. J. (2003b). Serial deployment of attention during visual search. *Journal of Experimental Psychology: Human Perception and Performance*, *29*, 121–138.

Xiao, Y., Wnag, Y., & Fellemen, D. J. (2003). A spatially organized representation of colour in macaque cortical area V2. *Nature*, *421*, 535–539.

Yabuta, N. H., & Callaway, E. M. (1998). Functional streams and local connections of layer 4C neurons in primary visual cortex of the macaque monkey. *Journal of Neuroscience*, *18*, 9489–9499.

Yamada, T., Kameyama, S., Fuchigami, Y., Nakazumi, Y., Dickins, Q. S., & Kimura, J. (1988). Changes of short latency somatosensory evoked potential in sleep. *Electroencpalography & Clinical Neurophysiology*, *70*, 126–136.

Yarrow, K., Haggard, P., Heal, R., Brown, P., & Rothwell, J. C. (2001). Illusory perceptions of space and time preserve cross-saccadic perceptual continuity. *Nature*, *414*, 302–305.

Yi, D.-J., Woodman, G. F., Widders, D., Marois, R., & Chun, M. M. (2004). Neural fate of ignored stimuli: Dissociable effects of perceptual and working memory load. *Nature Neuroscience*, *7*, 992–996.

Young, M. P. (1992). Objective analysis of the topological organization of the primate cortical visual system. *Nature*, *358*, 152–154.

Yuille, A. L., & Bülthoff, H. H. (1996). Bayesian decision theory and psychophysics. In D. C. Knill & W. Richards (Eds.), *Perception as Bayesian inference* (pp. 123–161). Cambridge, England: Cambridge University Press.

Zeki, S. (1991). Cerebral akinetopsia (visual motion blindness). *Brain*, *114*, 811–824.

Zeki, S. (1993). *A vision of the brain*. Oxford, England: Blackwell.

Zeki, S. (1997). The color and motion systems as guides to conscious visual perception. In K. S. Rockland, J. H. Kaas, & A. Peters (Eds.), *Cerebral cortex* (Vol. 12, pp. 777–809). New York: Plenum Press.

Zeki, S. (1998). Parallel processing, asynchronous perception, and a distributed system of consciousness in vision. *The Neuroscientist*, *4*, 365–372.

Zeki, S. (1999). *Inner vision*. Oxford, England: Oxford University Press.

Zeki, S., & Bartels, A. (1999). Toward a theory of visual consciousness. *Consciousness and Cognition, 8,* 225–259.

Zeki, S., & Marini, L. (1998). Three cortical stages of colour processing in the human brain. *Brain, 121,* 1669 1695.

Zeki, S., & Moutoussis, K. (1997). Temporal hierarchy of the visual perceptive systems in the Mondrian world. *Proceedings of the Royal Society of London, B, 264,* 1415–1419.

Zeki, S., & Shipp, S. (1988). The functional logic of cortical connections. *Nature, 335,* 311–317.

Zhaoping, L. (2003). V1 mechanisms and some figure–ground and border effects. *Journal of Physiology, Paris, 97,* 503–515.

Zhou, H., Friedman, H. S., & von der Heydt, R. (2000). Coding of border ownership in monkey visual cortex. *Journal of Neuroscience, 20,* 6594–6611.

Zihl, J., von Cramon, D., & Mai, N. (1983). Selective disturbance of movement vision after bilateral brain damage. *Brain, 106,* 313–340.

Zimba, L., & Blake, R. (1983). Binocular rivalry and semantic processing: Out of sight, out of mind. *Journal of Experimental Psychology: Human Perception and Performance, 9,* 807–815.

Zipser, K., Lamme, V. A. F., & Schiller, P. H. (1996). Contextual modulation in primary visual cortex. *Journal of Neuroscience, 16,* 7376–7389.

Contributors

Talis Bachmann
Institute of Law and Department of Psychology, University of Tartu, Tartu Tallinn, Estonia

Harold E. Bedell
College of Optometry, Center for Neuro-Engineering and Cognitive Science, University of Houston, Houston, Texas

Bruno G. Breitmeyer
Department of Psychology, Center for Neuro-Engineering and Cognitive Science, University of Houston, Houston, Texas

Jonathan S. Cant
Canadian Institutes of Health Research Group on Action and Perception, Department of Psychology, University of Western Ontario, London, Ontario, Canada

Yang Seok Cho
Department of Psychological Sciences, Purdue University, West Lafayette, Indiana

Susana T. L. Chung
College of Optometry, Center for Neuro-Engineering and Cognitive Science University of Houston, Houston, Texas

Vince Di Lollo
Department of Psychology, Simon Fraser University, Vancouver, British Columbia, Canada

James T. Enns
Department of Psychology, University of British Columbia, Vancouver, British Columbia, Canada

Gregory Francis
Department of Psychological Sciences, Purdue University, West Lafayette, Indiana

Melvyn A. Goodale
Canadian Institutes of Health Research Group on Action and Perception, Department of Psychology, University of Western Ontario, London, Ontario, Canada

Michael F. Green
Veterans Administration Greater Los Angeles Healthcare System, Department of Psychiatry and Biobehavioral Sciences, University of California at Los Angeles. Los Angeles, California

Fred Hamker
Allgemeine Psychologie, Psychologisches Institut II, Westfalische Wilhelms-Universität, Münster, Germany

Michael H. Herzog
Laboratory of Psychophysics, Brain Mind Institute, École Polytechnique Fédérale de Lausanne, Switzerland

Piotr Jaśkowski
Department of Cognitive Psychology, University of Finance and Management, Warsaw, Poland

Jacob Jolij
Department of Psychology, University of Amsterdam, Amsterdam, The Netherlands

Christof Koch
Division of Biology, California Institute of Technology, Pasadena, California

Grzegorz Króliczak
Canadian Institutes of Health Research Group on Action and Perception, Department of Psychology, University of Western Ontario, London, Ontario, Canada

Victor A. F. Lamme
Department of Psychology, University of Amsterdam, and The Netherlands Ophthalmic Research Institute, Amsterdam, The Netherlands

Alejandro Lleras
Department of Psychology, University of Illinois, Champaign, Illinois

Steven J. Luck
Department of Psychology, University of Iowa, Iowa City, Iowa

Wei Ji Ma
Division of Biology, California Institute of Technology, Pasadena, California

Haluk Öğmen
Department of Electrical & Computer Engineering, Center for Neuro-Engineering and Cognitive Science, University of Houston, Houston, Texas

Saumil S. Patel
Department of Electrical & Computer Engineering, Center for Neuro-Engineering and Cognitive Science, University of Houston, Houston, Texas

Mary C. Potter
Department of Brain and Cognitive Sciences, Massachusetts Institute of Technology, Cambridge, Massachusetts

Tony Ro
Department of Psychology, Rice University, Houston, Texas

Edmund T. Rolls
Department of Experimental Psychology, University of Oxford, Oxford, England

H. Steven Scholte
Department of Psychology, University of Amsterdam, Amsterdam, The Netherlands

Jens Schwarzbach
Neurocognitie, Universiteit Maastricht and F. C. Donders Centre for Cognitive Neuroimaging, Nijmegen, The Netherlands

Petra Stoerig
Institute of Experimental Psychology II, Heinrich Heine University, Düsseldorf, Germany

Rolf Verleger
Department of Neurology, University of Lübeck, Lübeck, Germany

Dirk Vorberg
Institut für Psychologie, Technische Universität Braunschweig, Germany

Jonathan K. Wynn
Department of Psychology, University of California at Los Angeles, Veterans Administration Greater Los Angeles Healthcare System, Los Angeles, California

Index